Inborn Errors of
Immunity and
Phagocytosis

Previous Symposia of the Society for the
Study of Inborn Errors of Metabolism*

1. Neurometabolic Disorders in Childhood. Ed. K. S. Holt and J. Milner 1963
2. Biochemical Approaches to Mental Handicap in Children. Ed. J. D. Allan and K. S. Holt 1964
3. Basic Concepts of Inborn Errors and Defects of Steroid Biosynthesis. Ed. K. S. Holt and D. N. Raine 1965
4. Some Recent Advances in Inborn Errors of Metabolism. Ed. K. S. Holt and V. P. Coffey 1966
5. Some Inherited Disorders of Brain and Muscle. Ed. J. D. Allan and D. N. Raine 1969
6. Enzymopenic Anaemias, Lysosomes and other papers. Ed. J. D. Allan, K. S. Holt, J. T. Ireland and R. J. Pollitt 1969
7. Errors of Phenylalanine Thyroxine and Testosterone Metabolism. Ed. W. Hamilton and F. P. Hudson 1970
8. Inherited Disorders of Sulphur Metabolism. Ed. N. A. J. Carson and D. N. Raine 1971
9. Organic Acidurias. Ed. J. Stern and C. Toothill 1972
10. Treatment of Inborn Errors of Metabolism. Ed. J. W. T. Seakins, R. A. Saunders and C. Toothill 1973
11. Inborn Errors of Skin, Hair and Connective Tissue. Ed. J. B. Holton and J. T. Ireland 1975
12. Inborn Errors of Calcium and Bone Metabolism. Ed. H. Bickel and J. Stern 1976
13. Medico-Social Management of Inherited Metabolic Disease. Ed. D. N. Raine 1977
14. The Cultured Cell and Inherited Metabolic Disease. Ed. R. A. Harkness and F. Cockburn 1977

The Society exists to promote exchanges of ideas between workers in different disciplines who are interested in any aspect of inborn metabolic disorders. Particulars of the Society can be obtained from the Editors of this Symposium.

* Symposia 1–10 published by E. & S. Livingstone

Inborn Errors of Immunity and Phagocytosis

Monograph based upon
Proceedings of the Fifteenth Symposium of
The Society for the Study of Inborn Errors of Metabolism

Edited by
F. Güttler
J. W. T. Seakins
and
R. A. Harkness

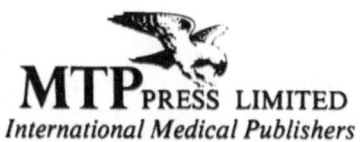

MTP PRESS LIMITED
International Medical Publishers

Published by
MTP Press Limited
Falcon House
Lancaster
England

ISBN-13: 978-94-011-6199-2   e-ISBN-13: 978-94-011-6197-8
DOI: 10.1007/978-94-011-6197-8

Contents

SECTION FOUR

Screening for Immunodeficiency

List of Contributors

O. BÄCK
Department of Dermatology, University of Umeå, S-901 85 Umeå, Sweden

R. L. BAEHNER
Division of Pediatric Hematology-Oncology, James Whitcomb Riley Hospital for Children, Indianapolis, Indiana 46202, USA

K. BAERLOCHER
Children's Hospital, CH-9000 St. Gallen, Switzerland

B. BECH
Department of Pediatrics TG, Rigshospitalet University of Copenhagen, Denmark

P. BELLAVITE
Department of General Pathology, University of Trieste, 34127 Trieste, Italy

V. BINDER
Department of Medical Gastroenterology C, Herlev Hospital, DIC-2730 Herlev, University of Copenhagen, Denmark

B. BJÖRKSTÉN
Department of Paediatrics, University of Umeå, S-901 85 Umeå, Sweden

L. A. BOXER
Division of Pediatric Hematology-Oncology, James Whitcomb Riley Hospital for Children, Indianapolis, Indiana 46202, USA

P. K. de BREE
University Children's Hospital, Het Wilhelmina Kinderziekenhuis, Utrecht, The Netherlands

D. A. CARSON
Division of Rheumatology, Department of Clinical Research, Scripps Clinic and Research Foundation, La Jolla, California 92037, USA

S. M. COCKLE
Division of Perinatal Medicine, MRC Clinical Research Centre, Harrow HA1 3UJ, Middlesex

B. COOK
Department of Pediatrics, Albany Medical College, Albany, New York 12208, USA

F. DAGUILLARD
INSERM U132, Groupe de Recherches d'Immunologie et de

ix

Rhumatologie Pédiatriques, Hôpital des Enfants Malades, 149 Rue de Sèvres, 75015 Paris, France

C. DAHLGREN
Department of Medical Microbiology, University of Linköping, S-581 85 Linköping, Sweden

E. DICKMEISS
The Tissue-Typing Laboratory of the Blood Grouping Department, State University Hospital, DK-2100 Copenhagen Ø, Denmark

P. DRI
Department of General Pathology, University of Trieste, 34127 Trieste, Italy

A. DURANDY
INSERM U132, Groupe de Recherches d'Immunologie et de Rhumatologie Pédiatriques, Hôpital des Enfants Malades, 149 Rue de Sèvres, 75015 Paris, France

O. FRIIS
Department of Pediatrics TG, Rigshospitalet, University of Copenhagen Denmark

R. A. GOOD
Department of Immunology, Sloan-Kettering Institute for Cancer Research, New York, NY 10021, USA

M. GRANT
Department of Paediatric Biochemistry, Royal Hospital for Sick Children, Edinburgh

C. GRISCELLI
INSERM U132, Groupe de Recherches d'Immunologie et de Rhumatologie Pédiatriques, Hôpital des Enfants Malades, 149 Rue de Sèvres, 75015 Paris, France

F. GÜTTLER
John F. Kennedy Institute, DK-2600 Glostrup, Denmark

B. HÄGGLÖF
Department of Paediatrics, University of Umeå, S-901 85 Umeå, Sweden

G. S. HANSEN
The Tissue-Typing Laboratory of the Blood Grouping Department, State University Hospital, DK-2100 Copenhagen Ø, Denmark

R. A. HARKNESS
Division of Perinatal Medicine, MRC Clinical Research Centre, Harrow HA1 3UJ, Middlesex

J. HED
Department of Medical Microbiology, University of Linköping, S-581 85 Linköping, Sweden

G. F. M. HENDRICKX
University Children's Hospital, Het Wilhelmina Kinderziekenhuis, Utrecht, The Netherlands

ROCHELLE HIRSCHHORN
Department of Medicine, New York University School of Medicine, New York, NY 10016, USA

T. HOVI
Department of Virology, University of Helsinki, F-00290 Helsinki, Finland

R. HULTBORN
University of Göteborg, Institute of Neurobiology, Fack, S-400 33, Göteborg 33, Sweden

K. S. JOHANSEN
Department of Clinical Microbiology, Statens Seruminstitut, Rigshospitalet, Copenhagen, Denmark

J. KAYE
Division of Rheumatology, Department of Clinical Research, Scripps Clinic and Research Foundation, La Jolla, California 92037, USA

J. A. LOOS
Central Laboratory of the Netherlands Red Cross Blood Transfusion Service, PO Box 9190, Amsterdam, The Netherlands

G. G. MacPHERSON
Sir William Dunn School of Pathology, University of Oxford, Oxford

I. MATTSBY-BALTZER
University of Göteborg, Department of Immunology, Institute of Medical Microbiology, Guldhedsgatan 10, S-413 46 Göteburg, Sweden

J. MEJER
Department of Internal Medicine C, Bispebjerg Hospital, DK-2400 Copenhagen, Denmark

H. J. MEUWISSEN
Department of Pediatrics, Albany Medical College, Albany, New York 12208, USA

L. MOLIN
Department of Dermatology, University of Linköping, S-581 85 Linköping, Sweden

P. NYGAARD
Department of Enzymology, Institute of Biological Chemistry, University of Copenhagen, Denmark

S. OLLING
University of Göteborg, Institute of Pathology and Department of

*Immunology, Institute of Medical Microbiology, Guldhedsgatan 10,
S-413 46 Göteborg, Sweden*

R. J. O'REILLY
*Department of Immunology, Sloan-Kettering Institute for Cancer
Research, New York, NY 10021, USA*

R. N. PAHWA
*Department of Immunology, Sloan-Kettering Institute for Cancer
Research, New York, NY 10021, USA*

S. G. PAHWA
*Department of Immunology, Sloan-Kettering Institute for Cancer
Research, New York, NY 10021, USA*

K. PARKER
*Department of Pediatrics, Albany Medical College, Albany, New York
12208, USA*

F. KARUP PEDERSEN
*University Clinic of Paediatrics, Department G, Rigshospitalet,
Blegdamsvej 9, 2100 Copenhagen Ø, Denmark*

P. PLATZ
*The Tissue-Typing Laboratory of the Blood Grouping Department,
State University Hospital, DK-2100 Copenhagen Ø, Denmark*

S. H. POLMAR
Rainbow Babies and Children's Hospital, Cleveland, Ohio 44106, USA

D. ROMEO
Department of Biochemistry, University of Trieste, 34127 Trieste, Italy

D. ROOS
*Central Laboratory of the Netherlands Red Cross Blood Transfusion
Service, P.O. Box: 9190, Amsterdam, The Netherlands*

J. ROSENKVIST
The Bloodbank, Rigshospitalet, Copenhagen, Denmark

F. ROSSI
*Department of General Pathology, University of Trieste, 34127 Trieste,
Italy*

L. P. RYDER
*The Tissue-Typing Laboratory of the Blood Grouping Department,
State University Hospital, DK-2100 Copenhagen Ø, Denmark*

MARGRIET L. J. van SCHAIK
*Central Laboratory of the Netherlands Red Cross Blood Transfusion
Service, PO Box 9190, Amsterdam, The Netherlands*

K. SCHOPFER
*Institute of Microbiology, Section of Immunology, CH-9000 St Gallen,
Switzerland*

J. W. T. SEAKINS
*Department of Chemical Pathology, Institute of Child Health, London
WC1N 1EH*

J. E. SEEGMILLER
*Department of Medicine, University of California, San Diego, La Jolla,
California 92037, USA*

A. W. SEGAL
*Division of Cell Pathology, MRC Clinical Research Centre, Harrow
HA1 3UJ, Middlesex*

ELIZABETH M. SMITHWICK
*Department of Immunology, Sloan-Kettering Institute for Cancer
Research, New York, NY 10021, USA*

G. E. J. STAAL
*University Children's Hospital, Het Wilhelmina Kinderziekenhuis,
Utrecht, The Netherlands*

O. STENDAHL
*Department of Medical Microbiology, University of Linköping, S-581
85 Linköping, Sweden*

J. W. STOOP
*University Children's Hospital, Het Wilhelmina Kinderziekenhuis,
Utrecht, The Netherlands*

A. SVEJGAARD
*The Tissue-Typing Laboratory of the Blood Grouping Department,
State University Hospital, DK-2100 Copenhagen Ø, Denmark*

A. TÄRNVIK
*Department of Clinical Bacteriology, University of Umeå, S-901 85
Umeå, Sweden*

W. J. M. TAX
*Department of Biochemistry, University of Nijmegen, Nijmegen,
The Netherlands*

M. THOMSEN
*The Tissue-Typing Laboratory of the Blood Grouping Department,
State University Hospital, DK-2100 Copenhagen Ø, Denmark*

I. TYGSTRUP
*Laboratory of Paediatric Pathology, Rigshospitalet, Copenhagen,
Denmark*

N. H. VALERIUS
*Department of Clinical Microbiology, Statens Seruminstitut,
Rigshospitalet, Copenhagen, Denmark*

J. H. VEERKAMP
*Department of Biochemistry, University of Nijmegen, Nijmegen,
The Netherlands*

S. K. WADMAN
*University Children's Hospital, Het Wilhelmina Kinderziekenhuis,
Utrecht, The Netherlands*

J. H. WANDALL
*Department of Medical Gastroenterology C, Herlev Hospital, DK-2730
Herlev, University of Copenhagen, Denmark*

R. S. WEENING
*Central Laboratory of the Netherlands Red Cross Blood Transfusion
Service, P.O. Box 9190, Amsterdam, The Netherlands*

B. J. M. ZEGERS
*University Children's Hospital, Het Wilhelmina Kinderziekenhuis,
Utrecht, The Netherlands*

Preface

The rapid growth of immunology has greatly increased our understanding of disease; this growth has also generated a subject which at times appears separated from some of the basic medical sciences. Recent studies in the areas of purine metabolism and of polymorphonuclear neutrophil phagocyte function have, however, linked immunology and clinical medicine with biochemistry. The precise defects of the inborn errors of metabolism have now provided good evidence for the importance of purine metabolism specifically the enzymes adenosine deaminase and nucleoside phosphorylase in lymphocyte function. In view of this and the steady advance of clinical and biochemical investigation of the polymorphonuclear neutrophil phagocyte, it appeared timely to review the inborn errors of immunity and phagocytosis at the fifteenth annual symposium of the Society for the Study of Inborn Errors of Metabolism at Elsinore, Denmark on September 11–14th, 1977.

The papers presented at that meeting form the basis of this volume which brings together contributions from immunologists, biochemists and clinicians. This interdisciplinary communication should be helpful to those concerned with immune function in their patients or in the laboratory.

The book is divided into four sections, One: defects of cell-mediated immunity, Two: enzyme defects and immunodeficiency, Three: disorders of non-specific immunity and Four: screening for immunodeficiency. Section One contains two reviews, one on immunodeficiency from Robert Good's group in New York and another on the genetics of the immune system from Arne Svejgaard of Copenhagen. Section Two contains eleven papers detailing the diagnosis, treatment and pathogenesis of adenosine deaminase and nucleoside phosphorylase deficiencies which both cause widespread defects of lymphocyte function. Dr Meuwissen presents the Milner lecture on this subject. In this section also many of the other leading groups in the field are represented. Section Three contains a series of reviews on different aspects of polymorphonuclear neutrophil phagocyte function as well as a series of clinical and laboratory medicine contributions on phagocyte function. This section is introduced by a major review by Baehner. Much recent European work including contributions from Scandinavia is included. Section Four on 'screening for immunodeficiency' was a round table discussion which distinguishes population screening from clinical diagnosis and discusses both, for the disorders described in this book.

Our main aim has been to provide a general view of those areas where well defined defects or deficiency of specific enzyme activities alter either specific or non-specific immune function. We hope that our attempt to provide a framework for interdisciplinary communication which has so ably been supported by the authors themselves will be of help in medical practice, research and possibly teaching.

We must express the thanks of all involved to our hosts the Danes, their Medical Research Council and their Ministry of Education as well as Nordisk Gjenforsikringselkabs Jubilaeumsfond and other Danish organizations which contributed to the costs of this meeting. We are especially grateful to Mr J. Milner of Milner Research and Scientific Ltd. and also the Scientific Hospital Services Ltd. for their generous support. We were privileged to have Dr E. Wamberg as our president during the meeting. It is also a pleasure to thank the City of Copenhagen for its usual warm and generous hospitality. The meeting would not have been possible but for the kindness and efficiency of so many members of staff of the John F. Kennedy Institute as well as the staff of the Biochemistry Department, Alder Hey Children's Hospital, Liverpool. Our special thanks are also due to the many people who have helped in the production of this book.

F. Güttler
J. W. T. Seakins
R. A. Harkness

SECTION ONE

Defects of Cell-mediated Immunity

1

Immunodeficiency diseases – a review*
R. N. Pahwa, S. G. Pahwa, R. O'Reilly, Elizabeth M. Smithwick and R. A. Good

Abbreviations

ADA	Adenosine deaminase	CVI	Common variable immunodeficiency
B cell	Bursal dependent lymphocyte	EBV	Epstein–Barr virus
BUDR	Bromodeoxyuridine	E rosettes	Rosettes with sheep erythrocytes
C	Complement		
cAMP	Cyclic adenosine monophosphate	HLA	Human lymphocyte antigen
CFU-C	Colony forming units in soft-agar culture	HTLA	Human T lymphocyte antigen
CGD	Chronic granulomatous disease	Ig	Immunoglobulin
		MHC	Major histocompatibility system
CMI	Cell-mediated immunity		
CSA	Colony stimulating activity	MLC	Mixed lymphocyte culture

* Aided by Public Health Service Research Grants CA–19267, CA–08748 and CA–17404 from the NCI; by the Zelda R. Weintraub Cancer Fund, the Judith Harris Selig Memorial Fund, and the Charles E. Merrill Trust.

MRBC	Mouse red blood cells	PWM	Pokeweed mitogen
NBT	Nitroblue tetrazolium	SCID	Severe combined
PC1	Plasma cell surface		immunodeficiency
	antigen		disease
PHA	Phytohaemagglutinin	SRBC	Sheep red blood cells
PMN	Polymorphonuclear	T cells	Thymus-dependent
	leukocyte		lymphocytes
Pt	Patient	WBC	White blood cells

Introduction

Recent years have witnessed a great surge in understanding immunological function in both cellular and molecular terms. This increased knowledge has permitted definition of the two major arms of the immunity system as cells that develop under thymic influence or under an alternative influence that is exercised by the bursa of Fabricius in birds (the T and B cell systems). Major aspects of the biological amplification systems by which the specific immunological adaptation can address the fundamental effector processes have also been recognized. Increasingly, these have been defined in precise molecular terms by chemical and immunological means. The fundamental effector processes are also beginning to be understood precisely in both cellular and molecular terms. Thus the complement system is now very well defined, lymphokines are increasingly well understood and the processes that underlie and effect phagocytosis, inflammation, vascular reactivity and blood coagulation are being analysed and defined with increasing precision.

This surge of new knowledge has permitted more frequent recognition, description and improved definition of the immunodeficiency diseases. It has also become possible to investigate and analyse the ongoing processes of immunological development and to use such analyses better to understand abnormalities of development when they exist. The specific immunological systems now can be shown to be featured by multiple subdivisions and to be characterized by both positive and negative controlling influences of the interacting components. From the new perspective made possible by the developing knowledge, it is challenging to look repeatedly at the primary immunodeficiency diseases. This is especially so since it is these inborn errors of metabolism which so frequently have pointed the directions for the fundamental inquiry and, on the other hand, have provided the most critical challenges to the developing knowledge. As our knowledge of immunity mechanisms becomes more complete and more precise, the opportunities to correct immunological abnormalities by cellular and/or macromolecular engineering can be expected to increase, and ability not only to predict but to control immunological function will improve.

Development of the lymphoid system

Ontogenetic studies in animals have shown that the stem cells originating in the yolk sac migrate initially to the fetal liver and later to the bone marrow where they divide and differentiate into myeloid, erythroid and lymphoid precursors[1-5]. Lymphoid precursors originating in both fetal liver and bone marrow may then circulate to the thymus, which provides for the differentiation of these cells into immunologically competent T cells. In birds, a parallel influence on differentiation of B lymphocytes is exercised by the bursa of Fabricius[4]. Since the bursa of Fabricius does not exist in mammals or in any animal except birds, the site of B cell differentiation has been perplexing. Recent evidence suggests that this influence may reside in the fetal liver[6] (see Figure 1.1). Both the T and B cells in the

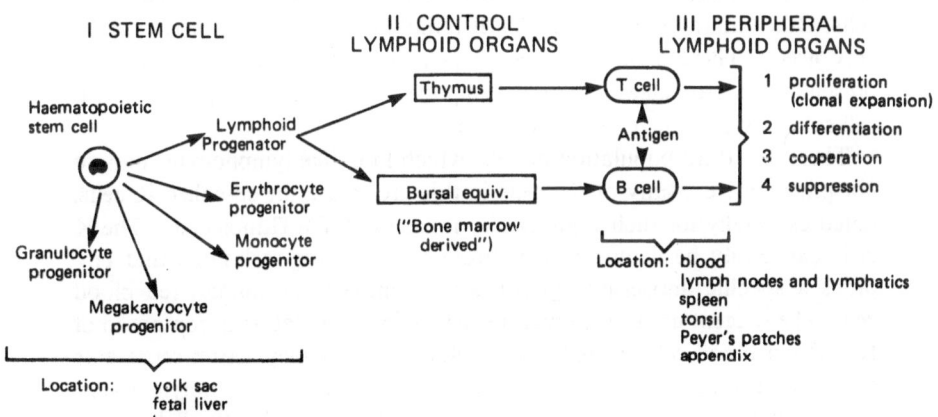

Figure 1.1 The two component scheme of the lymphoid system

peripheral lymphoid tissue and the circulation can now be defined by surface marker methodologies and by functional characteristics. Major markers of the T cells are the capacity to (a) form rosettes with SRBC; (b) respond to phytohaemagglutinin (PHA) and Concanavalin A (Con-A) in a solution (although non-T cells will respond to these lectins when they are presented in a polymerized or non-soluble form; (c) respond by proliferation to antigens against which the animals from which the cells are derived have already been immunized[7]; and (d) respond to allogeneic cells. T cells, furthermore, develop cell surface antigens very early in their differentiative process that permit us to define them in immunological terms. Antisera have also been prepared against human T lymphocytes, which are, after appropriate absorption, specific for T cells in tissues or in the peripheral blood[8-10].

B cells, of course, are those which have on their surface readily demonstrable surface immunoglobulin. The basis for specificity in the B cells is found in the antigen-combining site of the immunoglobulin molecule. This is probably true also of T cells. Whereas we know quite a lot about the immunoglobulin molecule on B cells in man and animals, the nature of the immunoglobulin or other molecule containing this site on T cells is still enigmatic. There are five different classes of surface immunoglobulin on different subpopulations of B cells: cells with surface IgM account for the greater proportion of the cells with surface immunoglobulins; some also have IgM + IgD, but present also in blood and lymphoid tissue are relatively small numbers of B cells with surface IgG, IgE, and IgA, as well as IgD alone. B cells, or a major subpopulation of B cells, have also been identified through their predisposition for rosetting with mouse red blood cells. Other markers once used for B lymphocytes have not proved to be very useful. These include F_c receptors and C_3 receptors, whch are also present on macrophages and other lymphocyte populations. Specific anti-B cell sera, however, have been developed[8].

There is a third population of cells which look like lymphocytes and do not phagocytize. Many of the cells in this group are the so-called K cells, noted especially for their high avidity receptors for IgG molecules. The K cells can easily be demonstrated through a rosetting technique that employs a specific antiserum against Rh(D) antigens on human red blood cells. The reagent used to enumerate cells of this population is composed of Rh(D) red blood cells coated with Ripley serum. Ripley serum represents an apparently monovalent anti-Rh(D) antiserum. K cells comprise a very significant proportion of the circulating lymphocytes. Like the B lymphocytes, K cells also have complement receptors, but they lack surface immunoglobulins and, as mentioned, do not phagocytize particulate matter[11].

Normally T lymphocytes comprise about 75% of circulating cells in the blood; B lymphocytes make up approximately 10% of the total lymphocyte population, and the third population approximately 12–15%. Within this last group, K, or so-called killer cells, account for as many as 8–10% of circulating white blood cells. Functionally, K cells have aroused interest because they participate as killer cells in antibody-mediated cytotoxicity reactions.

When we speak of T and B cells, we also must speak about the T and B

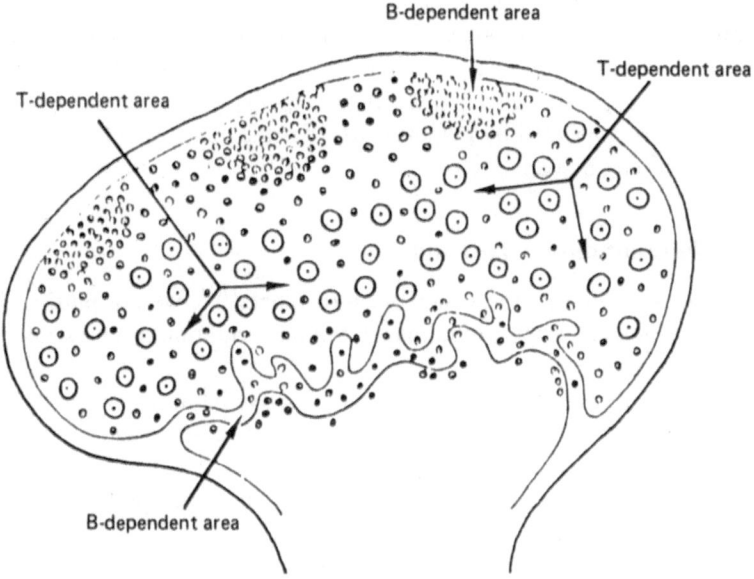

Figure 1.2 Stimulated lymph node. Antigen producing delayed allergy

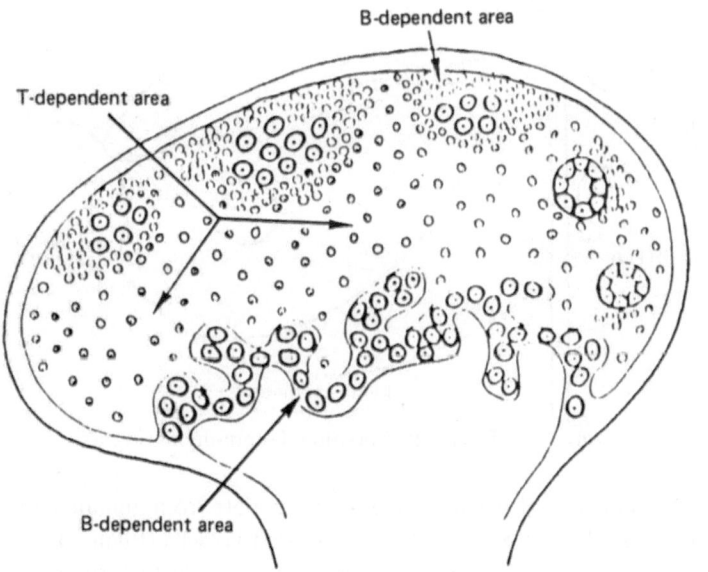

Figure 1.3 Stimulated lymph node. Antigen T-independent

regions in lymphoid tissue (Figures 1.2 and 1.3). B zones are classically found in the far cortical areas of the lymph node where germinal centres develop, and in the medullary cords where plasma cells develop. The deep cortical areas (or so-called paracortical regions) are thymus-dependent. These have been defined by Parrott *et al.*[12] for the mouse and by our group for chicken[4] and human[13].

T cell differentiation in humans

From our own observations and those of others[14-21], we are putting forward the following scheme of human T cell differentiation (Figures 1.4, 1.5, 1.6).

Lymphoid stem cells may produce an inductive influence on the thymus necessary for its maturation. The thymus may also produce inductive humoral factors which render stem cells susceptible to differentiative influences of the thymic microenvironment. Thus, the pre-thymic cells

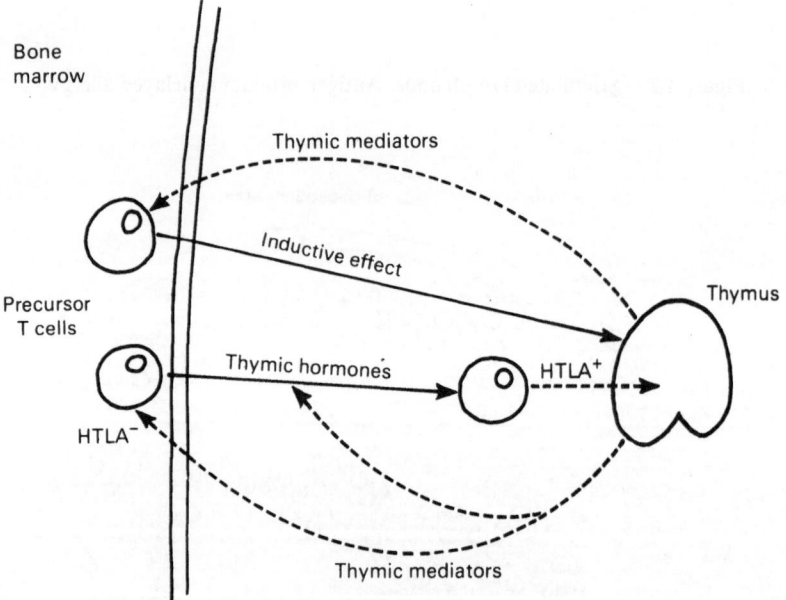

Figure 1.4   T-cell differentiation. I – pre-thymic events

under the influence of thymic factors differentiate from human T lymphocyte antigen (HTLA) negative to HTLA positive cells (Figure 1.4). These HTLA positive cells (Figure 1.5), which are unable to form E rosettes, mature under the influence of the thymic microenvironment into early post-thymic cells, which then become capable of rosetting with sheep red cells. Thus the thymus contains both populations of pre-T cells, i.e. HTLA$^+$ E rosettes$^-$ and HTLA$^+$ E rosettes$^+$ cells. These cells achieve some immunocompetence in the thymus and then recirculate, some cells going back to bone marrow whereas the other cells populate T zones of the peripheral lymphoid organs.

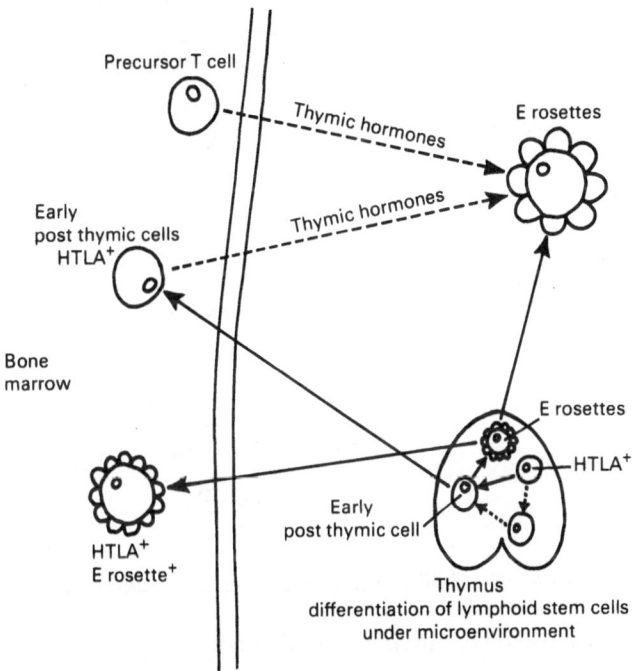

Figure 1.5   T-cell differentiation. II – thymic events

Thus, according to our working hypothesis (Figure 1.5), the bone marrow contains precursor T cells at all stages of differentation as well as post-thymic cells, that is, cells containing the following characteristic T cell markers:

(a) HTLA$^-$ E rosettes$^-$ mitogen$^-$ MLC$^-$
(b) HTLA$^+$ E rosettes$^-$ mitogen$^-$ MLC$^-$
(c) HTLA$^+$ E rosettes$^+$ mitogen$^-$ MLC$^-$
(d) HTLA$^+$ E rosettes$^+$ mitogen$^+$ MLC$^-$
(e) HTLA$^+$ E rosettes$^+$ mitogen$^-$ MLC$^+$

According to the studies of Touraine et al.[21] these post-thymic cells under the influence of thymic factors may then further differentiate into two subsets of lymphocytes, one responsible for GVH and MLC responses and the other for mitogen responses (Figure 1.6). Thus the sites of thymic

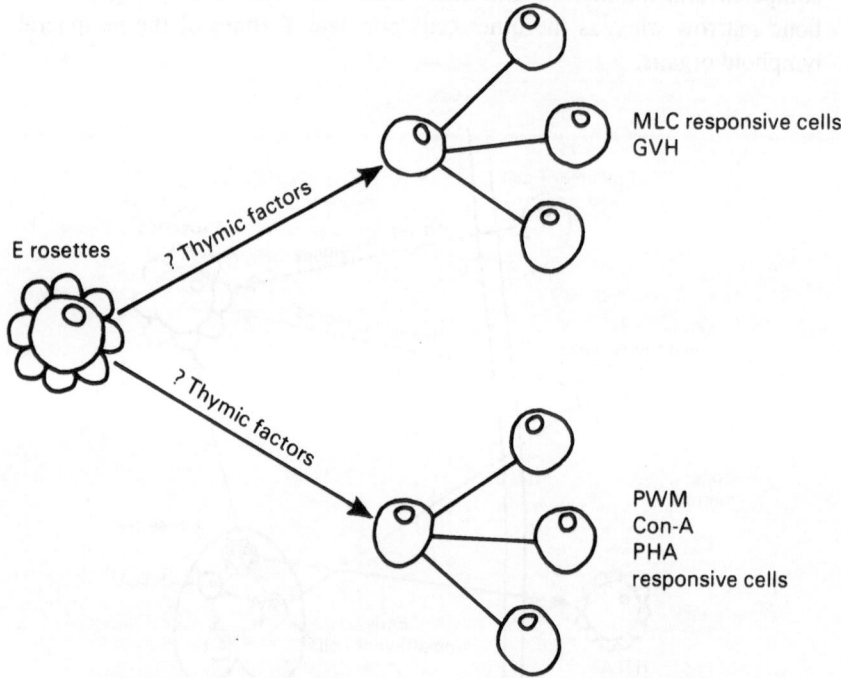

Figure 1.6   T-cell differentiation. III – terminal differentiation

influence may be (a) on pre-thymic cells, (b) on post-thymic cells, and (c) on the cells within the thymus where the intrathymic microenvironment may utilize both cell-to-cell contact and the thymic hormonal influences.

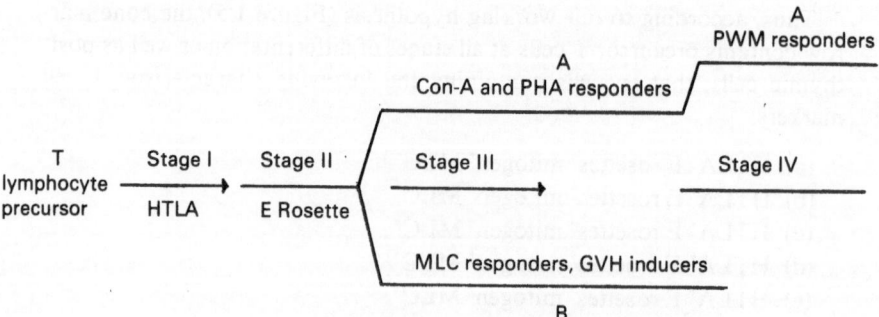

Figure 1.7   Differentiation of human T lymphocytes

In humans, the first step that seems to appear and on which the other steps depend is the appearance of human thymic lymphocyte antigen (HTLA) (Figure 1.7). Capacity to form E rosettes occurs during the second step, but not if HTLA-positive cells have been eliminated. If, however, either or both of these are eliminated, one cannot induce differentiation to Con-A responsive cells or PHA responsive cells. Interestingly, if one induces differentiation to Con-A responsive cells and then eliminates or inactivates the proliferating cells with bromodeoxyuridine (BUDR) and ultraviolet light, one eliminates also the PHA responding cells, but does not touch the MLC responses[19-21].

In experimental systems in mice, it has also been possible to show that graft-versus-host-inducing cells are linked to MLC responding cells.

B cell differentiation

Hämmerling et al.[22] have shown that in B cell differentiation, there is a sequence of differentiation reflected in the development of cell surface characteristics, which can be induced, step by step, by the influences of a molecule called ubiquitin[23]. This differentiative step is followed by a quantum proliferation and then development of Ia antigenicity. Subsequently, in a series of developmental steps, the complement receptor, F_c receptor, and the plasma cell surface antigen (PC 1) appear as the cell develops machinery for massive immunoglobulin synthesis and secretion and becomes what we have called a plasma cell. Although the definitions are surely incomplete, it is heartening to see that we are making progress toward defining these steps in B cell development and are actually beginning to be able to analyse the successive relationships of the various steps in the sequence.

In humans, based on study of the cell surface markers observed in various primary and secondary immunodeficiency diseases and in lymphoreticular neoplasia, the possible schemes of B cell differentiation are given in Table 1.1.

Vogler and Cooper et al.[24] have reported, in patients with Bruton's type agammaglobulinaemia and in those with common variable immunodeficiency, the presence of intracytoplasmic IgM postive cells in the bone marrow which may be the equivalent of the pre-B cell observed by Kincade et al.[25] in avian bursae and by Gathings et al.[26] in human fetal liver. These cells are absent in patients with thymoma with immunodeficiency. This marker is absent in subsets of B cells which form rosettes with mouse red cells. Gupta, Good and Siegal[27] provided definitive evidence that binding of mouse red blood cells to B lymphocytes is independent of surface Ig and

TABLE 1.1   Cellular differentiation markers applicable to immunodeficiency disorders

Bone marrow-derived (B) lymphocytes, their precursors and progeny

Precursors:	
lymphoid stem cell	B cell alloantigens
pre-B lymphocyte	cytoplasmic IgM
B lymphocytes	Surface IgM, IgD (IgA, IgG)
	Mouse erythrocyte rosette
	Receptors for immune complexes via IgG (sometimes aggregates used)
	C3d, C3b,
	B cell alloantigens
	EBV receptors
Plasmacytoid B cells:	Surface IgM
	Cytoplasmic Ig + other presumed antigenic markers,
Plasma cells:	Cytoplasmic Ig, J chains
	Plasma cell antigens
Other characteristics of B cells	Synthesis and secretion of Ig
	Response to mitogens (T cells and PWM)
	Localization to B cell areas of lymphoid tissue
	Tendency to aggregation

* Modified from 'Surface markers in leukemias and lymphomas'. F. P. Siegal *et al.*[245]

of receptors for IgG F_c and C3. During the ontogenetic process in human fetal liver, the receptors for mouse red blood cells are present at least as early as is surface IgM[28]. Mouse red blood cells appear to represent a marker for an early stage in the development of B lymphocytes. At this stage of B cell differentiation, these cells have on their surface characteristic B cell allo-antigens, receptors for EBV and immune complexes. The next two stages of differentiation are formation of plasmacytoid cells, then plasma cells, and ultimately synthesis and secretion of large amounts of Ig.

Suppressor cells, helper cells and subpopulations of T cells

Suppressor cells which inhibit B cell differentiation or Ig production in immunodeficiency were originally described by Waldmann *et al.*[29], and their existence confirmed and analysed by Siegal *et al.*[30], Broom *et al.*[31], Schwartz *et al.*[32], McKenzie and Paglieroni[33], and Waldmann *et al.*[34].

Suppression of blast transformation inducible by Concanavalin-A (Shou et al.[35]) was also observed. Assays for helper cells were proposed by Geha et al.[36] and by Cooper et al.[37]. Most recently, Broder et al.[38] showed that Sezary cells have helper activity and Safai et al.[39] have shown that sometimes they may have suppressor activity in vitro, while Keightley et al.[40] and Fauci et al.[41, 42] have reported that isolated B cells require T cells for pokeweed mitogen-induced terminal differentiation.

Siegal et al.[43] have recently found that even among normal T cells there is a functionally radiosensitive population which inhibits autologous B cell differentiation. Irradiated normal T cells have pronounced helper effect on the pokeweed mitogen-driven terminal differentiation of autologous B cells. Further, they have shown that normal persons possess among their blood cells both suppressor and helper lymphocytes.

Finally, one should consider among the regulatory cell interactions, the possible involvement of biologically active factors from T cells and/or macrophages, and the participation of both helper and suppressor T cells in the regulation of immune responses. The helper T cells interact with B cells to facilitate clonal expansion and differentiation of such cells to mature plasma cells which secrete immunoglobulin. The suppressor cells may interfere at any stage of B cell differentiation, e.g. preventing either helper T cell induction or function in interactions with B cells or by directly inhibiting B cell differentiation. Atwater et al.[44] and Schwartz et al.[45] have recently described class specific suppressor cells present in patients with IgA deficiency that are able selectively to suppress IgA synthesis and secretion.

Moretta, et al.[46, 47] and Gupta and Good[48] have demonstrated that human T lymphocytes under appropriate experimental conditions express receptors for IgM F_c designated as $T\mu$ and those with receptors for IgG F_c are designated as $T\gamma$. The latter are undoubtedly the same population studied also by Chiao et al.[49] among their so-called D lymphocytes. $T\mu$ cells are 'helpers' for the proliferation and differentiation of B cells to plasma cells, and $T\gamma$ cells[47], when activated with Concanavalin-A, appear to contain the 'suppressors' for B cell proliferation and differentiation to plasma cells. There remains a subpopulation of T cells which does not express receptors for either IgG or IgM, and, therefore, for those markers can be designated as 'null' T cells.

$T\mu$ cells are relatively resistant to the effect of corticosteroids, irradiation and thymopoietin influence[50], whereas $T\gamma$ cells are relatively sensitive to irradiation and to high doses of corticosteroids and their number increases upon exposure of peripheral blood lymphocytes to thymopoietin.

Kishimoto et al.[51] recently presented an additional important finding.

They investigated T cell lines and defined one as having helper and one as having suppressor capabilities. From the above observations and as in the mouse, helper and suppressor cells appear to be distinct entities. One can see why it is now necessary to talk in terms of a network theory rather than to think only about T and B cells as separate lineages of immunologically competent cells[52]. We must learn to contend with multiple subsets of T cells, multiple subsets of B cells, positive influences and negative influences as well, and any or all of these cells and their interactions may be disturbed in clinical immunodefiencies.

DISORDERS OF THE IMMUNE SYSTEM

Severe combined immunodeficiency

Some children are born without either T or B cell immunity systems. The tonsils of these children lack germinal centres, and have very few or no lymphocytes or plasma cells. The thymus, while present, is epithelial and very underdeveloped, having no cortex, no medulla, and no Hassall's corpuscles. Lymph nodes and spleen may lack both B and T cells. Developmentally, these patients are thought to be arrested at an early stage, at which point both T and B cell immunity systems are still one. The severe combined immunodeficiency diseases (SCID), however, have been found like all immunodeficiencies to be very heterogeneous. Patients having these defects have varying genetic backgrounds, in some the immunodeficiency is X-linked, in some autosomal recessive, and in some sporadic. A significant portion of SCID (about 10–20%) has occurred in conjunction with an adenosine deaminase (ADA) deficiency. In other cases, an apparent ADA deficiency seems to be due to the presence of an inhibitor of ADA activity[53,54]. SCID has also frequently been associated with bony abnormalities and may be reflected in the short-limbed dwarfism defined by Gatti et al.[55]. Nucleoside phosphorylase deficiency also has been shown to be associated with SCID or T cell immunodeficiency.

Increasing evidence exists that the differentiation potential of precursors of T cells is heterogeneous in patients with SCID[18,56,57], suggesting multiple potential sites of block in the T and B cell differentiations. Touraine et al.[14,15] have demonstrated induction of the HTLA marker in normal fractionated bone marrow cells after incubation with thymic extract. No induction of HTLA marker occurred in the marrow of several patients with severe combined immunodeficiency. Incefy et al.[16,18] confirmed this observation and demonstrated that normal fractionated bone marrow cells could be induced to express the HTLA marker and to form E rosettes when exposed to thymopoietin. This process was shown at first in human cells to depend upon transcription and translation, but not to involve replication[58,59]. When the technique has been applied to the analysis of severe combined immunodefiiency, at least two varients could be distinguished: in one group, no *in vitro* induction of HTLA marker could be demonstrated[17]; in a second group, there was induction of HTLA marker after the fractionated bone marrow cells had been treated with thymic extract or thymopoietin[18]. Thus, in two patients with the latter subtype of severe combined immunodeficiency, we demonstrated that fractionated marrow cells could be induced to bear the HTLA marker after incubation with human thymic extract or by thymopoietin. No receptors for SRBC (E rosettes) could be induced in the marrow cells of these patients after 15 h incubation with these inducing agents. This finding was in contrast to another group of SCID in which induction of HTLA and E rosetting failed to develop upon appropriate stimulation. This finding is consistent with the

TABLE 1.2 In vitro differentiation of bone marrow cells from SCID patient by normal thymic epithelial monolayers and supernatant from thymic monolayer culture

Additions	Percentage of large E rosettes Ficoll gradient			
	II	III	IV	V
Patient No. 1	I + II	III	IV + V	
Control	2.3	2.0	0.7	
Epi	22.0	22.3	6.7	
Sup	3.3	3.0	0	
Epi + Sup	17.3	32.3	15.5	
Patient No. 2				
Control	3.3	2.3	0.3	0.3
Epi	5.0	2.0	1.7	0.0
Sup	5.7	2.3	0.3	1.0
Epi + Sup	3.5	4.3	0.0	2.7
Patient No. 3				
Control	2.0	0.3	0.7	0.0
Epi	2.7	0.0	0.0	0.3
Sup	4.0	1.0	1.0	0.0
Epi + Sup	1.7	0.0	0.0	0.0

Control = cells cultured in medium alone
Epi = normal human thymic epithelial monolayer
Sup = normal human thymic epithelial supernatant

view expressed earlier that in ontogeny of T cell differentiation the HTLA marker is a marker for a cell stage earlier in differentiation than the capacity to form E rosettes.

Using a technique for culturing human thymic epithelium, as described by Pyke and Gelfand[60], we have initiated *in vitro* analysis of the differentiation of bone marrow cells and peripheral blood lymphocytes from normal volunteers and patients with primary immunodeficiency.

Normal bone marrow cells, when co-cultured with thymic epithelium and its supernatant, develop human T lymphocyte antigen (HTLA), capacity to form E rosettes with sheep red cells, and to yield a proliferative response to phytomitogens[56].

Results from co-culture of cells from five patients with severe combined immunodeficiency (SCID) with thymic epithelium and supernatant are shown in Tables 1.2 and 1.3. Two of these patients (numbers 4 and 5) were studied after fetal liver transplantation at a time when chimerism with cells derived from fetuses could be demonstrated, but prior to development of evidence of T cell functional reconstitution. The bone marrow cells of three patients (numbers 1, 4 and 5) when exposed to thymic epithelium, developed the capacity to form rosettes with sheep erythrocytes. By contrast, supernatant media from thymic epithelial cultures could be shown to induce this marker only in a single patient (number 5) who had received a fetal liver transplant and had chimerism for the donor cells. The induction

TABLE 1.3   In vitro differentiation of SCID bone marrow cells after fetal liver transplantation by normal thymic epithelium and thymic supernatant

	Percentage of large E rosettes Ficoll or BSA gradient			
Additions	II	III	IV	V
Patient No. 4				
Control	0.3	0	0	0.3
Epi	1.3	0.7	5.3	8.0
Sup	1.0	0	0.7	0
Patient No. 5				
Control	1.3	1.0	0.3	0.3
Epi	10.3	5.3	1.0	1.0
Sup	1.3	7.0	0.3	0.0

Control = cells cultured in medium alone
Epi = normal human thymic epithelial monolayer
Sup = normal human thymic epithelial supernatant

TABLE 1.4   In vitro differentiation of normal bone marrow cells by the epithelium and supernatants of cultured normal and SCID thymus

Type of thymus	Additions	Percentage of large E rosettes Ficoll gradient layers			
		II	III	IV	V
Normal thymus	Control	17	12	12	6
	Epi	13	35	13	5
	Sup	21	34	11	4
	Epi + Sup	—	32	13	2
SCID thymus	Control	3.5	7.7	9.0	26.0
	Epi	0	14.0	8.7	24.3
	Sup	16.7	18.7	12.0	22.3
	Epi + Sup	11.3	8.0	3.3	17.0

Control = cells cultured in medium alone
Epi = thymic epithelial monolayer
Sup = thymic epithelial supernatant

TABLE 1.5   In vitro differentiation of fetal liver cells by the epithelium and supernatants of cultured normal and SCID thymus

Type of thymus	Additions	Percentage of E-rosettes Ficoll hypaque separated fetal liver cells 11.0 weeks gestational age
Normal thymus	Control	2.2
	Epi	10.5
	Sup	9.7
	Epi + Sup	8.0
SCID thymus	Control	2.2
	Epi	8.3
	Sup	7.3
	Epi + Sup	8.0

Control = cells cultured in medium alone
Epi = thymic epithelial monolayer
Sup = thymic epithelial supernatant

of HTLA marker occurred in three patients (numbers 1, 2 and 4) studied. These results indicate the possibility that thymic supernatants are capable of inducing differentiation steps restricted to post-thymic cells which are absent in SCID patients or that these patients may be lacking one sub-population of precursor cells (thymus independent) which can be induced to develop E rosettes under the influence of thymic hormones.

TABLE 1.6   In vitro differentiation of SCID bone marrow cells by the epi-thelium and supernatants of cultured normal and SCID thymus

Type of thymus	Additions	Percentage of E-rosettes Ficoll gradient layers			
		II	III	IV	V
Normal thymus	Control	1.3	1.0	0.3	0.3
	Epi	10.3	5.3	1.0	1.0
	Sup	1.3	7.0	0.3	0
	Epi + Sup	nd	nd	nd	nd
SCID thymus	Control	1.0	0.7	0.0	0.0
	Epi	0.0	0	0	1.3
	Sup	0	0	0	0
	Epi + Sup	1.3	0	0	0

Control = cells cultured in medium alone
Epi = thymic epithelial monolayer
Sup = thymic epithelial supernatant
nd = no data

The interaction between lymphoid precursors and thymus in patients with SCID was examined in a unique *in vitro* study utilizing thymus from a patient with SCID (Tables 1.4, 1.5 and 1.6). This thymus was obtained at autopsy. Light microscopy showed the thymus to be embryonic in mor-phology. No lymphoid cells or Hassall's corpuscles were evident. The SCID cultured thymic epithelium and supernatant could also induce in normal bone marrow cells the capacity to form E rosettes (Table 1.4). Fetal liver cells (11 weeks gestational age) could be induced to form E rosettes when co-cultured with normal or with SCID thymic epithelium and its supernatant (Table 1.5). In striking contrast, the SCID patient-derived thymic epithelial cells failed to induce SCID bone marrow cells from another SCID patient[61, 62] (Table 1.6). These results suggest that in some variants of severe combined immunodeficiency, there may exist a communication defect between stem cells and the microenvironment of the thymus. The precursor T cell may normally produce a trophic effect on the thymus and be responsible, in part, for the development of the latter[63].

Evaluation of thymic function by quantitation of circulating serum thymopoietin level[63] and thymic factor[64] was carried out in patients with SCID, which is shown in Table 1.7. Thymopoietin was absent in the blood of all five patients studied. The level became normal, however, in three patients who had been successfully reconstituted with either bone marrow transplantation or with fetal liver plus thymus transplantation. In the remaining two patients, who were given fetal liver plus a cultured thymus transplant and who at present have no evidence of immunological reconstitution, the thymopoietin levels have remained low. In one patient (S.C.), who was given a bone marrow transplant, the thymopoietin levels were below demonstrable range before transplant but became normal after the bone marrow transplantation, suggesting that the bone marrow cells may exercise an inductive or trophic effect on the thymus for influencing its maturation. This apparently causes the thymus to start secreting thymopoietin *in vivo*.

Levels of the serum thymic factor of Bach[64] (Facteur thymique sérique – FTS) revealed heterogeneity in this syndrome. This factor was not detectable in one patient, but was present in normal or near normal concentrations in the remaining five patients with SCID. In one patient (M.W.), serum thymic factor was low or absent before transplantation, but became normal after successful immunological reconstitution with fetal liver and fetal thymus transplantation.

As seems true for the heterogeneity in the extent of T cell differentiation in SCID, there is now accumulating evidence of heterogeneity in B cell development, with a B cell defect being either primary or secondary to T cell abnormalities. Evidence of an abnormality intrinsic to B cells was demonstrated in one of our patients with SCID[65]. Antibody production was measured by a recently described direct plaque-forming cell (PFC) assay against sheep erythrocytes following polyclonal activation with pokeweed mitogen[41,42]. Before transplantation with bone marrow, mononuclear cells from the patient's peripheral blood and bone marrow could not form plaques against the sheep red blood cells even though helper cells had been provided as irradiated normal T cells. However after successful bone marrow transplantation, which corrected completely the immunodeficiency, we demonstrated that the lymphocytes from this patient's blood and bone marrow could now form plaques against sheep red cells. Similar evidence of primary B cell defect was found in a patient described by Geha[66]. In this case, following bone marrow transplant, a patient with SCID demonstrated T cell function with donor-derived T cells (karyotypic analysis), whereas B cells, which were of host origin, remained non-functional.

Of the two patients described by Griscelli[67], one was fully reconstituted by a matched sibling marrow transplantation, whereas the other who had been given fetal thymus exhibited only T-cell function. In the first patient, chromosome studies showed that the T cells were donor derived and immunoglobulins were synthesized by the host's B cells. The second patient, who was only reconstituted for T cells, had chimerism with donor-derived T cells with B cells of host origin. Similarly, our two patients of SCID with B cells who were given fetal liver and thymus transplants are immunologically reconstituted[68]. In both the cases T cells are donor derived whereas B cells are host derived. In one patient there is complete T and B cell reconstitution with normal immunoglobulins with evidence of atibody formation, whereas the second patient has only complete T cell reconstitution with partial B cell reconstitution, having low immuno-gobulins with no evidence of antibody formation. Seeger et al.[69] have recently demonstrated that lymphocytes from a patient with SCID which were incapable of synthesizing or secreting immunoglobulins following stimulation by mitogens could do so in the presence of normal purified T cells. These observations suggest that in some variants of SCID, the abnor-malities at the level of T helper cells can lead to failure of B lymphocytes to become immunoglobulin-producing cells.

The other possibility may be that full histocompatibility between T and B cells may be a necessary prerequisite for full T and B lymphocyte co-operation in vivo. This requirement may not always have to be met since one of our patients who was given fetal liver plus thymus transplants had T cells of donor origin and B cells of host origin. This patient has normal mitogen responses with normal serum immunoglobulins and shows clear evidence of antibody formation[68].

The presence of suppressor cells in some patients with SCID may also be responsible for the failure to achieve complete functional reconstitution after lymphoid cell transplantation. Schwartz et al.[70] have observed such suppressor cell activity in three patients with SCID in which lymphoid cell transplantation failed to achieve complete reconstitution of humoral immunity. No suppressor cells were observed in two other patients who were completely reconstituted by bone marrow transplantation. This devel-opment of suppressor cell activity may explain at least in part the pheno-menon of allogeneic resistance with particular regard to the difficulty in reconstituting B cell-derived function.

From the above observations, we proposed a classification of SCID based on possible pathogenetic mechanisms which could result in the final

TABLE 1.7 Serum thymopoietin and thymic factor activity in patients with severe combined immunodeficiency

Diagnosis	No. and type of transplant	Outcome of immunological reconstitution	Serum thymopoietin (ng) Normal 10.6 ng		Serum thymic factor activity Normal 1/32	
			Pre-trans.	Post-trans.	Pre-trans.	Post-trans.
M.R. Classical SCID autosomal recessive ADA⁺ without B cells	7 BMT	successful	—	—	1/16–1/32	1/16–1/32
S.C. SCID, ADA⁻ with inhibitor without B cells	3 BMT	successful	1.6	10.4	1/8–1/16	1/32–1/32
M.W. SCID, ADA⁺ with B cells Ig⁻	3 fetal liver / 1 irradiated fetal thymus	successful	0	12.0	1/2	1/16
K.M. SCID, ADA⁺ with B cells Ig⁺	3 fetal thymus / 2 fetal liver	successful	0	12.8	1/16–1/16	1/32–1/32
D.V. SCID, ADA⁺ with B cells Ig⁻	1 cultured thymus / 2 fetal liver	chimerism⁺⁺ immunologically no reconstitution	0	pending	1/16,1/32	1/16,1/32
J.J. SCID, ADA⁺ with B cells Ig⁺	fetal liver no. 1	no chimerism	—	0	—	1/2
	fetal liver no. 2	chimerism, no function	0	2.4	1/16	1/16
	1 cultured thymus	no function	2.4	pending	1/8–1/16	pending

BMT = bone marrow transplant
— = no data

TABLE 1.8   Classification of SCID based on possible pathogenetic mechanisms

A. *Defect in stem cells*
 1. Absence of stem cells
 2. Defective precursors of both T and B cells
 3. Defective precursors of T cells with normal precursors of B cells

The defect in T precursor cells may occur at one of several stages of differentiation leading to cells which are capable of becoming induced into any of the following by surface markers and functional criteria:

 (a) $HTLA^+$, E rosettes$^-$, mitogen responses$^-$, MLC responses$^-$
 (b) $HTLA^+$, E rosettes$^+$, mitogen responses$^-$, MLC responses$^-$
 (c) $HTLA^+$, E rosettes$^+$, mitogen responses$^-$, MLC responses$^+$
 (d) $HTLA^+$, E rosettes$^+$, mitogen responses$^+$, MLC responses$^-$

 4. Absence of a subpopulation of T cells

B. *Defect in thymus*
 1. Defective microenvironment with normal secretory activity of the thymus
 2. Defective secretory activity with normal microenvironment of the thymus
 3. Defect in both microenvironment and secretory activity

C. *Defect in communication between stem cells and thymus*, either of which in itself may or may not be normal

---

clinical expression of this disorder (Table 1.8). This classification based on our findings provides a working rationale for using selective fetal haemato-poietic tissue, fetal thymus or cultured postnatal thymus transplants in instances where an HLA identical MLC non-reactive marrow donor is not available.

Transplantation of bone marrow from an HLA genotypically identical sibling donor has been employed since the method was introduced in 1968 and remains the treatment of choice in SCID[71, 72]. The first indication that the terrible disease resulting from a combined immunodeficiency could be corrected through cellular engineering came 9 years ago when we studied a little patient with the X-linked recessive form of the disease, who was given a bone marrow transplant from his sister. She was found to be mismatched only at the HLA-A locus, HLA-D and B being the same in the patient and his sister. Marrow taken from his sister completely reconstituted the patient's immune system. However, because of an additional ABO mismatch, and perhaps also partially due to the HLA mismatch, the transplant produced an iatrogenic immunologically based aregenerative pancytopenia (aplastic anaemia).

We therefore had an opportunity in the same patient to treat, for the first time successfully, an aplastic anaemia by allogenic marrow transplantation, as well as to correct the SCID. Using the same donor, we completely changed the blood type of the patient, who remains today a fully vigorous child, blood group O instead of his own genetic blood group A. He is absolutely normal immunologically, with a normal haematopoietic system. All of the dividing cells in his bone marrow are of the female karyotype, and thus derived from the donor, and all of the cells in the peripheral blood which proliferate in response to stimulation by PHA are also of female karyotype[71, 72].

Soon after this initial success, Biggar, Park and Good[73] corrected, by a series of bone marrow transplantations, a little girl with a combined immunodeficiency which was associated with ADA deficiency. This patient lacked ADA entirely; both parents had half values of the enzyme, and a sister had normal values. This patient and her sister were matched at the major histocompatibility locus, facilitating the transplantation. Today, this girl also remains well and is an apparent chimera because her peripheral red cells still appear to lack the ADA, while all her lymphoid cells contain apparently normal amounts of the enzyme[73]. We have since cured another case of this form of SCID by marrow transplantation from a matched sibling donor, again creating the fascinating chimeric state revealed by the enzyme analysis of the red blood cells and leukocytes.

TABLE 1.9   **Therapeutic approaches for patients with SCID lacking an HLA genotypically identical sibling**

A. *Transplantation to replace defective lymphoid stem cells*
  1. Transplantation of marrow from other 'histocompatible' donors
     (a) HLA genotypically identical related donor
     (b) HLA phenotypically identical related donor
     (c) HLA non-identical, HLA-D matched related donor
     (d) HLA-D compatible unrelated donor
  2. Transplantation of histoincompatible marrow depleted of GVHD-inducing lymphocytes
     (a) Depletion of proliferating alloantigen responsive lymphocytes (suicide)
     (b) Pretreatment of marrow with antithymocyte serum
     (c) Marrow fractionation
  3. Transplantation of fetal tissues deficient in GVHD potential
     (a) Fetal thymus transplants
     (b) Fetal liver transplants

B. *Transplantation to replace defective tissues controlling lymphoid differentiation*
  1. Cultured thymus grafts

C. *Replacement of inducers or modulators of lymphoid differentiation*
  1. Enzyme replacement
  2. Thymosin
  3. Transfer factor

TABLE 1.10 Lymphoid reconstruction of SCID following transplantation of marrow from donors other than genotypically identical sibling

Patient	Donor	Degree of HLA compatibility	HLA incompatibility	Engraftment of donor cells	GVHD	T cell reconstruction	B cell reconstruction	Authors	References
1	Uncle	genotypic	none	T cells	none	+ (donor)	+ (host)	Vossen et al.	74
2	Father	genotypic	none	T cells	mild	+	−	Geha et al.	75
3	Father	phenotypic	none	full	severe	+	+	I. M. Anderson	76
4	Father	phenotypic	none	full	moderate	+	+ (delayed)	Polmar et al.	77
5	Uncle	non-identical	B7, B12	T cells	moderate	+	−	Copenhagen study group	78
6	Sibling	non-identical	BW 37	full	moderate	+	+	Gatti et al.	79
7	Mother	non-identical	A2	full	severe	+	+	D. Niethammer et al.	80
8	Father	non-identical	A2	full	none	+	+	Copenhagen study group	81

These children with transplanted bone marrow have survived more than 9 years following the transplantation, and the procedure has now been done in many centres throughout the world. Since this achievement, approximately 47 patients with this disorder have been successfully reconstituted. Consistent engraftment, reconstitution of both B and T cell functions and graft-versus-host disease (GVHD) of low intensity have been the rule in such transplants which have cured several genetic forms of the severe combined immunodeficiency.

Another great problem with bone marrow transplantation has been, of course, that a matched sibling donor is not always available. When a MHC-mismatched donor has been used to treat SCID, fatal graft-versus-host disease has been the rule. Other approaches designed to provide grafts of normal lymphoid stem cells with restricted potential for inducing lethal GVHD are summarized in Table 1.9.

Experience with transplantation of marrow from non-sibling related donors who are HLA genotypically or phenotypically identical or who are HLA-D compatible, but mismatched with respect to the HLA-A and/or HLA-B determinants, is still very limited[74-81], (Table 1.10). However, analysis of these cases reveals that GVHD has generally been more severe than when the matched HLA system has been complete and the reaction has frequently been associated with marrow suppression or aplasia[82]. In these reconstitutions, while lymphoid engraftment has been consistently achieved, it has frequently been functionally incomplete, resulting in only partial reconstruction, and often limited to the T cell system.

Transplantation of marrow from unrelated, histocompatible donors is another approach which has been proposed to reconstitute lymphoid function in patients with SCID. Horowitz et al.[83] have reported a patient with SCID who received a marrow transplant from an unrelated MLC compatible donor who differed from the patient on one HLA specificity. The patient died in the early stages of immunological reconstitution of interstitial pneumonia. The post-transplant course (30 days) in this patient was too short to allow full evaluation of immune competence or to assess the risk or consequences of GVHD. We have recently reported[84] a patient with SCID successfully reconstituted following seven transplants of marrow from an HLA-A non-identical but HLA-B and HLA-D compatible unrelated donor. The first four transplants resulted in a restricted engraftment principally demonstrable in the lymph nodes, which was associated with rudimentary evidence of functional reconstitution. A fifth transplant, administered after treating the patient with cyclophosphamide (25 mg/kg × 2), achieved durable engraftment of a functional T cell system. Marrow aplasia, probably secondary to GVHD, developed following recontamination. A subsequent transplant, administered after high dose cyclophosphamide (50 mg/kg × 4) achieved complete haematopoietic and immunological reconstitution. Seventeen months following transplantation, full functional engraftment persists; all haematopoietic and lymphoid elements are of donor origin. Graft-versus-host disease has been chronic and moderately severe in intensity but limited to the skin and oral mucosa. This case demonstrates a real potential for extending the application of marrow transplantation to those patients lacking a histocompatible sibling donor. Currently, the prospect of finding a compatible unrelated donor from existing donor pools is, however, very restricted.

Another approach for correcting this disorder is to use fetal tissue transplantation as shown in Table 1.11. Based on the predicted defects, we have treated two patients having SCID with fetal liver plus fetal thymus transplant[85]. The first of these was a 7-month old male with ADA-positive

TABLE 1.11   Predicted defects in SCID and suggested therapeutic approach

	In vitro *differentiation*				
Defects	*HTLA*	*E rosettes*	*Mitogen responses and MLC responses*	*Thymic hormones*	*Therapeutic* approach*
Absence of stem cells	−	−	−	present	BMT or fetal liver
Defective stem cells	+	±	−	present	BMT or fetal liver
Absence of stem cells with defective thymus	−	−	−	absent	BMT or fetal liver and thymus transplant
Defective stem cells with defective thymus	+	±	−	absent	BMT or fetal liver and thymus transplant
Thymus defect	+	+	+	absent	thymus transplant
Communication defect between stem cells and thymus	+	+	+	present	thymus transplant

BMT = bone marrow transplant
*Thymus = cultured for 3–4 weeks *in vitro* or fresh fetal thymus

SCID who lacked T cell functions, had B cells but did not produce Ig. Studies of his marrow prior to transplantation indicated a population of lymphoid precursors which, following stimulation with thymic extracts or thymopoietin, could be induced to bear a human thymic lymphocyte antigen (HTLA) but not to form E rosettes or to respond to mitogens. Two fetal liver transplants aimed at reconstitution were unsuccessful, despite evidence of chimerism. Serum concentrations of thymic factor and thymopoietin were found to be deficient. However, a population of lymphoid precursors was now detectable in the patient's marrow which, on coculture with normal thymic epithelium, could be differentiated to form E rosettes and to respond to mitogen. Accordingly, the patient received a transplant of an irradiated 18-week fetal thymus. No evidence of reconstitution of immune function was recorded, although thymic function had been restored, as evidenced by development of normal levels of thymic factor and thymopoietin[63, 64] (see Table 1.7). By the time of the thymus transplant, however, we were no longer able to demonstrate lymphoid elements derived from the second fetal liver graft in his circulation. A subsequent fetal liver transplant then achieved durable engraftment with full reconstitution of cell-mediated immune function; 18 months following this transplant, the patient is well at home. T lymphocytes are normal in number, representing 50% of the circulating pool. Lymphocyte responses to mitogens, bacterial antigens and allogeneic cells are normal. His immunoglobulins are low and antibody responses have not yet been seen. HLA typing of separated lymphocyte populations indicates that the circulating T lymphocytes are derived from the fetal liver graft and B lymphocytes are of host type. This, indeed, is a fascinating form of chimerism which may be responsible for failure of the full immunological reconstruction.

We therefore present evidence in this case of defects in both stem cell and thymus function. It would appear that the immunological reconstitution achieved required transplantation of both a fetal liver stem cell population and thymus.

The basis for the functional defects of the thymus demonstrable in this patient is unclear. The thymus might be intrinsically defective, either because of genetic abnormality or failure to undergo a critical differentiative event. Alternatively, functional differentiation may be blocked due to either a deficiency of extrinsic trophic factors necessary for development or the presence of inhibitory influences. Pyke et al.[86] recently demonstrated that the thymus of a patient with a variant of SCID similar in immunological characteristics to that of this patient (M.W.), was histologically embryonal and functionally defective in vivo but could develop more mature histological features and induce differentiation of lymphoid precursors normally after culture *in vitro*. Such data suggest that extrathymic influences may be in part responsible for the deficits in thymus function observed *in vivo* in some cases.

Our failure to achieve reconstitution despite engraftment of differentiable lymphoid precursors from a normal fetal liver also suggests the possibility that certain patients who present with what is termed SCID may have deficiencies correctable by thymus alone. We would postulate, then, that cellular and functional correction in such cases might be achieved only by transplantation of differentiated thymic tissue, such as an irradiated fetal thymus of 16 or more weeks' gestation as used in the present case, or thymus tissue derived from similarly aged fetuses or children that have been maintained *in vitro* for a period sufficient to insure loss of viable lymphocytes. We would expect transplantation of a prelymphoid thymus of less than 12 weeks' gestation to fail, in such reconstructions, even in those variants exclusively deficient in thymus function because of host-mediated restriction on the development of the thymic graft. Indeed, transplantation of early fetal thymus has failed to produce reconstitution in patients with SCID except in those instances in which fetal thymus-derived lymphocytes were also engrafted. Restoration of immune function attending grafts of the latter type has regularly been incomplete and GVH disease in some instances has been significant[87]. Conversely, transplants of developmentally mature thymus tissue (after prolonged culture *in vitro* to deplete viable lymphocytes) have recently been shown to induce the functional development of host-derived lymphoid populations in certain variants of SCID[88].

Hong *et al.*[89] recently presented clinical support for this hypothesis when they described a patient with SCID who was partially reconstituted with normal cultured human thymus. Four weeks after transplantation, immunoglobulins of host type were detected. An increase of *in vitro* reactivity to allogeneic cells and phytohaemagglutinin and a positive skin test to *Candida* antigen was also observed, but an increase in E rosettes was not clearly established. Thus, certain types of combined immunodeficiency may result from a defect involving the thymus as a primary or secondary event. It can be postulated that the thymus may be incapable of either accepting precursor cells or of differentiating these cells, and that this defect may lead to secondary defects of development and differentiation of B cells.

To date, 36 patients with SCID have received transplants of fetal liver; of this number 15 patients[90] were given frozen fetal liver cells with no evidence of immunological reconstitution, 21 patients have received trans-

TABLE 1.12 Successful fetal liver transplants in severe combined immunodeficiency

Diagnosis and age at transplant	Age of fetal donor	Nucleated cell dose	Route	Chimerism	GVHD	T Cell	B Cell	Survival after Tx	Cause of death	Reference
SCID (ADA^-) 3 months	8.5 weeks	2.5×10^8	i.p.	+	±	+	+	18 months	renal disease	87
SCID (ADA^-)*	12 weeks	1.2×10^9	i.v.		−	+	+	25 months	viral pneumonia	88
SCID (ADA^-)	8 weeks	8.4×10^7	i.p.	+	+	+	±	32.0 months		89
SCID (ADA^-) 5½ months	4–5 weeks	3.7×10^6	i.p.		+	+	0	30.5 months		90
SCID (ADA^-)* no.1 14 months	11.5 weeks	2.4×10^8	i.v.	−	−	0	0			
no.2 20 months	10.5 weeks	7.5×10^7	i.p.	+	−	+	(+)	19 months		90
SCID (ADA^-)* no.1 8 months	8 weeks	2.7×10^7	i.p.	−	−	0	0			
no.2 8.5 months	12.5 weeks	4×10^9	i.p.	+	−	0	0			
no.3 12 months	9.5 weeks	5.9×10^7	i.p.	+	(+)	+	−	15 months		91

* Fetal thymus also given

plants of freshly obtained fetal liver. In seven of the cases, definite immunological improvement occurred, manifested either as T cell reconstitution
alone in three patients, or as both T and B cell reconstitution in four
patients[68, 91-94] (Table 1.12). In 16 additional cases, evidence of functional immunological improvement in neither the B or T cell system was observed,
even though in two cases the percentage of E-rosetting cells increased
after transplantation; in one a temporary improvement in responsiveness was seen. After fetal liver transplantation the engraftment process is
very slow. Chimerism may not be detected until 6–10 weeks after transplantation. Functional reconstitution develops gradually over 3–4 months.

Engraftment of fetal liver transplants has not been consistently achieved.
The factors, such as cell dose, fetal age and route of transplantation, appear
to be important variables[95, 96]. For example, full T cell reconstitution has
not been observed in patients receiving fetal liver of more than 12 weeks'
gestation although GVH reactions in this group have been significant.
Regarding route of administration, durable engraftment has been achieved
in six, and transient engraftment in an additional two, out of ten fetal liver
transplants administered intraperitoneally, irrespective of cell dose.

Although graft-versus-host disease has been reported even in a patient
who received liver from a fetus of 5 weeks' gestation[94], GVH disease in
patients receiving fetal tissue grafts of less than 12 weeks' gestational age
has been mild, or has not occurred. The possibility of contaminating
maternal cells in the few instances of GVH disease, induced with fetal
tissues from fetuses under 12 weeks' embryonation, has not been excluded.

The contribution of the thymus to successful immunological reconstitution following fetal liver transplants deserves analysis. Five of the 13
evaluable patients who received fetal liver grafts also received transplants
of fetal thymus at some time in their course. Four of the five patients so
treated achieved durable T cell reconstitution. In contrast, only three out
of nine patients who received fetal liver alone have enjoyed lasting T
lymphocyte competence.

VARIANTS OF SEVERE COMBINED IMMUNODEFICIENCY

Immunodeficiency with generalized haematopoietic hypoplasia (reticular dysgenesis)[97]

Reticular dysgenesis is a severe, congenital cellular and antibody deficiency
with associated agenesis of the granulocyte precursors of the bone marrow.
Clinically these children present within the first few days of life with failure
to thrive, vomiting, diarrhoea, infection and if not treated they die within
a short time. The laboratory findings are similar to those described in

SCID. The treatment of choice for this disorder would be bone marrow transplantation from an HLA A, B, C and D-locus matched sibling. If no matched sibling is available prompt fetal liver transplantation would appear to be the method of choice.

Nezelof's syndrome

This syndrome was first described by Nezelof *et al.* in 1964[98]. It is a primary immunodeficiency characterized by autosomal recessive inheritance, lymphopenia, severe cell-mediated immunodeficiency with dysplastic thymus, normal levels of immunoglobulin with little or no antibody production. Clinical course and treatment of this disorder is the same as described in SCID.

Trace elements and immunodeficiency

One form of combined immunodeficiency is that associated with acrodermatitis enteropathica. The manifestations of this disease include severe skin lesions, devastating gastrointestinal malfunction with malabsorption and diarrhoea, bizarre behaviour often referred to as autism, and variable but often severe immunodeficiency involving functions of both T and B lymphocytes. Untreated, the disease has regularly been fatal. All manifestations of this disease have been found to be attributable to an inborn error of metabolism which prevents the normal absorption of zinc from the gastrointestinal tract. Treatment with zinc in sufficient amounts parenterally or large doses even by the oral route permits correction of all manifestations of this otherwise fatal disease. The central nervous system malfunctions are corrected most promptly, the T cell abnormality begins to return toward normal within a few days and the entire otherwise lethal syndrome disappears within weeks after initiating treatment with zinc. If, however, zinc therapy is interrupted, the entire syndrome reappears.

Experimentally in mice we have produced by restriction of zinc a model of this form of immunodeficiency, gastrointestinal malfunction and acrodermatitis. It can be anticipated that as we progress in our understanding of the functions and essential requirements of the immunological system, other forms of so-called primary immunodeficiency disease will be as readily, simply and completely correctable as has been the case in acrodermatitis enteropathica.

Already we and others have encountered severe combined immunodeficiency of adults associated with low zinc levels in blood that is correctable at least in part by the administration of zinc.

DiGeorge syndrome

The third and fourth pharyngeal pouch syndrome was called DiGeorge syndrome in the late 1960s after Dr Angelo DiGeorge, a paediatric endocrinologist, who described it as an immunodeficiency disease after encountering four children with profound hypoparathyroidism who at autopsy all lacked thymic tissue[99]. Interestingly, the first observation of the association between the thymus and parathyroid was made in 1829 by Harrington in a case description in a letter to the *London Medical Gazette*, and the earliest report in the American literature of such a patient was made by Lobdell, a pathologist in 1959[100].

TABLE 1.13   Characteristic features of DiGeorge syndrome

Facies: Hypertelorism, antimongoloid slant of eyes, shortened philtrum of the lip, fish mouth, low-set ears with notched pinnae and micrognathia
Associated anomalies include choanal atresia, oesophageal atresia, bifid uvula, tracheo-oesophageal fistula and hypothyroidism

Thymus: Completely absent or present but very small, often aberrant, histology normal. Chest X-ray: absence of thymic shadow

Parathyroids: Usually absent or rudimentary. Low serum calcium, high phosphorous, low-to-absent circulating parathormone

Cardiac: Mainly aortic arch and conotruncal anomalies

Immunological assessment: Total white cell and lymphocyte counts usually normal, depressed T cell numbers and function, elevated B cell numbers with normal function, depressed levels of circulating 'thymic factors' (thymopoietin, thymic hormone)

The characteristic features of this syndrome (shown in Table 1.13) are due to the anomalous development of the organs arising from and in close association with the third and fourth pharyngeal pouches and may result from an insult to the developing fetus during the 8th–10th week of gestation. These infants present soon after birth with hypocalcaemic convulsions and/or congenital heart disease. If they survive the neonatal period increased susceptibility to infection occurs that is manifested by chronic rhinitis, otitis, recurrent pneumonia, oral candidiasis, diarrhoea and failure to thrive.

Although one can arbitrarily classify DiGeorge syndrome as being partial or complete depending on the presence or absence of thymic tissue, it is often difficult to do so on clinical and laboratory evidence. At least three different modes of presentation are seen:

1. In the 'classical' DiGeorge syndrome, cell-mediated immunity is severely depressed and the immunodeficiency persists as such. An attempt at immunological correction is clearly indicated in such cases.

2. Cell-mediated immunity which is initially depressed may slowly and spontaneously recover in rare instances[101]. This kind of presentation has led to much controversy in the treatment of DiGeorge syndrome, as some people feel that given the time most cases will recover. Undoubtedly, these cases would fall in the category of 'partial' DiGeorge syndrome. If the defects observed initially are not severe it would be considered reasonable to observe such patients. However, if CMI is severely depressed, to with-hold specific therapy is possible only at great risk to the patient.

3. Substantial thymic-dependent lymphoid function may be present initially[102, 103] and may later be depressed. Many theories have been advanced as to why in some cases the CMI is normal or near normal initially, the most accepted being that maternal 'thymic hormones' transferred via the placenta induce maturation in the pre-thymic cells of the offspring or a small piece of thymus functions at first and later ceases to do so. The exact pathogenetic mechanism of this deficiency remains open to question. Suffice it to say for this time that these are the cases at the greatest risk of being neglected. Two such cases[102, 103] at autopsy had no evidence of thymus tissue despite careful search with serial sections of the neck, mediastinum and adjacent areas.

Based on a questionnaire sent out to immunologists in the US and Europe and on a thorough review of literature[104] we have found 63 cases of DiGeorge syndrome. Of these eight were given thymus transplants and in seven of these evidence of either partial or complete restoration of immunity was recorded. Two of these cases died, one 9 days post-transplant with pneumocystis and the other 2 years later due to cardiac cause. Only 13 of the 55 non-transplanted cases are living, most of whom had only partial defects of thymic-dependent lymphoid function. The primary causes of death have been those associated with cardiac malformation, infections, seizures, aspiration and sudden death of unknown cause.

Listed in Table 1.14 are the eight cases of DiGeorge syndrome who received thymus transplants. The points of importance are as follows:

1. Restoration of T cell function occurred in all cases.

2. Recovery of thymic-dependent lymphoid function was rapid in most instances, occurring within 10 days in four cases (number 2, 4, 5 and 6) and within 3 weeks in one (number 1). In the other two cases (numbers 3 and 7), there was a delay in the recovery requiring more than 4 months before clear evidence of immunological recovery was recorded.

TABLE 1.14 Thymus transplant in DiGeorge syndrome

Author	Age of patient		Fetal thymus		Recon-stitution	Result	
	Diagnosis	Transplant	Age	Route†		How soon after transplant	Current status
Cleveland	5 weeks	7 months	13 weeks	i/m	yes	3 weeks	alive, 9 years neurolog. deficit
August	9 months	21 months	16 weeks	i/m	yes	4 days	alive, 9 years
Gatti	10 days	1.5 months	10–12 weeks	i/m	yes	4–7 months	alive, 5 years
Steele	12 days	10 weeks	13 weeks	d.c.	yes	6 hours	died, 9 days post-transplant pneumocystis
Biggar	2 months	5 months	1) 14 weeks 2) 15 weeks	i/p i/p	yes	1 week	alive, 4 years
*Touraine	6 months	7 months	1) 13 weeks 2) 12 weeks	i/m i/p	yes	10 days	alive, 2 years
*Pahwa	1 week	3 months	2) 14 weeks	i/p	yes	7 months	died, 2 years sudden death
*Dooren	1 week	1 month 3 months	1) 17 weeks 2) 12 weeks	i/m i/m	no	—	alive?

* Personal communication
† i/m = intramuscular, usually into rectus abdominis muscle; i/p = intraperitoneal: d.c. = diffusion chamber
Table modified from 'Review of thymus transplants',[104]

3. No GVHD or chimerism was noted in any case. Eosinophilia occurred in the first case 2 to 5 weeks post-transplant.

Regarding the mechanism by which the thymus restores immunity, a hormonal induction, causing maturation and expansion of already present precursor cells, is the most favoured explanation. Evidence to support this hypothesis included the following:

1. Serum levels of thymopoietin and thymic factor have been low prior to transplantation becoming normal following successful thymus transplant[63, 64].

2. Normal induction of bone marrow precursors into E rosette-forming and HTLA⁺ cells occurs following incubation with various thymus extracts[105], and with cultured human thymic epithelium monolayers[106].

It is quite possible that in cases where some thymic tissue is present all that is needed is an extra push into maturation of cells which have already been influenced by the thymus and that the process of maturation is quite delayed if the precursors have never been exposed to thymic tissue.

Defects of B cell line

The pertinent features of various conditions in which B cell function is impaired are listed in Table 1.15.

Bruton-type agammaglobulinaemia

The classic agammaglobulinaemia[107] is the congenital sex-linked recessive form; some sporadic cases have also been identified in boys. A few girls with similar clinical and cell marker deficits have also been described[108, 109] and recently Hoffman and Good[110] have described in detail two sisters who had total lack of B cells in blood and lymph nodes. Clinically these patients completely lack antibody function but have normal cell-mediated immunity[110, 111]. Germinal centres and plasma cells are lacking in their peripheral lymphoid tissue[112-115]; and follicular structure is absent in the tonsils and in Peyer's patches[111, 112]. The thymus is usually normal. Circulating lymphocyte levels are usually within normal limits but these patients totally lack cells bearing definitive markers of B cells in their peripheral blood and bone marrow. Vogler and Cooper et al.[24] have recently reported intracytoplasmic IgM positive cells in the bone marrow in these patients, the presence of which may be the human equivalent of the pre-B cell observed by Kincade et al.[25] in avian bursae and by Gathings

TABLE 1.15 Defects of B cell line

Disease	Bruton's X-linked infantile agammaglobulinaemia	Thymoma agammaglobulinaemia	Common variable immunodeficiency	Severe combined immunodeficiency
Intracytoplasmic Ig	+	−	+	nd
Mouse rosettes	−	−	v	v
Surface Ig+	−	−	v	v
Cell-mediated immunity	normal	v	v	absent
Suppressor cells	usually + +	usually + +	v	+ (3 pt) − (2 pt)
Helper cells				
Tμ	usually + +	usually + +	+	→
Tγ	v	↑	v	→
Patient's cells + normal helper cells	no differentiation	no differentiation	±	usually no differentiation
Possible defect	stem cells	stem cells with or without suppressor cells inhibiting RBC development or both B cell and RBC differentiation	80% B cell defect with or without defect in T–B cooperation; 20% attributable to suppressor effect	heterogeneous; usually stem cell defect

v = variable
− = absent
+ = present
nd = no data

et al.[26] in human fetal liver. However, these patients lack cells which bear surface IgM or IgD[108, 116-119] or cells with Epstein–Barr (E–B) virus receptors[120] or mouse erythrocyte rosette-forming cells[121]. Further, they lack cells that possess antigens characteristic of the B cell line. This observation indicates that congenitally agammaglobulinaemic patients can synthesize intracytoplasmic Ig molecules but cannot generate B cells beyond this very early precursor cell. Further studies to confirm the presence of these B cell precursors are very much needed.

Siegal and Good[30] first described in these patients the presence of cells that are capable of suppressing normal B cell differentation. Suppressor cell activity in these patients has been confirmed by Waldmann *et al.*[34], Dosch and Gelfand[122] and Schwartz *et al.*[32]. Furthermore removal of suppressors by adherence columns or depletion of T cells does not release B cells to normal differentiation. Helper cells are regularly found among the peripheral blood lymphocytes when suppressor cells have been ablated by irradiation. B cells of these patients do not differentiate to plasmacytoid elements in the presence of either autologous or allogeneic T cells from normals. So the primary defect in this disorder resides in the B cells or in the receipt of helper function by the B cells. Suppressor cells seen in this disease are probably not the cause of the immunodeficiency. By contrast the irradiated lymphocytes from patients with X-linked agammaglobulinaemia exert vigorous helper function when mixed with normal B lymphocytes[43].

Thymoma with immunodeficiency

This syndrome, first described by Good[123], has been held by many to be an acquired defect in stem cells[124]. The immune defects seen in these patients have ranged from pure B cell abnormalities to a pattern of severe combined immunodeficiency, with most patients having abnormalities in both of the major cellular immunity systems. Their lymphoid tissues have most often shown extreme atrophy with no discernible germinal centres and few or no plasma cells. Many of these patients have had other haematological abnormalities: pure red cell aplasia, pancytopenia, leukopenia and lymphopenia. A few cases with profound eosinopenia have been described[124]. Histologically about 75% of the thymomas are spindle cell in type. All of them however appear to be stromal cell neoplasia. These patients are lacking B cells which bear surface IgM or IgD[108, 125] and also lack mouse erythrocyte rosette-forming cells[121]. Vogler and Cooper *et al.*[24] have demonstrated a complete absence of the putative precursor B cells in the bone marrow of these patients. These are the small lymphocyte-like cells mentioned above which possess intracytoplasmic Ig. This finding appears to indicate that the defect in these patients occurs very early in B cell differentation (although few patients have been described who have early B cells – mouse rosette-forming cells) in their bone marrow[126].

Siegal and Good[30] and Waldmann et al.[34] have observed cells suppressing Ig synthesis in some patients with thymoma and immunodeficiency. These suppressor cells may, however, represent a secondary phenomenon brought on by the absence of B cells, and may be autoimmune lymphocytes activated against antigens specific to particular stages of B cell differentiation. The helper cells are regularly found when suppressor cells have been ablated by X-irradiation[43].

In patients with thymoma and pure red cell aplasia, Zanjani et al.[127] have described in the blood the presence of suppressor T cells which inhibit the erythroid differentiation in vitro.

Common variable immunodeficiency (CVI)

According to the current WHO classification[128], this includes all the poorly defined and 'new syndrome' cases of immunodeficiency. Clinical and immunological status may change in the same patient from time to time and during infection. Most patients with these diseases, unlike those with thymoma or Bruton-type agammaglobulinaemia, have B lymphocytes. The T and B lymphocytes have functions which are quite variable.

Most have their greatest clinical difficulties residing at the level of antibody deficiency disease. Despite quite severe evidence of T cell defects, according to in vitro tests of T cell function which is sometimes seen, these patients are normally capable of handling viral and fungal infections quite well. The clinical problem reflects a general inability of the mature B cells in their natural environment to differentiate terminally into plasma cells which secrete Ig.

Recent developments may indicate that the chief derangement in some patients is one of control mechanisms for Ig secretion and B cell differentiation. Waldmann et al.[20] first reported the presence of suppressor cells in some patients with CVI, and their observations have been confirmed by several other groups[30-33]. Particularly interesting is the finding that relative class-specific suppression can occur[33] in certain patients, providing a possible explanation for certain peculiar patterns of Ig class deficiency which might not be understood in terms of a more fundamental block in differentiation. Wu, Lawton and Cooper[129] have demonstrated that cells of most of these patients cultured with PWM are capable of transforming into plasma cells, despite their failure to do so in vivo, whereas other investigators[29-32] have observed that very few or no plasma cells and no synthesis and secretion of immunoglobulin were seen when the patients' lymphocytes are cultured with PWM. However in a few cases when sheep rosetting cells or adherent cells were removed from the mononuclear cells of patients with CVI, plasma cell development proceeded quite normally. Geha et al.[130] have described patients with this syndrome who could make intracellular Ig but who were severely immunoglobulin-deficient indicating a secretory block that prevents Ig escape from fully formed plasma cells. This finding has not turned up in any of our cases. However Choi and Good[131] showed that some patients with CVI can synthesize Ig in nearly normal amounts, but do not secrete the Ig presumably because the B cells do not take a final step and differentiate to plasma cells. Further analysis of these patients[132] described by Geha et al. has demonstrated an inability of their cells to incorporate sugars into the cytoplasmic Ig, a step known to be a concomitant of Ig secretion from plasma cells.

Cooper et al.[133] have described in these patients considerable heterogeneity in helper functions. Some have T lymphocytes which help poorly both the patient's B cells and normal B cells. Some have B cells that do not respond to the helper influences of their own or normal T cells, and some have T cells which help normal persons' B cells but cannot cooperate with their own. Siegal et al.[43] have found that irradiation of normal T cells removes a suppressor influence, but does not inhibit the ability of the normal lymphocyte or lymphocytes of patients with CVI to help autologous B cells differentiation in vitro. When this system was applied to a large group of CVI patients, at least two variants could be distinguished. In our experience, rather at variance with Cooper et al., the T cells of all patients studied have been able to provide helper effects in vitro, but B cells of some patients evidently cannot be helped to differentiate terminally, despite mixing with irradiated normal T cells. One should, however, surely consider especially from the analysis of Cooper et al. defects in T–B cooperation which could lead to clinical immunodeficiency.

Immunodeficiency with ataxia–telangiectasia

Ataxia–telangiectasia is an autosomal recessive disorder, characterized by telangiectasia of conjunctivae, skin and other organs, progressive cerebellar ataxia and a variable immunodeficiency involving the antibody or the cellular immune system or both. The disease was first clearly described as an entity by Louis-Bar in 1941, and later Boder and Sedgwick in 1957[134] defined the disease in detail and termed it 'ataxia telangiectasia'.

There is considerable variability in the onset of symptoms[135, 136]. The majority of the patients develop ataxia during infancy when they first begin to walk. Speech is also involved and becomes increasingly slurred. Telangiectasias occur initially on the bulbar conjunctivae and may be present as early as 1 year of age or appear as late as 6 years. Recurrent sinopulmonary infections leading to bronchiectasis are present in more patients. Numerous malignancies have been reported. The most common is lymphosarcoma[136-138], but Hodgkin's disease[135], leukaemia[139], adenocarcinoma[140], reticulum cell carcinoma[141], medulloblastoma[138] and dysgerminoma[138] have also been reported.

The very high frequency of malignancy and possibly the complex immunodeficiency as well have recently been attributed to a chromosomal instability[142]. Abnormalities especially of ring chromosome in group 14 have repeatedly been encountered. Just how the chromosomal abnormality accounts for the immunodeficiency or the susceptibility to malignancies has not yet been elucidated. Members of the families of patients with ataxia–telangiectasia also experience a high frequency of malignancies and both patients and family members often have absent or lower than normal levels of IgE[143].

The most consistent findings of surface marker analysis in these patients is the presence of normal or elevated numbers of IgA bearing cells in the absence of serum IgA[119, 144]. Studies of antibody response to specific viral and bacterial antigen show variable degrees of deficiency[145] and they have increased incidence of autoantibodies[146].

Cell-mediated immunity is abnormal in most of the patients, as demonstrated by delayed hypersensitivity skin tests[132, 147, 148], skin allograft rejection and responses of peripheral blood lymphocytes to stimulation with phytomitogens, antigens or allogeneic cells[149]. In cell surface markers, some investigators have found low proportions or low absolute numbers of T cells to parallel depressed PHA responses[150-152], and others[121] have found T cell numbers to be either normal or only slightly depressed. These differences may simply reflect different degrees of immune defect in the various cases studied. Boumsell et al.[153] demonstrated the presence of blood cells capable of expressing T cell markers when incubated with thymic extracts in some patients. Studies of the thymus have shown abnormalities[136, 145]. In some, the thymus was thought to be atrophic; but in most, the thymus was hypoplastic, underdeveloped or atrophic in appearance and lacked Hassall's corpuscles and corticomedullary differentiation. Waldman et al. described the frequent presence of elevated serum concentrations of α-fetoprotein in the blood of patients with this disease[154].

Immunodeficiency with Wiskott–Aldrich syndrome

This syndrome is characterized by thrombocytopenia, eczema, recurrent infection and an inability to form antibodies to polysaccharide antigens. Krivit and Good[155] first showed that these patients are unable to form isohaemagglutinins. The most consistent immunoglobulin pattern is that of normal IgG, decreased IgM, increased IgA and IgE[156-159] in spite of hyper-metabolism of IgG[160]. These patients consistently fail to respond with antibody production to polysaccharide antigens, while they respond better to certain protein antigens[161-163]. However Blaese et al.[164] showed that their responses in vivo to certain classical protein antigens is also defective. It has proved difficult to define precisely the location of the immune defect. Much evidence locates the defect on the afferent limb of immune response but a precise definition is still needed[162].

Diminished in vitro responses of lymphocytes to phytohaemagglutinin and certain antigens have been described[164]. Some patients with this disease may have defective F_C receptor activity on monocytes, which may be responsible for defective antigen processing leading to the ill-defined immunodeficiency in this disorder. Poplack et al.[165] have also found that the capacity of monocytes to cooperate in the antibody-dependent killing of target cells is quite regularly deficient in these patients.

Nine years ago Bach et al. in Wisconsin transplanted a 2-year-old with this disease, using marrow from a HLA-matched sibling donor. The immunodeficiency has been largely corrected and the child remains chi-meric[166]. His haematopoietic abnormalities have not been corrected, e.g. his platelets are still low, but he is living as a normal healthy child and seems to be immunologically reconstituted. Here is another previously fatal disease which has been corrected, at least in part, by bone marrow transplantation. More recently full correction of both haematological and immunological abnormalities appears to have been accomplished by total body irradiation plus antithymocyte globulin administration followed by bone marrow transplantation from a HLA matched sibling donor[167].

Selective IgA deficiency

The incidence of selective IgA deficiency in the general population is between 1 : 500 and 1 : 1000[168,169]. In some patients total absence of IgA occurs while others have detectable amounts in serum and secretions[170]. Patients with other immunodeficiencies may lack IgA but show no other Ig defects, e.g. in ataxia–telangiectasia or in some cases of chronic mucocutaneous candidiasis[171]. In these patients, IgA-bearing B cells are regularly present and sometimes this number is increased[118, 144].

Cooper, Keightley and Lawton[37] and Delespesse et al.[172] have shown that terminal differentiation of IgA B cells into IgA-containing plasma cells occurs under the influence of PWM. Waldmann et al.[34] have recently demonstrated that T cell help may facilitate IgA plasma cell differentiation in vitro in IgA-deficient patients' cells. Recently Atwater et al.[44] and Schwartz et al.[45] have demonstrated class-specific suppression of IgA synthesis and secretion in about 20% of the patients with selective IgA deficiency. The suppressor cells reported in this disease are probably not the cause of the immunodeficiency.

Lymphocytes and haematopoiesis

Next we should also consider the interaction between lymphocyte and the haematopoietic system. It has been shown[173] that mitogen-stimulated lymphocytes can generate factors which help in the differentiation of colony-forming cells of granulocytes (CFU-C) in soft-agar culture. Similarly these lymphocytes under certain circumstances can also suppress CFU-C in soft-agar culture.

Exciting recent evidence suggests that lymphocytes in the bone marrow or even lymphocytes present in the peripheral blood may play an important part in pathogenesis of aplastic anaemia[174, 176], Blackfan–Diamond syndrome[177], thymoma immunodeficiency and red cell aplasia[127], and a variety of neutropenias including congenital and cyclic neutropenia[178, 179]. We first demonstrated in the bone marrow of patients with aplastic anaemia, the existence of suppressor lymphocytes which inhibit proliferation, differentiation and growth in soft-agar culture of committed granulocyte stem cells (CFU-C). Further analysis[175] revealed three probable pathogenetic bases for aplastic anaemia. Approximately one-third of the patients have suppressor lymphocytes of this type, capable of inhibiting differentiation of leukocytes, two-thirds of the patients have a basic stem cell defect and one patient in our series was defined as a patient having normal stem cells and having no suppressor cells. In this patient it appears that an environmental defect exists in the marrow. These findings have been repeatedly confirmed by others[180, 181]. Hoffman et al.[176] have also observed a presence of lymphocyte suppressor of erythroid colony formation in the blood of patients with aplastic anaemia. There are several reports of patients with aplastic anaemia who have received bone marrow transplants after preconditioning with cytoxan, total body irradiation, or horse antihuman thymocyte globulin. Some of these patients reject their allografts and then recover from their aplasia with complete regeneration of their own marrow[182,183]. Recently patients who do not have a matched sibling for bone marrow transplantation have been treated with either cytoxan[184,185] or antilymphocyte serum[180,181] and have recovered from their aplastic anaemia. Similarly certain patients with Blackfan–Diamond syndrome in whom lymphocyte suppression for erythroid colony formation was demonstrated, recovered partially after being treated with prednisone[186].

We have recently[178] described the presence of lymphocyte suppressor cells in patients with neutropenia including congenital and cyclic neutropenia. Extracts of conditioned media obtained from non-rosetting lymphocytes of patient's marrow and peripheral blood regularly exhibited inhibitory activity against autologous and allogeneic granulocyte stem cells in a soft-agar culture assay. The characteristic of these cells in the patients with neutropenia are: density less than 1.070 g/cm^3, they are not granulocytes or monocytes, they sediment from 2–4 mm/h at unit gravity and they are small lymphocytes which do not rosette with SRBC. This inhibitory activity is absent in lymphocytes of normal persons and is different from that elaborated by normal neutrophils and by leukaemic cells[187]. The site of action of this inhibitory activity is at CFU-C level and it does not inhibit colony stimulating activity (CSA) production by normal monocytes. Further it does not inactivate preformed CSA.

Complement system

The complement system consists of a group of normal serum proteins that act as an extraordinary biological amplification system for the immune response[188,189]. Activation of the complement helps to enhance phagocytosis, vascular permeability, chemotaxis of polymorphonuclear cells and monocytes. Its action leads to membrane damage and production of immunopathogenic lesions in immune complex disease. It is now possible to define inherited deficiences of each of the separate components of the complement cascade, with the exception of C9[189]. Increasing evidence that illness and diseases are frequently associated with each of the specific component abnormalities or deficiencies[189] has been presented. A summary of known disorder associated with individual complement component deficiencies is given in Table 1.16. The argument as to whether infection is associated with complement component deficiencies in addition to C3 has been overwhelmingly settled in the affirmative.

One well-defined disease of complement abnormality is hereditary angioneuroticoedema also known as Osler's syndrome. This is due to the lack of or abnormality of C1 esterase inhibitor in the serum, which was described by Donaldson, Rosen and co-workers[190-192]. In this disease,

TABLE 1.16   Complement deficiency in man

C Component deficiency	Associated diseases
C1s	Systemic lupus erythematosus (SLE); lupus-like syndrome
C1s 1NH	Hereditary angioneurotic oedema
C1r	Recurrent infections and chronic glomerulonephritis; LE-like syndrome, necrotizing skin lesions, arthritis
C1q	Agammaglobulinaemia; severe combined immunodeficiency
C2	SLE; SLE-like syndrome; discoid lupus; membranoproliferative glomerulonephritis; dermatomyositis; synovitis; purpura; anaphylactoid purpura; hypertension and recurrent septic meningococcal infection; Hodgkin's disease; chronic lymphatic leukaemia and dermatitis herptiformis; healthy individuals
C3	Recurrent infections; skin rash, arthralgias, fevers
C3b 1NH	Recurrent infection
C4	LE-like syndrome; healthy individual
C5	SLE and recurrent infection
C5 dysfunction	Leiner's syndrome, Gram-negative skin and bowel infection
C6	Recurrent meningococcal meningitis, mild Raynaud phenomenon
C7	Raynaud's phenomenon; renal disease, disseminated gonococcal infection
C8	Disseminated gonococcal infections; *Xeroderma pigmentosum*

For review of complement deficiency diseases in man, see [189]

affected individuals are prone to experience sudden attacks of circumscribed painless non-pitting oedema, which may cause disfigurement of the affected part and usually subsides within 2–3 days. Sometimes, even after minor trauma, oedema may involve hypopharynx and pharynx resulting in sudden death from asphyxia. Abdominal pain and skin rash resembling erythema marginatum are also seen in this syndrome. Of the affected individuals, about 15% possess a biologically inactive form of C1 esterase inhibitor which is immunologically identical to the normal protein[193]. Pickering et al.[194] showed that attacks of the disease, and thus the major hazard of fatal laryngeal oedema, can be promptly aborted by intravenous injection of fresh normal plasma which contains the C1 esterase inhibitor in large amount. Such therapy is not hazardous and has been most helpful in management of this disease. Frank et al.[195] have very recently shown that by treatment with anabolic steroids (Danazol), which are substituted androgens, one can in most of these patients induce the production of the inhibitor and prevent the dangerous attacks. This treatment seems to be able to prevent completely the life-threatening consequences of this immunologically based disorder. Further study of treated patients shows that the normal C1 esterase inhibitor appears in the plasma after treatment in patients lacking the inhibitor and both normal and abnormal inhibitor are present in patients who have the inhibitor-like molecule which is non-functional.

C1q deficiency has been observed in some patients with severe combined immunodeficiency[196], and agammaglobulinaemia[197]. Ballow et al.[198] showed that C1q was reconstituted after bone marrow transplantation, whether or not the marrow transplantation corrected the immunodeficiency. In one patient in whom there was no evidence of successful engraftment, C1q remained very low.

Pickering et al.[199] and Day et al.[200] have described patients in whom C1r deficiency caused serious disease and destruction of the kidney. We now know that a deficiency of any of the early components of complement is, in fact, often associated with kidney disease[199]. In the same patient, studied by Pickering et al.[201] and Day et al.[202], a kidney transplant corrected the complement abnormality, since cells in the transplanted organ were able to produce the missing complement and correct the immunodeficiency disease.

A disorder which deserves mention is Leiner's disease or C5 dysfunction syndrome. The clinical entity was first described by Leiner in 1908 and later on Miller et al.[203-205] demonstrated deficient opsonic activity for yeast particles in such a patient's serum, and associated this deficiency with an abnormality of C5 function. Measurement of total haemolytic complement was normal, as was the patient's C5 on immunochemical measurement. Clinically, this syndrome is characterized by seborrhoeic dermatitis, persistent diarrhoea, recurrent infections and marked wasting and dystrophy. In these cases, administration of appropriate plasma from normal donors has allowed the patients to recover from an otherwise frequently fatal disease and to grow and develop normally.

Disorders of the phagocytic system

One of the critical host defence mechanisms found in man is the ability of both polymorphonuclear leukocytes (PMN) and monocytes to eliminate foreign material. Failure in either or both of these systems invariably results in increased susceptibility to infections. Only a few years ago it was estimated that phagocyte disorders account for less than 5% of all primary immunodeficiences. However, recently, increasing numbers of patients with defects in phagocytic cells are being described in the literature.

TABLE 1.17 Functional properties of granulocytes in different disorders of the phagocytic system

	CGD	Myeloperoxidase deficiency	Chediak–Higashi syndrome	HyperIgE recurrent skin infection
I. *Inflammatory responses*				
(a) Granulocytopoiesis	normal	normal	reduced	reduced
(b) Skin window response	normal	normal	reduced	?reduced
(c) Chemotaxis	usually normal	?	reduced	reduced
II. *Microbicidal activities*				
(a) Phagocytosis	normal	normal	normal to increased	normal
(b) Killing of:				
Catalase-positive organisms	impaired	delayed	delayed	normal
Catalase-negative organisms	normal	?slight delay	delayed	normal
(c) Metabolic activities during phagocytosis	reduced; no H_2O_2 release	increased; protein iodination reduced	normal to increased	normal

The six serial physiological steps involved in phagocytosis and killing of the bacteria are (a) random movement, (b) chemotaxis, (c) opsonization and bacterial fixation, (d) ingestion, (e) activation of the phagocytes and (f) destruction of foreign material. The defect in microbicidal activity can occur at any step, leading to increased susceptibility to infection. A summary of functional properties of granulocytes in different disorders of the phagocytic system is given in Table 1.17. Of all phagocytic disorders described, the most thoroughly studied is chronic granulomatous disease of childhood.

Chronic granulomatous disease (CGD)

In 1957, Berendes, Bridges and Good[206] first defined the distinct clinical entity of fatal chronic granulomatous syndrome of childhood. In 1968, Windhorst et al.[207] and Carson and his co-workers[208] confirmed this finding and strengthened the evidence for an X-linked transmission of one form of the disease. Holmes et al.[209] discovered that these patients fail to show the oxidative burst, H_2O_2 formation and hexose monophosphate shunt activity that accompanies ingestion of micro-organisms by the polymorph and monocytes of normal persons. Clinically this syndrome consists of recurrent purulent granulomatous infection of the skin, reticuloendothelial organs and lungs. Lymphadenopathy and pulmonary infections associated with an inability of patient's phagocytes to kill catalase-positive bacteria establish the diagnosis. The most common catalase-positive organisms are *Staphylococcus aureus, Klebsiella, Escheriscia coli, Serratia marscesens, Pseudomonas, Asperigillus, Candida albicans, Proteus, Salmonella, Mycobacteria, Nocardia* and other enteric bacteria. Pneumocystis infection in this disease has not been described. However at least two patients with CGD have had pneumocystis[210,211], one of which was studied in our own institution. This patient had, however, been placed on prednisone by his family doctor. Clinically our patient presented with fever, respiratory distress and chest X-ray showed infiltration in the lung. The diagnosis of pneumocystis was made from closed lung biopsy and was effectively treated with trimethoprim-sulpha. The basic enzymatic defect in the most common form of this disease has not yet been defined. It has been attributed to deficiency of various enzymes necessary for the oxidative metabolic activity of the cell for the final production of H_2O_2 which helps in the final killing of bacteria. These enzyme defects are NADH oxidase[212,213] and NADPH oxidase[214]. However, levels of these enzymes are normal in the resting cells of the patients. Recently a defective function of an NADH dehydrogenase enzyme which is normally located in the plasma membrane has been described[215]. There seems no longer any question that generation of H_2O_2, important in halogenation of the bacteria and the activated forms of oxygen, superoxide (O_2^-), singlet oxygen ($'O$) and OH^- radicals are involved in killing of ingested micro-organisms. These substances are not generated in the abnormal leukocytes of the patients with the X-linked form of CGD, Marsh et al.[216,217] have described an antigen which is associated with generation of Kell specificities that may be the key to understanding the fundamental abnormality of the leukocytes in this disease. This antigen is called Kx. It is lacking from the red cells of the Kell negative mutant called McLeod mutant. This antigen is present on the leukocytes but lacking from the red cells in persons with this genetic variant and they have no defect of leukocyte function. Normal persons have Kx antigen in both their red cells and white blood cells. Patients with CGD are Kell negative too frequently[218]. Such patients lack Kx on both red cells and white blood cells. Patients with the X-linked form of CGD who are Kell positive, however, also lack the Kx antigen on their white blood corpuscles even though they possess it on their red blood corpuscles. This abnormality of the surface of the cells of the patients with X-linked CGD seems to us to be very proximally related to the essential defect inherited in these patients.

Clinical manifestations of chronic granulomatous septic disease have been related to at least three other genetically determined abnormalities. There is an autosomal recessive form of the disease first recognized as a separate entity when it turned up in female patients. These patients lack the enzyme glutathione reductase and their parents frequently show half values of this enzyme in their leukocytes[219,220]. Another variant also inherited as an autosomal recessive is observed in patients with complete absence of glucose-6-phosphate dehydrogenase[221-223]; a final form also apparently autosomally inherited is not associated with any defined enzyme abnormality as yet but is clearly a different entity from the X-linked disease[224]. We postulate that in the X-linked recessive form of the disease the membrane abnormality is somehow related to failure of the internalized membrane to trigger the metabolic events that so characterize phagocytic cells. Exactly how this trigger mechanism works is still a moot point but it and the nature of the Kx antigens now seems to us to be the central issue in the further analysis of this fascinating inborn error of metabolism. The surface Kx antigen as might be expected is not abnormal or lacking on the leukocytes of patients with the autosomal recessive forms of the disease. The genetic analysis of patients with the X-linked forms of CGD has been extensively studied by Windhorst et al.[225] who established that carrier mothers, sisters and grandmothers have defective ability to kill catalase-positive organisms. This deficiency is intermediate between the normal and patients with CGD. Further the leukocytes of the carrier females appear to be of two separate populations as might be expected from the hypothesis of Lyon. Approximately half of the granulocytes for example reduce the tetrazolium dye to formazan while half do not. Baehner and Nathan[226] also showed the usefulness of nitroblue tetrazolium (NBT) in the diagnosis and detection of the carrier stage of CGD. Quantitative determinations of reduction of NBT in male and female CGD patients demonstrated deficient reduction of NBT by their PMN both at rest and during phagocytosis. The mothers of male patients had intermediate reduction of NBT supporting the theory that the disease is due to a genetic defect on the X-chromosome. Studies by Quie *et al.*[227] and Macfarlane *et al.*[228] also suggested that the X-linked carrier state can be detected by an intermediate degree of bacterial killing as well as intermediate abnormalities in oxygen consumption or activity of the hexose monophosphate shunt activity.

Since at the present time we cannot find a way to achieve a continuous supply of hydrogen peroxide and/or the agitated states of oxygen to the phagocytic vacuoles of the PMN, the treatment of this disorder remains inadequate. During the course of an active infection, identification of the organism and vigorous antibiotic therapy even using the intravenous route should be administered. Granulocyte transfusion along with antibiotics may be beneficial during a course of severe infection. Long-term, or continuous administration of sulphonamide[229] or anti-staphylococcal drugs[230] has appeared to decrease infections in most patients in whom it has been tried, but controlled trial of these drugs in chronic CGD has not been performed. Bone marrow transplantation may turn out to be the treatment of choice when an HLA-identical matched sibling is available. Recently Hobbs *et al.*[231] have treated a GCD patient with bone marrow transplantation from a fully compatible unrelated donor. After marrow transplantation, this patient demonstrated clinical improvement with definite evidence of engraftment and improved neutrophil function especially during infection. This direction of therapy development must be extended.

Disorders of mobility

The syndromes associated with disorders of mobility are lazy leukocyte syndrome, Chediak–Higashi syndrome, familial chemotactic defect, Wiskott–Aldrich syndrome, the hyperimmunoglobulinaemia E syndrome and acrodermatitis enteropathica.

Lazy leukocyte syndrome

This syndrome was described by Miller et al. in 1971[232]. It is characterized by severe peripheral neutropenia, recurrent bacterial infections, dermatitis, periodontitis and impaired random migration and chemotaxis of the polymorphonuclear leukocytes. These patients are unable to mobilize an apparently normal store of PMN as detected by epinephrine stimulation of the marginal pool.

Chediak–Higashi syndrome

This syndrome is characterized by partial oculocutaneous albinism, neutropenia, recurrent pyogenic infections, giant lysosomes in all lysosomal-containing cells and autosomal recessive pattern of inheritance. Although phagocytosis of bacteria is normal in this disorder intracellular killing is delayed[233]. Both neutrophil and monocyte chemotaxis are abnormal in this disease[234-236], but Smithwick and Pahwa et al.[237] have observed normal neutrophil and monocyte chemotaxis in a patient with Chediak–Higashi syndrome who also had Hodgkin's disease and was getting vitamin C as part of therapy. A primary defect in PMN deformability has been suggested to be the cause for depressed chemotaxis in these patients. Unusually high levels of cyclic adenosine monophosphate (cAMP) have been found in the neutrophil and ultrastructural studies have suggested that impaired neutrophil function may be related to abnormal microtubule assembly which was associated with the increased levels of cAMP. Boxer et al.[238] have corrected the cellular defect in chemotaxis, phagocytosis, cAMP levels and defective microtubules by exposing the cells to ascorbic acid in vitro. They have treated a patient of this disorder with oral ascorbic acid and were able to reverse the chemotactic, bactericidal and degranulation defects by treatment with vitamin C. Neutrophil defects which were present before the onset of treatment with vitamin C also decreased the level of cAMP in the neutrophil after in vivo treatment. It remains to be determined whether this rather simple therapy will prevent the infections and malignancies which otherwise cause the early death of these children.

The hyperimmunoglobulinaemia E syndromes

In recent years disorders of neutrophil mobility associated with recurrent staphylococcal infection have been observed in several clinical entities. Five clinical variants have been described, but all have in common elevated serum IgE levels and very frequently defective chemotaxis.

1. Buckley et al.[239] have described two adolescent boys who had recurrent cutaneous, pulmonary, and joint abscesses, growth retardation, coarse facies, chronic dermatitis, high serum concentration of IgE, eosinophilia, defective PMN chemotaxis and depressed in vivo cellular immunity and antibody formation. These patients do not show pulmonary allergy or atopic dermatitis. Later Snyderman and Buckley and associates[240] studied monocyte chemotaxis in these patients and found variable defects in some patients.

2. Clark et al.[241] and Hill and Quie[242] have reported patients who had mucocutaneous candidiasis and lifelong history of pyogenic infections. They had elevated serum IgE level and eosinophilia.

3. Hill and Quie[243] then described three patients with chronic atopic dermatitis and elevated serum IgE level, accompanied by recurrent superficial and deep abscesses of the scalp, buttocks, thighs and trunk, suppurative lymphadenitis, cellulitis, and marked pruritus.

4. Hill and Quie et al.[242] re-evaluated the patients described as having Job's syndrome, who had similar elevated serum IgE levels, atopic-like eczema and recurrent cold staphylococcocal abscess, red hair and fair skin. These patients also were found to have defective PMN chemotaxis.

5. Finally, we have observed[244] three patients with hyperIgE, eosinophilia, recurrent skin infections, and associated boney abnormalities, such as craniosynostosis. Monocyte chemotaxis was defective in two and a granulocyte chemotactic defect was found in the other.

The mechanisms of faulty chemotaxis in patients with elevated serum IgE level is not yet known. IgE from these patients does not inhibit chemotaxis of normal PNMs, but histamine did inhibit chemotaxis in a study carried out by Quie[242].

Listed in Table 1.18 are some immunodeficiency diseases, which can be effectively corrected by cellular engineering. In Figure 1.8 are summarized some suggestions for the effective treatment of immunodeficiency diseases.

In this dissertation we have attempted to analyse the immunodeficiency diseases of man from the perspective of our ever-increasing knowledge of the specific immunological systems, biological amplification processes and fundamental effector mechanisms of immunity. From this perspective new primary immunodeficiencies can rapidly be recognized and definition of immunodeficiencies constantly improved. Although many of these diseases can already be defined in genetic terms and a few now even defined in terms of the fundamental enzymatic deficiencies or abnormalities, none is as yet fully understood. However our progress has been

TABLE 1.18   Diseases corrected by cellular engineering

1. DiGeorge syndrome
2. SCID, X-linked recessive
3. SCID, autosomal recessive ADA⁻
4. SCID, autosomal recessive ADA⁺
5. SCID, inhibitor ADA, autosomal recessive
6. Wiskott–Aldrich syndrome, autosomal recessive
7. Aplastic anaemia
    (a) suppressor⁺
    (b) suppressor⁻
8. Leukaemia, AML, ALL
9. Chronic granulomatous disease, X-linked form
10. C1r deficiency

sufficient to permit us increasingly to approach treatment using measures that replace missing components and sometimes even cure the disease. Cellular engineering is developing rapidly and experimental studies

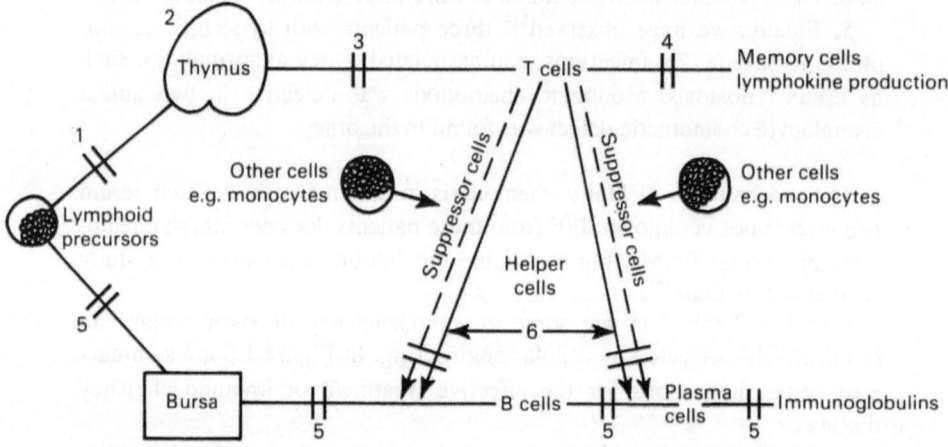

1. Replacement of lymphoid cells
2. Thymus transplant
3. ? Thymic factors
4. Transfer factor
5. Replacement therapy with immunoglobulin or plasma
6. Normal B cells with – suppressor cells – immunosuppression; replacement therapy
   lack of helper cells – ??? helper factors; replacement therapy
5. and 6. Together – replacement therapy

Figure 1.8   Treatment of immunodeficiency

encourage ambitions to extend this approach much further, even beyond immunobiology to correction of many inborn and acquired deficiencies. Substitution therapy is being improved and we are beginning to use effectively what might be called macromolecular engineering and differentiation therapy to address some of our problems.

From all of these studies, therapeutic efforts and analyses, it is clear that the primary immunodeficiencies, which are not the rare diseases we once thought them to be, continue to be the most incisive teachers of immunology. In addition they present the most effective challenges to our developing knowledge. Although the primary, generally genetically determined immunodeficiencies are not common diseases, many of the immunological lessons they teach are applicable to considerations of the most common diseases of man. Immunodeficiencies are now known to exist in the neonate and the aged, and with nutritional deprivation be produced by infections with viruses, bacteria, fungi, and parasites. Immunodeficiencies have been associated with autoimmunity and mesenchymal disease. There are very likely lacunar immunodeficiencies that are consequent to genetic differences at the major histocompatibility region of chromosome six. Immunodeficiencies are surely associated or produced by many efforts at drug therapy; even cancer is frequently associated with immunodeficiency. All of these will be better understood as a consequence of analysis focused by studies in patients with the primary immunodeficiencies. We feel certain that because of the complexity of the immunological system and the positive and negative interactions of the many components that we are just beginning to describe and understand the immunodeficiency diseases. Continued study from these great teachers should give us an increasing ability to address common diseases of man with increasingly effective tools and ultimately to be able efficiently to correct the immunodeficiency diseases of man in whatever situation they are found.

References

1. Good, R. A. and Papermaster, B. W. (1964). Ontogeny and phylogeny of adaptive immunity. *Adv. Immunol.*, 4, 1
2. Moore, M. A. S. and Owen, J. J. T. (1967). Experimental studies on the development of the thymus. *J. Exp. Med.*, 126, 715
3. Moore, M. A. S. and Metcalf, D. (1970). Ontogeny of the hemopoietic system: Yolk sac origin of *in vivo* and *in vitro* colony forming cells in the developing mouse embryo. *Br. J. Haematol.*, 18, 279
4. Cooper, M. S., Peterson, R. D. A., South, M. A. and Good, R. A. (1966). The function of the thymus system and the bursa system in the chicken. *J. Exp. Med.*, 123, 75
5. Tyan, M. L. and Herzenburg, L. A. (1968). Studies on the ontogeny of the

mouse immune system. II. Immunoglobulin producing cells. *J. Immunol.*, 101, 446

6. Owen, J., Cooper, M. D. and Raff, M. (1974). *In vitro* generation of B lymphocytes in mouse foetal liver, a mammalian bursa equivalent. *Nature (London)*, 249, 361

7. Aiuti, F. and Wigzell, H. (1974). A study on human T lymphocytes, their function and frequency in some diseases. In B. D. Jankovic and B. Isakovic (eds.), *Microenvironmental Aspects of Immunity*, p. 307. (New York: Plenum Press)

8. Greaves, M. F., Owen, J. J. T. and Raff, M. C. (1973). *T and B Lymphocytes Origins, Properties and Roles in Immune Responses.* (Amsterdam: Excerpta Medica; New York: American Elsevier Publishing Co. Inc.)

9. Touraine, J. L., Incefy, G. S., Touraine, F. Traeger, J. and Good, R. A. (1976). Antilymphocyte antibodies: an approach to dissecting the heterogeneity of the immune system. *Post. Med. J.*, 52 (suppl 5), 41

10. Good, R. A., Incefy, G. S. and Touraine, J. L. (1976). Human anti-T-cell cytotoxic sera as an approach to dissection of immunological systems. *Post. Med. J.*, 52 (suppl 5), 35

11. Froland, S. S. and Natvig, J. B. (1973). Identification of three different lymphocytes populations by surface markers. *Transplant Rev.*, 16, 114

12. Parrott, D. M., DeSousa, M. A. B. and East, J. (1966). Thymus-dependent areas in the lymphoid organs of neonatally thymectomized mice. *J. Exp. Med.*, 123, 191

13. Peterson, R. D. A., Cooper, M. D. and Good, R. A. (1965). The pathogenesis of immunologic deficiency diseases. *Am. J. Med.*, 38, 579

14. Touraine, J. L., Incefy, G. S., Touraine, F., Rho, Y. M. and Good, R. A. (1974). Differentiation of human bone marrow cells into T lymphocytes by *in vitro* incubation with thymic extracts. *Clin. Exp. Immunol.*, 17, 151

15. Touraine, J. L., Incefy, G. S., Touraine, F., L'Espérance, P., Siegal, F. P. and Good, R. A. (1974). T lymphocyte differentiation *in vitro* in primary immunodeficiency diseases. *Clin. Immunol. Immunopathol.*, 3, 228

16. Incefy, G. S., L'Espérance, P. and Good, R. A. (1975). *In vitro* differentiation of human marrow cells into T lymphocytes by thymic extracts using the rosette technique. *Clin. Exp. Immunol.*, 19, 475

17. Incefy, G. S., Boumsell, T., Touraine, J. L., L'Espérance, P., Smithwick, E., O'Reilly, R. and Good, R. A. (1975). Enhancement of T-lymphocyte differentiation *in vitro* by thymic extracts after bone marrow transplantation in severe combined immunodeficiencies. *Clin. Immunol. Immunopathol.*, 4, 258

18. Incefy, G. S., Grimes, E., Kagan, W. A., Goldstein, G., Smithwick, E., O'Reilly, R. and Good, R. A. (1976). Heterogeneity of stem cells in severe combined immunodeficiency. *Clin. Exp. Immunol.*, 25, 462

19. Touraine, J. L., Touraine, F., Hadden, J. W., Hadden, E. M. and Good, R. A. (1976). 5-Bromodeoxyuridine-light inactivation of human lymphocytes stimulated by mitogens and allogeneic cells: evidence for distinct T lymphocyte subsets. *Int. Arch. Allergy Appl. Immunol.*, 52, 105

20. Touraine, J. L., Hadden, J. W., Touraine, F., Hadden, E. M., Estensen, R. and Good, R. A. (1977). Phorbolmyristate acetate: a mitogen selective for a T lymphocyte subpopulation. *J. Exp. Med.*, 145, 460

21. Touraine, J. L., Hadden, J. W. and Good, R. A. (1977). Sequential stages of human T lymphocyte differentiation. *Proc. Natl. Acad. Sci. USA*, 73, 3414
22. Hämmerling, U., Chin, A. F. and Abbott, J. (1976). Ontogeny of murine B lymphocytes: sequence of B cell differentiation from surface immunoglobulin negative precursors to plasma cells. *Proc. Natl. Acad. Sci. USA*, 73, 2008
23. Goldstein, G., Scheid, M., Hämmerling, U., Boyse, E. A., Schlesinger, D. H. and Wiall, H. D. (1975). Isolation of a polypeptide which has lymphocyte-differentiating properties and is probably represented universally in living cells. *Proc. Natl. Acad. Sci. USA*, 72, 11
24. Vogler, L. B., Pearl, E. R., Gathings, W. E., Lawton, A. R. and Cooper, M. D. (1976). B lymphocyte precursors in bone-marrow in immunoglobulin deficiency diseases. *Lancet*, ii, 376
25. Kincade, P. W., Lawton, A. R., Bockman, D. E. and Cooper, M. D. (1970). Suppression of immunoglobulin-G synthesis as a result of antibody-mediated suppression of immunoglobulin-M synthesis in chickens. *Proc. Natl. Acad. Sci. USA*, 67, 1918
26. Gathings, W. E., Cooper, M. D., Lawton, A. R. and Alford, C. A. Jr. (1976). B cell ontogeny in humans. *Fed. Proc.*, 35, 276
27. Gupta, S., Good, R. A. and Siegal, F. P. (1976). Rosette-formation with mouse erythrocytes. II. A marker for human and B and non-T lymphocytes. *Clin. Exp. Immunol.*, 25, 319
28. Gupta, S., Pahwa, R., O'Reilly, R., Good, R. A. and Siegal, F. P. (1976). Ontogeny of lymphocyte subpopulations in human fetal liver. *Proc. Natl. Acad. Sci. USA*, 73, 919
29. Waldmann, T. A., Broder, S., Blaese, R. M., Durm, M., Blackman, M. and Strober, W. (1974). Role of suppressor T cells in pathogenesis of common variable hypogammaglobulinaemia. *Lancet*, ii, 609
30. Siegal, F. P., Siegal, M. and Good, R. A. (1976). Suppression of B cell differentiation by leukocytes from hypogammaglobulinemic patients. *J. Clin. Invest.*, 58, 109
31. Broom, B. D., de la Concha, E. G., Webster, A. D. B., Janossy, G. J. and Asherson, G. L. (1976). Intracellular immunoglobulin production *in vitro* by lymphocytes from patients with hypogammaglobulinemia and their effect on normal lymphocytes. *Clin. Exp. Immunol.*, 23, 77
32. Schwartz, S. A., Choi, Y. S., Shou, L. and Good, R. A. (1977). Modulatory effects on immunoglobulin synthesis and secretion by lymphocytes from immunodeficient patients. *J. Clin. Invest.*, 59, 1176
33. McKenzie, M. R. and Paglieroni, T. (1975). Class specific Ig suppression in variable immunodeficiency. *Blood*, 46, 1019
34. Waldmann, T. A., Broder, S., Krakauer, R., MacDermott, R. P., Durm, M., Goldman, C. and Meade, B. (1976). The role of suppressor cells in the pathogenesis of common variable hypogammaglobulinemia and the immunodeficiency associated with myeloma. *Fed. Proc.*, 35, 2067
35. Shou, L., Schwartz, S. A. and Good, R. A. (1976). Suppressor cell activity after concanavalin A treatment of lymphocytes from normal donors. *J. Exp. Med.*, 143, 1100
36. Geha, R. S., Schneeberger, E., Merler, E. *et al.* (1974). Synthesis of an M component by circulating B lymphocytes in severe combined immunodeficiency. *N. Engl. J. Med.*, 290, 726

37. Cooper, M. D., Keightley, R. G. and Lawton, A. R. (1975). Defective T and B cells in primary immunodeficiencies. In M. Seligmann, J. L. Preud'homme, and F. M. Kourilsky (eds.), *INSERM Symposium I*, p. 431. (New York: American-Elsevier)

38. Broder, S., Edelson, R. L., Lutzner, M. A. *et al.* (1976). The Sézary syndrome: A malignant proliferation of helper T cells. *J. Clin. Invest.*, **58**, 1297

39. Safai, B. *et al.* Personal communication

40. Keightley, R. G., Cooper, M. D. and Lawton, A. R. (1976). The T cell dependence of B cell differentiation induced by pokeweed mitogen. *J. Immunol.*, **117**, 1538

41. Fauci, A. S. and Pratt, K. S. (1976). Polyclonal activation of bone-marrow-derived lymphocytes from human peripheral blood measured by a direct plaque-forming cell assay. *Proc. Natl. Acad. Sci. USA*. **73**, 3676

42. Fauci, A. S., Pratt, K. S. and Whalen, G. (1976). Activation of human B lymphocytes II. Cellular interactions in the PFC response of human tonsillar and peripheral blood B lymphocytes to polyclonal activation by pokeweed mitogen. *J. Immunol.*, **117**, 2100

43. Siegal, F. P. and Siegal, M. (1977). Enhancement by irradiated T cells of human plasma cell production: dissection of helper and suppressor functions *in vitro*. *J. Immunol.*, **118**, 642

44. Atwater, J. S. and Tomasi, T. B. (1977). Suppressor cells in selective IgA deficiency. In *American Congress of Allergy and Immunology, New York, 1977*. Abstracts of Scientific Papers (Library of Congress Catalogue No. 77-79345). Abstract 133

45   Schwartz, S. Personal communication

46. Moretta, L., Ferrarini, M., Durante, M. L. and Minari, M. C. (1975). Expression of a receptor for IgM by human T cells in vitro. *Europ. J. Immunol.*, **5**, 565

47. Moretta, L., Webb, S. R., Grossi, C. E., Lydyard, P. M. and Cooper, M. D. (1976). Functional analysis of two subpopulations of human T cells and their distribution in immunodeficient patients. *Clin. Res.*, **24**, 448A

48. Gupta, S. and Good, R. A. (1977). Subpopulations of human T lymphocytes. 1. Studies in immunodeficient patients. *Clin. Exp. Immunol.*, **30**, 222

49. Chiao, J. W., Pantic, V. S. and Good, R. A. (1974). Human peripheral lymphocytes bearing both B-cell complement receptors and T-cell characteristics for sheep erythrocytes detected by a mixed rosette method. *Clin. Exp. Immunol.*, **18**, 485

50. Gupta, S. and Good, R. A. (1977). Subpopulations of human T lymphocytes. II. Effect of thymopoietin, corticosteroids and irradiation. *Cell. Immunol.*, **34**, 10

51. Kishimoto, T., Ralph, P. and Good, R. A. (1978). Stimulation of a human B lymphocyte line by anti-immunoglobulin and its concanavalin A induced suppression by a T cell line. *Clin. Exp. Immunol.* (In press)

52. Jerne, N. K. (1974). Towards a network theory of the immune system. *Ann. Immunol.* (*Paris*), **125C**, 373

53. Trotta, P. P., Smithwick, E. M. and Balis, M. E. (1976). A normal level of adenosine deaminase activity in the red cell lysates of carriers and patients with severe combined immunodeficiency disease. *Proc. Natl. Acad. Sci. USA*, **73**, 104

54. Trotta, P. P., Smithwick, E. M., Good, R. A. and Balis, E. M. (1976). Characterization of adenosine deaminase from red cell lysates of carriers and patients with severe combined immunodeficiency. *Fed. Proc.*, 35, 733

55. Gatti, R. A., Platt, N., Hong, R., Langer, L. O., Kay, H. E. M. and Good, R. A. (1969). Hereditary lymphopenic agammaglobulinemia associated with a distinctive form of short-limbed dwarfism and ectodermal dysplasia. *J. Pediatr.*, 75, 675

56. Pahwa, R. (Unpublished observation)

57. Buckley, R., Gilbertsen, B., Schiff, R. I., Ferreira, E., Sanal, S. and Waldmann, R. A. (1976). Heterogeneity of lymphocyte subpopulations in severe combined immunodeficiency. *J. Clin. Invest.*, 58, 130

58. Incefy, G. S. and Good, R. A. (1976). The need for transcription and translation for differentiation of bone marrow cells by thymic factors in man. In M. Feldman and A. Globerson, (eds.), *Immune Reactivity of Lymphocytes: Development, Expression and Control*, p. 41. (New York: Plenum)

59. Storrie, B., Goldstein, G., Boyse, E. A. and Hämmerling, U. (1976). Differentiation of thymocytes: evidence that induction of the surface phenotype requires transcription and translation. *J. Immunol.*, 116, 1358

60. Pyke, K. W. and Gelfand, E. M. (1974) Morphological and functional maturation of human thymic epithelium in culture. *Nature (London)*, 251, 421

61. Pahwa, R. N., Pahwa, S. G. and Good, R. A. (1979). T.-lymphocyte differentiation in severe combined immunodeficiency: defects of the thymus. *Clin. Immunol. Immunopathol.* (In press)

62. Pahwa, R., O'Reilly, R., Pahwa, S. and Good, R. A. (1977). Possible defect of communication between precursor cells and thymus in severe combined immunodeficiency. *Clin. Res.*, 25, 486A

63. Lewis, V., Twomey, J., Goldstein, G., O'Reilly, R., Smithwick, E., Pahwa, R., Pahwa, S., Good, R. A., Schulte-Wissermann, H., Horowitz, S., Hong, R., Jones, J., Sieber, O., Kirkpatrick, C., Polmar, S. and Bealmear, P. (1977). Circulating thymic hormone activity in congenital immunodeficiency. *Lancet*, ii, 471

64. Incefy, G. S., Dardenne, M., Pahwa, S., Grimes, E., Pahwa, R., Smithwick, E. M., O'Reilly, R. J. and Good, R. A. (1977). Thymic activity in severe combined immunodeficiency diseases. *Proc. Natl. Acad. Sci. USA*, 74, 1250

65. Pahwa, S. (Unpublished observations)

66. Geha, R. S. (1976). Is the B cell abnormality secondary to T cell abnormality in severe combined immunodeficiency? *Clin. Immunol. Immunopathol.*, 6, 102

67. Griscelli, C., Durandy, A., Virelizier, J. L., Ballet, J. J. and Daguillard, F. (1978). Selective defect of precursor T cells associated with apparently normal B lymphocytes in severe combined immunodeficiency disease. *J. Pediatr.*, 93, 404

68. O'Reilly. (Unpublished cases)

69. Seeger, R. C., Robins, R. A., Stevens, R. H., Klein, R. B., Waldmann, D. J., Zeltzer, P. M. and Kessler, S. W. (1976). Severe combined immunodeficiency with B lymphocytes: *in vitro* correction of defective immunoglobulin production by addition of normal T lymphocytes. *Clin. Exp. Immunol.*, 26, 1

70. Schwartz, S. A., Shou, L. and Good, R. A. (1977). Suppressor cell activity in severe combined immunodeficiency. In *American Congress of Allergy and Immunology, New York, 1977*. Abstracts of Scientific Papers (Library of Congress Catalogue No. 77–79345) (abstract 133)

71. Gatti, R. A., Meuwissen, H. J., Allen, H. D., Hong, R. and Good, R. A. (1968). Immunologic reconstitution of sex-linked lymphopenic immunologic deficiency. *Lancet*, ii, 1366

72. Good, R. A. (1969). Immunologic reconstitution: the achievement and its meaning. *Hosp. Prac.*, 4, 41

73. Biggar, W. D., Park, B. H. and Good, R. A. (1975). Compatible bone marrow transplantation and immunologic reconstitution of combined immunodeficiency disease. In D. Bergsma, ed., R. A. Good, and J. Finstad, scientific eds. *Immunodeficiency in Man and Animals*, p. 385. Sinauer Associates, Inc., Sunderland, Mass., 1975. (Birth Defects: Original Article Series, Vol. XI, no. 1, 1975)

74. Vossen, J. M., Dekoning, J., Van Bekkum, D. W., Dicke, K. A., Eijsvoogel, P. P., Hijams, W., Van Logem, E., Radl. J., Van Rood, J. J., Van Der Waay, D. and Dooren, L. J. (1973). Successful treatment of an infant with severe combined immunodeficiency by transplantation of bone marrow cells from an uncle. *Clin. Exp. Immunol.*, 13, 20

75. Geha, R. S., Malakian, A., Le Franc, G., Chayban, D. and Serre, J. L. (1976). Immunologic reconstitution in severe combined immunodeficiency following transplantation with parental bone marrow. *Pediatrics*, 58, 451

76. Anderson, I. M. (1975). Bone marrow transplants. *Proc. Roy. Soc. Med.*, 68, 577

77. Polmar, S. and Sorensen, R. U. (1976). Personal communication

78. Copenhagen Study Group of Immunodeficiencies (1973). Bone marrow transplantation from an HL-A-non-indentical but mixed-lymphocyte-culture identical donor. *Lancet*, i, 1146

79. Gatti, R. A., Meuwissen, H. J., Allen, H. D., Hong, R. and Good, R. A. (1968). Immunological reconstitution of sex-linked lymphopenic immunological deficiency. *Lancet*, ii, 1366

80. Niethammer, D., Goldman, S. F., Haas, R. J., Dietrich, M., Flad, H. B., Fliedner, R. M. and Kleihaver, E. (1976). Bone marrow transplantation for severe combined immunodeficiency with the HLA-A incompatible but MLC identical mother as a donor. *Transplant. Proc.*, 8, 623

81. Copenhagen Study Group of Immunodeficiencies (1976). Bone marrow transplantation from parent to child (both DW-2-homozygous). Personal communication

82. Dupont, B., Hansen, J., Good, R. A. and O'Reilly, R. J. (1977). Histocompatibility testing for clinical bone marrow transplantation. In G. B. Ferrara (ed.) *HLA System—New Aspects*, p. 153. (New York: Elsevier/North-Holland Biomedical Press)

83. Horowitz, S. D., Bach, F. H., Groshong, T., Hong, R. and Yunis, E. J. (1975). Treatment of severe combined immunodeficiency with bone marrow from an unrelated, mixed-leukocyte-culture-non-reactive donor. *Lancet*, ii, 431

84. O'Reilly, R. J., Dupont, B., Pahwa, S., Grimes, E., Smithwick, E. M., Pahwa, R., Schwartz, S., Hansen, J. A., Siegal, F. P., Svejgaard, A., Jersild, C.,

Thomsen, M., L'Esperance, P. and Good, R. A. (1978). Successful hematologic and immunologic reconstitution of severe combined immunodeficiency and secondary asplasia by transplantation of bone marrow from an unrelated HLA-D compatible donor. *N. Engl. J. Med.*, 297, 1311

85. Pahwa, R., Pahwa, S., Good, R. A., Incefy, G. S. and O'Reilly, R. J. (1977). Rationale for combined use of fetal liver and thymus for immunological reconstitution in patients with variants of severe combined immunodeficiency. *Proc. Natl. Acad. Sci. USA*, 74, 3002

86. Pyke, K. W., Dosch, M. M., Ipp, M. M. and Gelfand, E. W. (1975). Demonstration of an intrathymic defect in a case of severe combined immunodeficiency disease. *N. Engl. J. Med.*, 293, 424

87. Ammann, A. J., Wara, D. W., Salmon, S. and Perkins, H. (1973). Permanent reconstitution of cellular immunity in a patient with sex-linked combined immunodeficiency. *N. Engl. J. Med.*, 289, 5

88. Gelfand, E. W., Dosch, H. M., Huber, J. and Shore (1977). *In vitro* and *in vivo* reconstitution of severe combined immunodeficiency disease with thymic epithelium. *Clin. Res.*, 25, 358A

89. Hong, R., Santosham, M., Schulte-Wissermann, H., Horowitz, S., Hsu, S. H. and Winkelstein, J. A. (1976). Reconstitution of B and T lymphocytes function in severe combined immunodeficiency disease after transplantation with thymic epithelium. *Lancet*, ii, 1270

90. Buckley, R. H. (1976). Personal communication

91. Keightley, R. G., Lawton, A. R., Cooper, M. D. and Yunis, E. J. (1975). Successful fetal liver transplantation in a child with severe combined immunodeficiency. *Lancet*, ii, 850

92. Ackert, C., Plüss, H. J. and Hitzig, W. H. (1976). Hereditary severe combined immunodeficiency and adenosine deaminase deficiency. *Pediatr. Res.*, 10, 67

93. Buckley, R. H., Whisnant, J. K., Schiff, R. I., Gilbertsen, R. B., Huang, A. T. and Platt, M. S. (1976). Correction of severe combined immunodeficiency by fetal liver cells. *N. Engl. J. Med.*, 294, 1076

94. Rieger, C. H. L., Lustig, J. V., Hirschhorn, R. and Rothberg, R. (1977). Reconstitution of T cell function in severe combined immunodeficiency disease following transplantation of early embryonic liver cells. *J. Pediatr.*, 90, 707

95. Lowenberg, B. (1975). *Fetal Liver Cell Transplantation*, p. 56. (The Netherlands: Radiobiological Inst. Rijswijk)

96. Lowenberg, B., Dicke, K. A., van Bekkum, D. W., and Dooren, L. J. (1976). Quantitative aspects of fetal liver cell transplantation in animals and man. *Transplant. Proc.*, 8, 532

97. DeVaal, O. M. and Seynhaeve, U. (1959). Reticular dysgenesis. *Lancet*, ii, 1123

98. Nezelof, C., Jammet, M. L., Lortholary, P., Labrune, B. and Lamy, M. (1964). L'hypoplasie héréditaire du thymus. Sa place et sa responsabilité dans une observation d'aplasie lymphocytaire, normoplasmocytaire et normoglobulinémique du nourrisson. *Arch. Fr. Pédiatr.*, 21, 897

99. DiGeorge, A. M. (1968). Congenital absence of the thymus and its immunologic consequences: Concurrence with congenital hypoparthyroidism. *Birth Defects: Original Article Series*, 4, 116

100. Lobdell, D. H. (1969). DiGeorge's syndrome. *Arch. Pathol.*, 87, 353

101. Sieber, O. F., Durie, B. C., Hattler, B. C. et al. (1974). Spontaneous evolution of immune competence in DiGeorge syndrome. Pediatr. Res., 8, 418

102. Lischner, H. W., Valdes-Dapena, M. A., Biggin, J. et al. (1973). Proliferative responsiveness of human B and T lymphocytes to phytohaemagglutinin and pokeweed mitogen. In: Leucocyte Culture Conference, 7th; Proceedings, p. 547

103. Pabst, H. F., Wright, W. C., LeRiche, J. and Stiehm, E. R. (1976). Partial DiGeorge syndrome and substantial cell-mediated immunity. Am. J. Dis. Child., 130, 316

104. Pahwa, S. (1976). (Unpublished observation)

105. Incefy, G. S., et al. (Unpublished observation)

106. Pahwa, R., et al. (Unpublished observation)

107. Bruton, O. C. (1952). Agammaglobulinemia. Pediatrics, 9, 722

108. Siegal, F. P., Pernis, B. and Kunkel, H. G. (1971). Lymphocytes in human immunodeficiency states: a study of membrane-associated immunoglobulins. Europ. J. Immunol., 1, 482

109. Afuti, F., LaCava, V., Garofalo, J. A., D'Amelio, R. and D'Asero, C. (1973). Surface markers on human lymphocytes: studies of normal subjects and of patients with primary immunodeficiencies. Clin. Exp. Immunol., 15, 43

110. Hoffman, T., Winchester, R., Schulkind, M., Frias, J. L., Ayoub, E. M. and Good, R. A. (1977). Hypoimmunoglobulinemia without B lymphocytes in female siblings. Clin. Immunol. Immunopathol., 7, 364

111. Gitlin, D., Janeway, C. A., Apt, L., and Craig, M. (1959). Agammaglobulinemia. In H. S. Lawrence (ed.) Cellular and Humoral Aspects of the Hypersensitive States, p. 375. (New York: Hoeber-Harper)

112. Good, R. A., Kelly, W. D., Rötstein, J. and Varco, R. L. (1962). Immunological deficiency diseases. Agammaglobulinemia, hypogammaglobulinemia, Hodgkin's disease and sarcoidosis. Progr. Allergy, 6, 187

113. Craig, J. M., Gitlin, D. and Jewett, T. C. (1954). The response of lymph nodes of normal and congenitally agammaglobulinemic children to antigenic stimulation. Am. J. Dis. Child., 88, 626

114. Good, R. A. (1954). Agammaglobulinemia: an experimental study. Am. J. Dis. Child., 88, 625

115. Good, R. A. (1955). Studies on agammaglobulinemia. II. Failure of plasma cell formation in the bone marrow and lymph nodes of patients with agammaglobulinemia. J. Lab. Clin. Med., 46, 167

116. Cooper, M. D., Lawton, A. R. and Bockman, D. E. (1971). Agammaglobulinemia with B lymphocytes. Specific defect of plasma cell differentiation. Lancet, ii, 791

117. Grey, H. M., Rabellino, E. and Pirofsky, B. (1971). Immunoglobulins on the surface of lymphocytes. IV. Distribution in hypogammaglobulinemia, cellular immune deficiency, and chronic lymphatic leukemia. J. Clin. Invest., 50, 2368

118. Geha, R. S., Rosen, F. S. and Merler, E. (1973). Identification and characterization of subpopulations of lymphocytes in human peripheral blood after fractionation on discontinuous gradients of albumin. The cellular defect in X-linked agammaglobulinemia. J. Clin. Invest., 52, 1726

119. Preud'homme, J. L., Griscelli, C. and Seligmann, M. (1973). Immunoglobulins on the surface of lymphocytes in fifty patients with primary

immunodeficiency diseases. *Clin. Immunol. Immunopathol.*, 1, 241

120. Hayward, A. R. and Greaves, M. F. (1975). Central failure of B-lymphocyte induction in pan-hypogammaglobulinemia. *Clin. Immunol. Immunopathol.*, 3, 461

121. Gupta, S., Good, R. A. and Siegal, F. P. (1976). Rosette-formation with mouse erythrocytes. III. Studies in patients with primary immunodeficiency and lympho-proliferative disorders. *Clin. Exp. Immunol.*, 26, 204

122. Dosch, H. M. and Gelfand, E. W. (1976). *In vitro* antibody synthesis and suppression in humoral immunodeficiency states. *Clin. Res.*, 24, 481A

123. Good, R. A. (1954). Agammaglobulinemia: a provocative experiment of nature. *Bulletin of the University of Minnesota Hospital and Minnesota Medical Foundation*, 26, 1

124. Jeunet, F. S. and Good, R. A. (1968). Thymoma, immunologic deficiencies and hematological abnormalities. In D. Bergsma and R. A. Good (eds.). *Immunologic Deficiency Diseases in Man* p. 192. *Birth Defects Original Article Series*, Vol. IV, No. 1

125. Cooper, M. D. and Lawton, A. R. (1972). Circulating B-cells in patients with immunodeficiency. *Am. J. Pathol.*, 69, 513

126. Siegal, F. P., Wernet, P., Dickler, H. B., Fu, S. M. and Kunkel, H. G. (1975). B lymphocytes lacking surface Ig in patients with immune deficiency: initiation of Ig synthesis in culture in cells of a patient with thymoma. In D. Bergsma, R. A. Good and J. Finstad (eds.). *Immunodeficiency in Man and Animals* p. 40. *Birth Defects Original Article Series*, Vol. XI, No. 1

127. Zanjiani, E. D., Litwin, S. D. and Zalusky, R. (1975). Impairment of erythroid colony function by lymphocytes from patients with variable immunodeficiency. *Blood*, 46, 1038

128. Fudenberg, H. H., Good, R. A., Goodman, H. C., Hitzig, W., Kunkel, H. G., Roitt, I. M., Rosen, F. S., Rowe, D. S., Seligman, M. and Soothill, J. R. (1971). Primary immunodeficiencies. *Bull. World Health Organization*, 45, 125

129. Wu, L. Y. F., Lawton, A. R. and Cooper, M. D. (1973). Differentiation capacity of cultured B lymphocytes from immunodeficient patients. *J. Clin. Invest.*, 52, 3180

130. Geha, R. S., Schneeberger, E., Merler, E. and Rosen, F. S. (1974). Heterogeneity of 'acquired' or common variable agammaglobulinemia. *N. Engl. J. Med.*, 291, 1

131. Choi, Y. S., Biggar, W. D. and Good, R. A. (1972). Biosynthesis and secretion of immunoglobulins by peripheral blood lymphocytes in severe hypogammaglobulinaemia. *Lancet*, i, 1149

132. Ciccimarra, F., Rosen, F. S., Schneeberger, E. and Merler, E. (1976). Failure of heavy chain glycosylation of IgG in some patients with common, variable agammaglobulinemia. *J. Clin. Invest.*, 57, 1386

133. Cooper, M. D., Moretta, L., Webb, S. R., Pearl, E. R., Okos, A. J. and Lawton, A. R. (1976). Analysis of defects in human B cell differentiation and in development of two T-cell subpopulations. In *Symposium on Immunodeficiency, Tokyo, Japan, September 13–15*

134. Boder, E. and Sedgwick, R. P. (1957). Ataxia–telangiectasia: A familial syndrome of progressive cerebellar ataxia, oculocutaneous telangiectasia and frequent pulmonary infection. *Univ. S. Cal. Med. Bull.*, 9, 15

135. Boder, E. and Sedgwick, R. P. (1962). Ataxia–telangiectasia: A review of 101 cases. In G. Walsh (ed.). *Cerebellum, Posture and Cerebral Palsy* (London: Heinemann Medical Books Ltd.)

136. Peterson, R. D. A., Cooper, M. D. and Good, R. A. (1966). Lymphoid tissue abnormalities associated with ataxia–telangiectasia. *Am. J. Med.*, **41**, 342

137. Sineby, B. (1966). Ataxia–telangiectasia. *Acta Paediatr. Scand.*, **55**, 239

138. Solitare, G. B. (1968). Louis-Bar's syndrome (ataxia–telangiectasia). *Neurology*, **18**, 1180

139. Harley, R. D., Baird, H. W. and Craven, E. M. (1967). Ataxia–telangiectasia. *Arch. Ophthalmol.*, **77**, 582

140. Haerer, A. F., Jackson, J. F. and Evers, C. G. (1969). Ataxia–telangiectasia with gastric adenocarcinoma. *J. Am. Med. Assoc.*, **210**, 1884

141. Feigin, R. D., Vietti, T. J., Wyatt, R. G., Kaufman, D. G. and Smith, C. H. (1970). Ataxia–telangiectasia with granulocytopenia. *J. Pediatr.*, **77**, 431

142. Hecht, F. and McCau, B. K. (1977). Chromosome instability syndromes. in J. Mulvihill, R. W. Miller and F. Fraumeni (eds.). *Genetics of Human Cancer*, p. 105. (New York: Raven Press)

143. Mcfarlin, E. D., Strober, W. and Waldmann, T. A. (1972). Ataxia-telangiectasia. *Medicine*, **51**, 281

144. Cooper, M. D. and Lawton, A. R. (1972). Circulating B cells in patients with immunodeficiency. *Am. J. Pathol.*, **69**, 513

145. Peterson, R. D. A., Kelly, W. D. and Good, R. A. (1964). Ataxia-telangiectasia: its association with defective thymus, immunological deficiency disease and malignancy. *Lancet*, **i**, 1189

146. Ammann, A. J. and Hong, R. (1971). Autoimmune phenomena in ataxia-telangiectasia. *J. Pediatr.*, **78**, 821

147. Eisen, A. H., Karpati, G., Laszlo, T., Andermann, F., Robb, J. P. and Bacal, H. L. (1965). Immunologic deficiency in ataxia–telangiectasia. *N. Engl. J. Med.*, **272**, 18

148. Epstein, W. L., Fudenberg, H. H., Reed, W. B., Boder, E. and Sedgwick, R. P. (1966). Immunologic studies in ataxia–telangiectasia. *Int. Arch. Allergy*, **30**, 15

149. Biggar, W. D. and Good, R. A. (1975). Immunodeficiency in ataxia-telangiectasia. In *Immunodeficiency in Man and Animals*, p. 271. *Birth Defects: Original Article Series*, Vol. XI, No. 1

150. Gajl-Peczalska, K., Park, B. H., Biggar, W. and Good, R. A. (1973). B and T lymphocytes in primary immunodeficiency disease in man. *J. Clin. Invest.*, **52**, 919

151. Luckasen, J. R., Sabad, A., Gajl-Peczalska, K. and Kersey, J. H. (1974). Lymphocytes bearing complement receptors, surface immunoglobulins and sheep erythrocyte receptors in primary immunodeficiency diseases. *Clin. Exp. Immunol.*, **16**, 535

152. Wara, D. W., Goldstein, A. L., Doyle, N. E. and Ammann, A. J. (1975). Thymosin activity in patients with cellular immunodeficiency. *N. Engl. J. Med.*, **292**, 70

153. Boumsell, L., Incefy, G. S., Bernard, A., Schwartz, S., Smithwick, E. M. and Good, R. A. (1975). T lymphocyte differentiation *in vitro* in ataxia-telangiectasia associated with lymphosarcoma. *J. Pediatr.*, **87**, 435

154. Waldmann, T. A. and McIntire, K. B. (1972). Serum alpha-fetoprotein levels

in patients with ataxia–telangiectasia. *Lancet*, ii, 1112

155. Krivit, W. and Good, R. A. (1959). Aldrich's syndrome (thrombocytopenia, eczema and infection in infants). *Am. J. Dis. Child.*, 97, 137

156. West, C. D., Hong, R. and Holland, N. H. (1962). Immunoglobulin levels from the newborn period to adulthood and in immunoglobulin deficiency states. *J. Clin. Invest.*, 41, 2054

157. Eitzman, D. V. and Smith, R. T. (1960). Immunological studies on a patient with Aldrich's syndrome. *Southern Med. J.*, 53, 1593

158. Palmgren, B. and Lindberg, T. (1963). Immunological studies in Wiskott–Aldrich syndrome. *Acta Paediatr. (Stockholm) (suppl)*, 146, 116

159. Amiet, A. (1963). Aldrich–Syndrom. Beobachtung zweir Fälle. *Ann. Paediatr. Basel*, 201, 315

160. Blaese, R. M., Stober, W., Levy, A. L. and Waldmann, T. A. (1971). Hypercatabolism of IgG, IgA, IgM, and albumin in Wiskott–Aldrich syndrome. *J. Clin. Invest.*, 50, 2331

161. Blaese, R. M., Strober, W., Brown, R. S. and Waldmann, T. A. (1968). The Wiskott–Aldrich syndrome: A disorder with a possible defect in antigen processing or recognition. *Lancet*, i, 1056

162. Cooper, M. D., Chase, H. P., Lowman, J. T., Krivit, W. and Good, R. A. (1968). Wiskott–Aldrich syndrome: an immunologic deficiency disease involving the afferent limb of immunity. *Am. J. Med.*, 44, 499

163. Ayoub, E. M., Dudding, B. A. and Cooper, M. D. (1968). Dichotomy of antibody response to group A streptococcal antigens in Wiskott–Aldrich syndrome. *J. Lab. Clin. Med.*, 72, 971

164. Blaese, R. M., Strober, W. and Waldmann, T. A. (1975). Immunodeficiency in the Wiskott–Aldrich syndrome. In *Immunodeficiency in Man and Animals*, p. 250. *Birth Defects: Original Article Series*, Vol. XI, No. 1

165. Poplack, D. G., Bonnard, G. D., Moliman, B. J. and Blaese, M. R. (1976). Monocyte mediated antibody-dependent cellular cytotoxicity. *Blood*, 48, 809

166. Bach, F. H., Albertini, R. J., Joo, P., Anderson, J. J., and Bortin, M. M. (1968). Bone marrow transplantation in a patient with Wiskott–Aldrich syndrome. *Lancet*, i, 1364

167. Parkman, R., Rappaport, J., Greha, R. *et al.* (1978). Correction of the Wiskott–Aldrich syndrome by bone marrow transplantation. *N. Engl. J. Med.*, 248, 921

168. Bachmann, R. (1965). Studies on the serum γ-A-globin level. III. The frequency of a γ-A-globulinemia. *Scand. J. Clin. Lab. Invest.*, 17, 316

169. Berg, T., and Johansson, S. G. O. (1969). Immunoglobulin levels during childhood with special regard to IgE. *Acta Pediatr. Scand.*, 58, 513

170. Ammann, A. J., and Hong, R. (1971). Selective IgA deficiency: presentation of 30 cases and a review of the literature. *Medicine*, 50, 223

171. Schlegel, R. J., Bernier, G. M., Bellanti, J. A., Maybee, D. A., Osborne, G. B., Stewart, J. L., Pearlman, D. S., Quellette, J. and Biehusen, F. C. (1970). Severe candidiasis associated with thymic dysplasia, IgA deficiency, and plasma anti-lymphocyte effects. *Pediatrics*, 45, 926

172. Delespesse, G., Gausset, P., Cauchie, C. and Govaerts, A. (1976). Cellular aspects of selective IgA deficiency. *Clin. Exp. Immunol.*, 24, 273

173. Cline, M. J. and Golde, D. W. (1974). Production of colony-stimulating

activity of human lymphocytes. *Nature (London)*, **248**, 703

174. Ascensao, J., Pahwa, R., Kagan, W. *et al.* (1976). Aplastic anaemia: evidence for an immunological mechanism. *Lancet*, i, 669

175. Kagan, W. A., Ascensao, J., Pahwa, R. *et al.* (1976). Aplastic anaemia. Presence in human bone marrow of cells that suppress myelopoiesis. *Proc. Natl. Acad. Sci. USA*, **73**, 2890

176. Hoffman, R., Zanjani, E. D., Lutton, J. D. *et al.* (1977). Suppression of erythroid colony formation by lymphocytes from patients with aplastic anaemia. *N. Engl. J. Med.*, **296**, 10

177. Hoffman, R., Zanjani, E. D., Vila, J. *et al.* (1976). Diamond–Blackfan syndrome: lymphocyte-mediated suppression of erythropoiesis. *Science*, **193**, 899

178. Broxmeyer, H. E., Pahwa, R., Jacobsen, N., Grossbard, E., Good, R. A. and Moore, M. A. S. (1977). Inhibitory activity obtained from cells of patients with neutropenia directed against granulocyte colony forming cells. *Exp. Hematol.*, **5 (Supp. No. 2)**, 96

179. Pahwa, R., O'Reilly, R. J., Broxmeyer, H. E., Smithwick, E. M., Pahwa, S. G., Kapadia, A. and Good, R. A. (1977). Partial correction of neutrophil deficiency in congenital neutropenia. *Exp. Hematol.*, **5 (Supp. No. 2)**, 45

180. Speck, B., Cornu, P., Nissen, C., Groff, P. and Jeannet, M. (1977). On the immune pathogenesis of aplastic anaemia. *Exp. Hematol.*, **5 (Supp. No. 2)**, 2

181. Gluckman, E. Personal communication.

182. Jeannet, M., Rubenstein, A., Pelet, B. and Kummer, H. (1974). Prolonged remission of severe aplastic anaemia after ALG pretreatment and HLA semi-compatible bone marrow cell transfusion. *Transplant. proc.*, **6**, 359

183. Thomas, E. D., Storb, R., Giblet, E. R., Longpre, B., Welden, P. L., Fefer, A., Witherspoon, R., Clift, R. A. and Buckner, C. D. (1976). Recovery from aplastic anemia following attempted marrow transplantation. *Exp. Hematol.*, **4**, 97

184. Baran, D. T., Griner, P. F. and Klemperer, M. R. (1976). Recovery from aplastic anaemia treated with cyclophosphamide. *N. Engl. J. Med.*, **295**, 1522

185. O'Reilly, R. J., Pahwa, R., Kagan, W., Kapoor, N., Sorell, M., Meyers, P. and Good, R. A. (1977). Reconstitution of hematopoietic function in post-hepatic aplasia following high dose cyclophosphamide and allogenic fetal liver transplantation. *Exp. Hematol.*, **5 (Supp. No. 2)**, 46

186. Miller, D. Personal communication.

187. Broxmeyer, H. E., Baker, F. L. and Galbraith, P. R. (1976). *In vitro* regulation of granulopoiesis in human leukemia. Application of an essay for colony inhibiting cells. *Blood*, **47**, 389

188. Müller-Eberhard, H. J. (1975). Complement. *Am. Rev. Biochem.*, **44**, 679

189. Day, N. K., Moncada, B. and Good, R. A. (1977). Inherited deficiencies of the complement system. In N. K. Day and R. A. Good (eds.). *Biological Amplification Systems in Immunology*, p. 229. (New York: Plenum Press), (*Comprehensive Immunology, Vol. 2*)

190. Donaldson, V. H. and Evans, R. R. (1963). A biochemical abnormality in hereditary angioneurotic edema: absence of serum inhibitor of C1 esterase. *Am. J. Med.*, **35**, 37

191. Donaldson, V. H. and Rosen, F. S. (1964). Action of complement in heredi-

tary angioneurotic edema; the role of C'1 esterase. *J. Clin. Invest.*, **43**, 2204

192. Rosen, F. S. and Alper, C. A. (1973). Disorders of the complement system. In E. R. Stiehm and V. A. Fulginiti (eds.). *Immunologic Disorders in Infants and Children*, p. 289. (Philadelphia: W. B. Saunders, Co.)

193. Rosen, F. S., Charache, P., Pensky, J. and Donaldson, V. (1965). Hereditary angioneurotic edema: two genetic variants. *Science*, **148**, 957

194. Pickering, R. J., Kelly, J. R., Good, R. A. and Gewurz, H. (1969). Replacement therapy in hereditary angioedema: successful treatment of two patients with fresh frozen plasma. *Lancet*, **i**, 326

195. Gelfand, J. A., Sherins, R. J., David, W. A. and Frank, M. M. (1976). Treatment of hereditary angioedema with Danozal. Reversal of clinical and biochemical abnormalities. *N. Engl. J. Med.*, **296**, 1444

196. O'Connell, E. J., Enriquez, P., Linman, J. W., Gleich, G. J. and McDuffie F. C. (1967). Absence of activity of first component of complement in man: Association with thymic alymphoplasia and defective inflammatory response. *J. Lab. Clin. Med.*, **70**, 715

197. Müller-Eberhard, H. J. and Kunkel, H. G. (1961). Isolation of a thermolabile serum protein which precipitates γ-globin aggregates and participates in immune hemolysis. *Proc. Soc. Exp. Biol. Med.*, **106**, 291

198. Ballow, M., Day, N. K., Biggar, W. D., Park, B. H., Yount, W. J. and Good, R. A. (1973). Reconstitution of $C1_q$ following bone marrow transplantation in patients with severe combined immunodeficiency. *Clin. Immunol. Immunopathol.*, **2**, 28

199. Pickering, R. J., Naff, G. B., Stroud, R. M., Good, R. A. and Gewurz, H. (1970). Deficiency of $C1_r$ in human serum: effects on the structure and function of macromolecular C1. *J. Exp. Med.*, **141**, 803

200. Day, N. K., Geiger, H., Stroud, R., deBracco, M., Moncada, B., Windhorst, D. and Good, R. A. (1972). $C1_r$ deficiency: an inborn error associated with cutaneous and renal disease. *J. Clin. Invest.*, **51**, 1102

201. Pickering, R. J., Michael, A. F., Herdman, R. C., Good, R. A. and Gewurz, H. (1971). The complement system in chronic glomerulonephritis in three newly-associated aberrations. *J. Pediatr.*, **78**, 30

202. Day, N. K. and Good, R. A. (1975). Deficiencies of the complement system in man. In D. Bergsma (ed.)., R. A. Good and J. Finstad (scientific eds.). *Immunodeficiency in Man and Animals*, (Sunderland, Mass., Sinauer Associates), (*Birth Defects: Original Article Series*, Vol **XI**, *No. 1*)

203. Miller, M. E., Seals, J., Kaye, R. and Levitsky, L. C. (1968). A familial plasma-associated defect of phagocytosis; a new cause of recurrent bacterial infections. *Lancet*, **i**, 60

204. Miller, M. E. and Nilsson, U. R. (1970). A familial deficiency of the phagocytosis-enhancing activity of serum related to a dysfunction of the fifth component of complement (C5). *N. Engl. J. Med.*, **282**, 354

205. Miller, M. E. and Koblenzer, P. J. (1972). Leiner's disease and deficiency of C5. *J. Pediatr.*, **80**, 879

206. Berendes, H., Bridges, R. A. and Good, R. A. (1957). Fatal granulomatous disease of childhood: Clinical study of a new syndrome. *Minn. Med.*, **40**, 309

207. Windhorst, D. B., Page, A. R., Holmes, B., Quie, P. G. and Good, R. A.

(1968). The pattern of genetic transmission of the leukocyte defect in fatal granulomatous disease of childhood. *J. Clin. Invest.*, **47**, 1026

208. Carson, M. J., Chadwick, D. L., Brubaker, C. A., Cleland, R. S. and Landing, B. H. (1968). Thirteen boys with progressive septic granulomatosis. *Pediatrics*, **35**, 405

209. Holmes, B., Quie, P. G., Windhorst, D. B. and Good, R. A. (1966). Fatal granulomatous disease of childhood, an inborn abnormality of phagocytic function. *Lancet*, i, 1225

210. Smithwick, E. M. Personal communication.

211. Pedersen, F. K., Johansen, K. S., Rosenkvist, J., Tygstrup, I. and Valerius, N. H. (1977). *Pneumocystis carinii* infection in a girl with chronic granulomatous disease treated with transfusions of granulocytes. In *15th Annual Symposium of the Society for the Study of Inborn Errors of Metabolism, Elsinore, Denmark*

212. Baehner, R. L. and Nathan, D. G. (1967). Leukocyte oxidase: defective activity in chronic granulomatous disease. *Science*, **155**, 835

213. Baehner, R. L. and Karnovsky, M. L. (1968). Deficiency of reduced nicotinamide-adenine dinucleotide oxidase in chronic granulomatous disease. *Science*, **162**, 1277

214. Hohn, D. C. and Lehrer, R. I. (1975). NADPH-oxidase deficiency in X-linked chronic granulomatous disease. *J. Clin. Invest.*, **55**, 707

215. Segal, A. W., Peters, T. J. (1976). Characterization of the enzyme defect in chronic granulomatous disease. *Lancet*, i, 1364

216. Marsh, W. L., Øyen, R., Nichols, M. E. *et al.* (1975). Chronic granulomatous disease and the kell blood groups. *Br. J. Hematol.*, **29**, 247

217. Marsh, W. L., Uretsky, S. C. and Douglas, S. D. (1975). Antigens of the kell blood group system on neutrophils and monocytes: their relation to chronic granulomatous disease. *J. Pediatr.*, **87**, 1117

218. Marsh, W. L. (1977). The kell blood group, Kx antigen, and chronic granulomatous disease. *Mayo Clin. Proc.*, **52**, 150

219. Holmes, B., Park, D. H., Malawista, S. E. *et al.* Chronic granulomatous disease in females: A deficiency of leukocyte glutathione peroxidase. *N. Engl. J. Med.*, **283**, 217

220. Malawista, S. E. and Gifford, R. H. (1975). Chronic granulomatous disease of childhood with leukocyte glutathione peroxidase deficiency in a brother and sister: A likely autosomal recessive inheritance. *Clin. Res.*, **23**, 416A

221. Cooper, M. R., Dechâtelet, L. R., Metcall, I. R., LaVia, C. E., Spurr, C. F. and Baehner, R. L. (1970). Leucocyte GCPD deficiency. *Lancet*, ii, 110

222. Bellanti, J. A., Cantz, B. E. and Schlegel, R. J. (1970). Accelerated decay of glucose-6-phosphate-dehydrogenase activity in chronic granulomatous disease. *Pediatr. Res.*, **4**, 405

223. Gray, G. R., Stamatoyannopoulos, G., Naiman, S. C. *et al.* (1973). Neutrophil dysfunction, chronic granulomatous disease, and non-spherocytic haemolytic anaemia caused by complete deficiency of glucose-6-phosphate dehydrogenase. *Lancet*, ii, 530

224. Quie, P. G., Kaplan, E. L., Page, A. R., Gruskay, F. L. and Malawista, S. E. (1968). Defective polymorphonuclear leukocyte function and chronic granulomatous disease in two female children. *N. Engl. J. Med.*, **278**, 976

225. Windhorst, D. B., Page, A. R., Holmes, B., Quie, P. G. and Good, R. A.

(1968). The pattern of genetic transmission of the leukocyte defect in fatal granulomatous disease of childhood. *J. Clin. Invest.*, **47**, 1026

226. Baehner, R. L. and Nathan, D. G. (1968). Quantitative nitroblue tetrazolium test in chronic granulomatous disease. *N. Engl. J. Med.*, **278**, 971

227. Quie, P. G., White, J. G., Holmes, B. and Good, R. A. (1967). *In vitro* bactericidal capacity of human polymorphonuclear leukocytes: Diminished activity in chronic granulomatous disease of childhood. *J. Clin. Invest.*, **46**, 668

228. Macfarlane, P. S., Speirs, A. L. and Sommerville, R. G. (1967). Fatal granulomatous disease of childhood and benign lymphocytic infiltration of the skin. *Lancet*, **i**, 408

229. Johnston R. B. Jr., Wilbert, C. M., Buckley, R. H. *et al.* (1975). Enhanced bactericidal activity of phagocytes from patients with chronic granulomatous disease in the presence of sulphisoxazole. *Lancet*, **ii**, 824

230. Philippart, A. I., Colodny, A. H. and Baehner, R. L. (1972). Continuous antibiotic therapy in chronic granulomatous disease. Preliminary communication. *Pediatrics*, **50**, 923

231. Foroozonfar, N., Hobbs, J. R. *et al.* (1977). Bone marrow transplant from an unrelated donor for chronic granulomatous disease. *Lancet*, **i**, 210

232. Miller, M. E., Oski, F. A. and Harris, M. B. (1971). Lazy Leucocyte syndrome. *Lancet*, **i**, 665

233. Root, R. K., Rosenthal, A. S. and Balestra, D. J. (1972). Abnormal bactericidal, metabolic and lysosomal functions of Chediak–Higashi syndrome leukocytes. *J. Clin. Invest.*, **51**, 649

234. Clark, R. A. and Kimball, H. R. (1971). Defective granulocyte chemotaxis in the Chediak–Higashi syndrome. *J. Clin. Invest.*, **50**, 2645

235. Gallin, J. I., Klimerman, J. A., Padgett, G. A. *et al.* (1975). Defective mononuclear leukocyte chemotaxis in the Chediak–Higashi syndrome of human, cattle and mink. *Blood*, **45**, 863

236. Wolff, S. M., Dale, D. C., Clark, R. A. *et al.* (1972). The Chediak–Higashi syndrome: studies of host defense. *Ann. Intern. Med.*, **76**, 293

237. Smithwick, E. M., Pahwa, S. G. *et al.* Personal communication.

238. Boxer, L. A., Wantanabe, A. M., Rister, M. *et al.* (1976). Correction of leukocyte function in Chediak–Higashi syndrome by ascorbate. *N. Engl. J. Med.*, **295**, 1041

239. Buckley, R. H., Wray, B. B. and Belmaker, E. Z. (1972). Extreme hyperimmunoglobulinemia E and undue susceptibility to infection. *Pediatrics*, **49**, 59

240. Synderman, R. and Buckley, R. H. (1975). Defects of monocyte chemotaxis in patients with hyperimmunoglobulinemia E and undue susceptibility to infection. *Clin. Res.*, **23**, 25A

241. Clark, R. A., Root, R. K., Kimball, H. R. and Kirkpatrick, C. H. (1973). Defective neutrophil chemotaxis and cellular immunity in a child with recurrent infections. *Ann. Intern. Med.*, **78**, 515

242. Hill, H. R. and Quie, P. G. (1975). Defective neutrophil chemotaxis associated with hyperimmunoglobulinemia E. In J. A. Bellanti and D. H. Dayton (eds.) *The Phagocytic Cell in Host Resistance*, p. 249. (New York: Raven Press)

243. Hill, H. R. and Quie, P. G. (1974). Raised serum IgE levels and defective

neutrophil chemotaxis in three children with eczema and recurrent bacterial infections. *Lancet*, i, 183

244. Good, R. A. *et al.* Personal communication

245. Siegal, F. P., Filippa, D. A. and Koziner, B. (1978). Surface markers in leukemia and lymphomas. *Am. J. Pathol.*, 90, 451

2

Genetics of the immune system

A. Svejgaard, E. Dickmeiss, G. S. Hansen, P. Platz, L. P. Ryder and M. Thomsen

Apart from the brain, the immune system is perhaps the most complex 'organ' in vertebrates[1]. In contrast to most other organs, it shares with the brain the ability to react in a specific way to a large variety of 'unforeseen' events imposed by an everchanging environment. Although most metabolic pathways are able to adjust their activities within large environmental variations, these adjustments are mainly quantitative and much more simple than the flexibility shown by the reactions of the immune system. Accordingly, the genetic background of this system must be much more complex than those controlling more classic metabolic systems, and our knowledge about this background is still at a very early stage. However, within the last two decades a large amount of information has been accumulated and provided us with some insight into the marvellous immune machinery which allows each individual to react specifically to an almost endless number of different antigenic stimuli.

In this survey, we shall concentrate on two major fields relating to the genetics of the immune systems: (1) the genetics of immunoglobulins, which are the most well known of all the products of the immune organ, and (2) the genetics of the immune response in relation to the major histo-compatibility complex (MHC). Other aspects of the genetics of the immune response are described elsewhere in this volume by Simonsen[2], Pahwa *et al.*[3], and Meuwissen[4] among others. It should be noted that the references quoted in this paper are mainly reviews since we have not attempted to quote all the original findings.

IMMUNOGLOBULINS

As discussed by Simonsen[2] and Pahwa *et al.*[3], the immune system consists mainly of lymphocytes, monocytes, and a variety of soluble mediators, e.g. immunoglobulins, lymphokines, and complement factors. The lymphocytes may be divided into at least two major subclasses: B lymphocytes which are the precursors of antibody secreting plasma cells, and T lymphocytes which are responsible not only for delayed hypersensitivity but also for helping B lymphocytes to elicit a humoral immune response. Most recently, the monocytes have attained an increasing interest by immunologists as these cells seem to be necessary for a normal T lymphocyte activation to take place. Thus, it would appear that many immune responses start with the monocytes which then activate T lymphocytes which in turn trigger B lymphocytes. One of the final steps of this series of interactions is the production of humoral antibodies – immunoglobulins – capable of reacting specifically with the antigen initiating the process. Thanks to the work of Porter[6] and Edelman[5] among others, we have quite a detailed knowledge about the structure of immunoglobulins, which is essential for the understanding of the genetics of the immune system. The following overview is based mainly on a number of recent reviews[1, 7-10], which should be consulted in case more detailed information is required. Most of the information on immunoglobulin structure has been obtained from studies of myeloma proteins.

Immunoglobulin structure

Basically, all immunoglobulins (Igs) consist of four polypeptide chains which are pairwise identical (Figure 2.1), i.e. each Ig molecule contains at least two sets of two different polypeptides: a heavy (H) chain (mw about 50 000) and a light (L) chain (mw about 25 000). These chains are bound together by interchain disulphide bonds, and in addition there are intra-chain disulphide bonds within the chains which create a number of loops (domains) in each chain. The H chain has four or more and the L chain two domains. One of the domains in each chain is particularly interesting

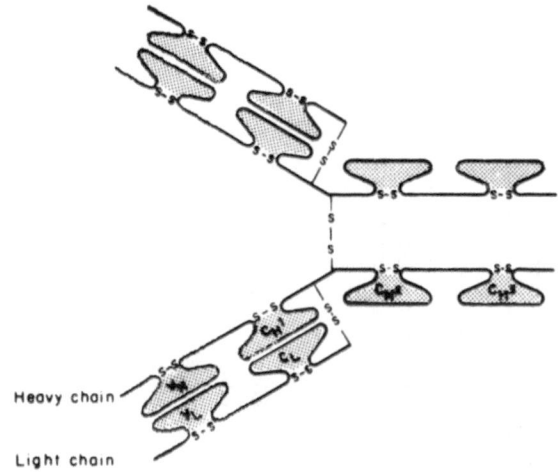

Heavy chain

Light chain

Figure 2.1 Schematic presentation of the basic Ig subunit with the two heavy and two light chains. The various domains are shown: V_L and V_H – the variable domains of the light and heavy chain, respectively – compose the antigen binding site; C_L is the constant part of the light chain and C_{H1}, C_{H2}, and C_{H3} are the constant domains of the heavy chain. Disulphide bridges are indicated by S–S. Molecules of the IgG class consist of one such subunit, while, for example, IgM consists of five. The heavy chain of IgM, however, has one more C-domain: C_{H4} (modified from Roitt[10])

because it makes up the part of the Ig molecule which combines with antigen. These domains are called the variable (V_H and V_L) parts of H and L chains, respectively. The remaining parts of the chains are called constant (C_H and C_L) as they show little or no variation within each immunoglobulin class. The subdivision of Ig molecules into Ig classes (Table 2.1) is, on the other hand, due to differences in the constant parts – and more specifically the C_H parts. Thus, there at least five different Ig classes: IgG, IgA, IgM, IgD, and IgE, each with its own C_H part. These C_H parts determine some general properties of the entire Ig molecule, e.g. its capacity to bind complement (IgG and IgM), to combine with the so-called secretory component and thus to be present in excretions (IgA), and to bind to mast cells and thus to elicit atopic allergy (IgE). The IgG class can be further subdivided into subclasses which are separable by antigenic and biochemical properties, and these subclasses have been found to have different biological activities and they have different allotypes of the so-called Gm system which is a serum group system recognizable by means of alloantibodies.

The constant part of the L chains shows less variation as there seems to

TABLE 2.1 Classes and subclasses of immunoglobulins and some of their properties

Class	Subclass	Molecular weight	Heavy chains	Light chains	Gm allotypes	Major properties
IgG	IgG1	150 000	γ ⎰γ1	κ λ	a, y, f, x	⎰complement fixation
	IgG2		⎱γ2		n	⎱placenta transport
	IgG3		γ3		b, b₃, b₄, s, t, c, g	
	IgG4		γ4			
IgM		900 000	μ			⎰complement fixation
IgA		160 000	α			⎱early immune response
IgE		200 000	ε			secretory Ig
IgD		185 000	δ			atopic Ig

Modified from ref. 10

be only two major types of L chains: kappa (κ) and lambda (λ) chains. Each of these may combine with each of the various H chains mentioned above. In man, the Inv serum allotype serves to distinguish different allelicly controlled C_L domains of kappa chains.

Although each Ig molecule consists of at least two H and two L chains, it is a striking fact that the two H chains within the subunit (Figure 2.1) of a given Ig molecule are completely identical not only as regards the constant but also with respect to the variable part. The same is true for the two L chains within an Ig molecule. This phenomenon has very important implications for our understanding of the genetic expression of Ig genes.

Whereas amino acid sequence studies have revealed striking constancy within the C parts of each of the various Ig classes and subclasses, similar studies of the V domains of both H and L chains have unravelled the most extraordinary variability. Naturally, this is to be expected since it is just these parts of the molecule which build the antigen-binding site which accordingly must show great variation between different Ig molecules each of which can combine with 'its own' specific antigen. Nevertheless, even within the V domains some constancy has been found at a number of amino acid positions. These relatively invariant segments of the V parts probably serve to keep the very variable regions in the right position for combination with antigen.

Immunoglobulin genes

Although Ig molecules contain varying amounts (3–13%) of carbohydrate, there is no doubt that the genetic material responsible for antibody diversity and Ig subclasses resides mainly or exclusively in the genes coding for H and L polypeptide chains. Our knowledge concerning these genes derives from the study of a variety of animals (including man), but as the homologies between species have so far proved to be rather striking, it seems justifiable to make some generalizations when discussing this subject.

The immunoglobulins are controlled by three different autosomal genetic systems: the H (heavy chains), the κ (kappa chain) and the λ (lambda chain) systems each consisting of a multigene family. Rabbits have proven particularly useful in the clarification of the relationship between these three systems because there is information of allotypic markers on all three chains (H, κ and λ), which has made it possible to determine that the three corresponding genetic systems are non-linked[8]. In man, it has been shown that H and κ genes are non-linked, whereas linkage between κ and λ has not yet formally been excluded as no polymorphic markers have yet been found on λ chains. However, homology studies of amino acid sequences have revealed considerable differences between κ and λ chains.

When combining the information available from various species, it becomes clear that all the genes coding for the constant parts of the H chains are closely linked. Thus, the constant parts of heavy chains of IgG, IgA, IbM, IgD and probably IgE are controlled by closely linked genes. Moreover, in rabbits, genetic markers have been found for both the constant and the variable parts of heavy chains (C_H and C_V), – the latter in the relatively invariant portion of V, and these have been demonstrated to be closely linked. Accordingly, Edelman and co-workers[5] and others[9] have suggested the scheme of genetic arrangement of C_H and V_H genes illustrated in Figure 2.2. The crucial point is that there is a set of closely linked C_H

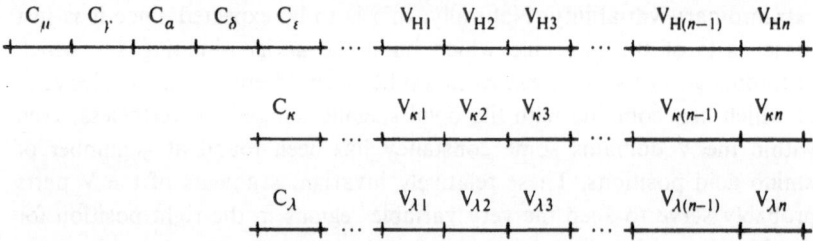

Figure 2.2 Hypothetical arrangement of Ig genes in the three different genetic systems controlling heavy, κ and λ chains. Within each system, one or more genes controlling constant Ig parts are linked to an array of V genes. The order of C_H genes shown is arbitrary (modified from Gally and Edelman (1977)[5] and Hood, Campbell and Elgin (1975)[9])

genes (γ, a, μ, δ, and ε), and linked to these there is an array of V_H genes. It seems likely that the situation is similar for the genetic systems controlling κ and λ chains. In the production of Ig chains one must therefore conclude that *one* polypeptide chain (H, κ or λ) is coded for by *two* genes: this is the 'two genes one polypeptide chain' concept. It is not clear whether the C and V genes are brought together in the chromosome by some rearrangement of genes or whether the genes remain apart during transcription, but the former possibility seems most likely.

There is another concept which is unique in relation to the genetics of immunoglobulins. This is the phenomenon, known as 'allelic exclusion', which derives from the observation that one cell only produces one antibody. Although each cell has two sets of genes (haplotypes) for each of systems (H, κ, and λ) only two of these six haplotypes are expressed in the individual cell: one H and either a κ or a λ haplotype. This is analogous to the Lyon hypothesis for the X chromosome: only one of a pair of

X-linked alleles is expressed in each cell but with Ig autosomal genes are involved. Moreover, only one class or subclass of C_H genes are expressed and either the κ or the λ system is totally repressed. The only exceptions to this rule is seen (1) in immature B lymphocytes which may carry IgM and IgD on the cell surface simultaneously, and (2) early in the immune response where there is a shift from IgM to IgG production. In this shift, it is the same V_H gene which is translated (assuring identical combining sites) while a C_γ gene becomes activated at the expense of a C_μ gene. In the mature Ig-secreting plasma cells the repression is complete. The biological reason for these restrictions is obvious: if all Ig genes were expressed in a given cell, it would produce a variety of different antibodies only one of which might correspond to the antigen which had induced the antibody formation.

One of the most debated phenomena within the field of immunology concerns the problem as to how every individual can respond immunologically with antibody formation to each of the multitude of foreign antigens which surround us. Two different theories have been advanced to explain the origin of antibody diversity: (1) according to the *germ line theory*[11], all the V genes present in the immunologically mature individual are inherited via the germ cells, whereas (2) various *somatic theories*[12] postulate that only limited number of V genes are inherited and that the majority of diversity arises by special mechanisms – e.g. somatic mutation – during ontogeny. Both of these theories have much to support them, and at the present time it is not possible to decide which of them is correct However, it may be worth noting that if there are about 1000 different V genes within each of the systems, H, κ, and λ, this may give rise to $2 \times 1000^2 = 2$ million different antibody combining sites. Nevertheless, this calculation is probably much too simple, and at the present time, somatic theories are gaining support[1].

'Inborn errors' of immunoglobulins seem to be extremely rare, although deficiencies of IgG subclasses have been described[13]. However, few – if any – of the known inherited immunodeficiencies of man seem to be due to malfunctioning or lacking Ig genes: most of them – including Bruton's agammaglobulinaemia and the more common IgA deficiency – seem to be due to maturation defects or to suppression of various precursors of antibody-forming cells. Nevertheless, the existence of malfunctioning Ig genes has by no means been excluded and should be kept in mind. In particular, if most of the antibody diversity is present in the germ line, it would appear that humoral immunodeficiencies against one or a few foreign antigens might be good candidates for such abnormalities. Indeed, such deficiencies are now being discovered in mice (Möller and Möller, personal communication).

However, the ability of an individual to respond well or poorly to a given antigen has been found to be at least to some extent genetically determined, and the immune response (Ir) genes responsible for this genetic variation are usually not linked to the Ig genes, but have surprisingly been found to be closely linked to the major histocompatibility complex (MHC) of the species in question[14].

The rest of this survey will be devoted to a discussion of this relationship.

IMMUNE RESPONSE GENES ASSOCIATED WITH THE MAJOR HISTOCOMPATIBILITY SYSTEM[15-20]

Each vertebrate species investigated has been found to possess one very complex genetic system coding for strong transplantation antigens. These major histocompatibility complexes (MHCs) contain a number of closely linked loci with genes controlling not only (1) transplantation antigens, but

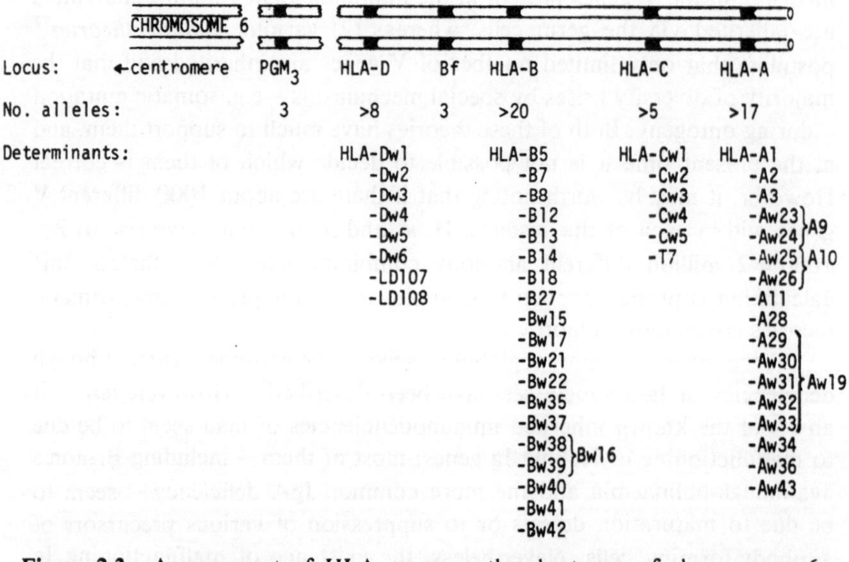

Locus:	←centromere	PGM$_3$	HLA-D	Bf	HLA-B	HLA-C	HLA-A
No. alleles:		3	>8	3	>20	>5	>17
Determinants:			HLA-Dw1		HLA-B5	HLA-Cw1	HLA-A1
			-Dw2		-B7	-Cw2	-A2
			-Dw3		-B8	-Cw3	-A3
			-Dw4		-B12	-Cw4	-Aw23 }A9
			-Dw5		-B13	-Cw5	-Aw24
			-Dw6		-B14	-T7	-Aw25 }A10
			-LD107		-B18		-Aw26
			-LD108		-B27		-A11
					-Bw15		-A28
					-Bw17		-A29
					-Bw21		-Aw30
					-Bw22		-Aw31 }Aw19
					-Bw35		-Aw32
					-Bw37		-Aw33
					-Bw38 }Bw16		-Aw34
					-Bw39		-Aw36
					-Bw40		-Aw43
					-Bw41		
					-Bw42		

Figure 2.3 Arrangement of HLA genes on the short arm of chromosome 6. Alleles of the HLA-A, B and C loci control the HLA-A, B and C determinants (antigens) while the HLA-D (MLC) antigens are controlled by HLA-D genes. These genes are identical with or very closely linked to the immune response (Ir) genes. The genes controlling the second (C2) and fourth (C4) components of the complement cascade are also closely linked to the HLA. PGM$_3$ refers to phosphoglucomutase-3 and Bf to properdin factor Bf. The distance between HLA-A and -B is approximately 1 centimorgan

also (2) some components of the complement cascade, and (3) a variety of immune responses. For example, the MHC of man, the HLA system (Figure 2.3), contains three loci, HLA-A, B, and C, which control antigens present on most cells except red cells. The HLA-D locus controls another group of HLA antigens with a different molecular structure and they are mainly present on monocytes and B lymphocytes. The HLA-D antigens are responsible for the stimulation seen in mixed leukocyte cultures (MLCs) of allogeneic cells. These antigens seem to be closely associated with and may indeed be identical with the HLA-DR antigens which can be recognized on the same cells by means of serological methods. In mice, the analogues of DR antigens are the so-called Ia (immune region-associated) antigens. In addition to the HLA-ABCD loci, this system also contains genes controlling the second (C2) and the fourth (C4) component of complement as well as the properdin factor, Bf, of the alternative complement pathway. Formal proof for the existence of immune response (Ir) genes within the HLA system is still lacking, but such genes have been found within the MHCs of all other vertebrates studied from mice to monkeys and as there are striking homologies between all these MHCs, there is little doubt that HLA also contains Ir genes.

Immune responses related to HLA-ABC antigens

Recently, there has been an important advance in our knowledge about how the MHC may control the immune responsiveness and our defence against viral infections. The breakthrough was the 'altered self' theory advanced by Doherty and Zinkernagel[21] to explain some peculiar observations seen when lymphocytes from virus-infected animals were investigated for their ability to kill virus-infected cells. It has long been known that mice infected with, for example, LCM (lymphocyte choriomeningitis) virus develop 'killer' cells which can lyse virus-infected cells. Doherty and Zinkernagel also observed that lysis only took place when the infected target cells shared MHC antigens with the animal in which the killer cells had been educated. They interpreted this finding by postulating that the specificity of the killer cells was directed not solely against the virus, but against the virus in combination with autologous MHC antigens (altered self). Similar observations have now been made for a variety of other viruses and also for more well-defined antigens[22, 23] and the same mechanism has been shown to operate in man too[24-26].

Dinitrofluorobenzene (DNFB) is a so-called 'hapten' which when applied to the skin can elicit a cell-mediated immunity detectable as a delayed-type skin reaction upon subsequent application of DNFB. This reaction is due to activation of effector T lymphocytes specific against DNFB-coated cells in the skin. The reaction between effector T cells and DNFB-coated cells can also be demonstrated *in vitro*[25]: when ^{51}Cr-labelled DNFB-coated lymphocytes are exposed to DNFB-sensitized lymphocytes they will lyse and release ^{51}Cr to the medium. However, this lysis only occurs if the DNFB-coated lymphocytes share HLA-A, B, and possibly C antigens with the sensitizing lymphocytes[25]. Similar findings have been made with influenza virus-infected cells[26], and the 'altered self' phenomenon also operates in women who are sensitized against the male H–Y minor transplantation antigen controlled by the Y chromosome[24]. Perhaps one of the most interesting observations made in the human experiments was that while killing of DNFB-coated or H–Y antigen-bearing cells was preferentially restricted to the HLA-A2 antigen, the restriction seen for influenza virus-infected cells concerned mainly the HLA-B7 antigen. Similar preferential restrictions (Figure 2.4) have been observed in some mouse experiments[27, 28], and the obvious importance of this phenomenon is that some HLA (and H2) antigens apparently are superior to others in

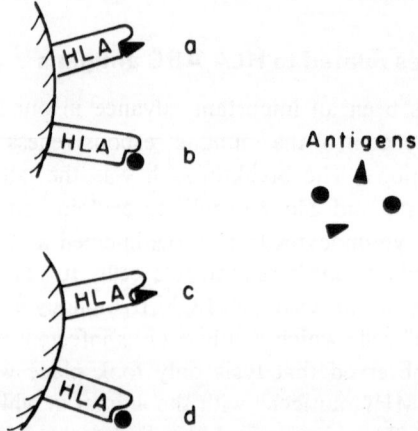

Figure 2.4 Simplified illustration of the 'preferential restriction' phenomenon. The HLA antigen on the upper cell shows a good fit (a) with the 'triangular' foreign antigen but reacts not as well with the 'circular' one (b). The opposite is true for the lower cell (c and d). Situations (a) and (d) would give a good presentation of the foreign antigen to the immunocompetent T lymphocytes. Accordingly, individuals having the upper HLA antigen would be high responders to the triangular and low responders to the circular antigen, while the opposite would hold for individuals having the lower HLA antigen. Heterozygous individuals having both HLA antigens would be high responders to both foreign antigens

the 'altered self' mechanism, i.e. there is a certain specificity already in the combination between foreign antigen and HLA antigen. This may be an important clue to our understanding of the pronounced polymorphism of these genetic systems.

When trying to explain the mechanism behind the 'altered self' phenomenon, the following scheme, which we shall call the 'presentation mechanism', seems most likely at the present time: HLA-A, B, and C antigens combine with and may even have a special affinity for some foreign antigens (e.g. virus and some haptens such as DNFB). The complex between foreign antigen and HLA antigen is then 'presented' to some members of a subclass of T lymphocytes (analogous to the Ly2,3-positive T lymphocytes in mice[2]), which recognize the complex by means of receptors specific for altered HLA-ABC (Figure 2.5). This recognition triggers these

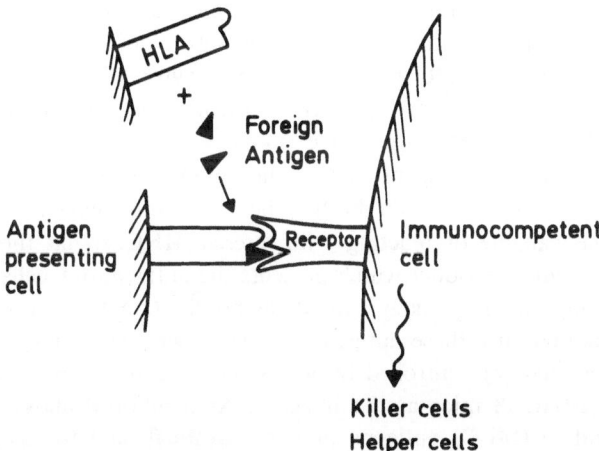

Figure 2.5   Schematic illustration of the presentation mechanism: HLA antigen on the 'antigen presenting cell' combines with foreign antigen and this coxplex is recognized by a receptor on an immumocompetent T lymphocyte which subsequently develops into helper or an effector (killer, suppressor or delayed-type hypersensitivity) T cell depending on (1) the presenting antigen, and (2) the receptor on the T cell (cf. text)

T lymphocytes to develop into cytotoxic killer cells which upon close contact can lyse cells carrying the same foreign antigen complexed with the HLA antigens in question. It is likely that T helper lymphocytes related to those discussed below are necessary for this triggering process.

Immune response related to HLA-D antigens

The function of Ir genes has been studied most extensively in mice and guinea-pigs[14,29-31]. These genes control the specific immune responses to a variety of synthetic and naturally occurring antigens – in general the antigens for which B lymphocytes need T lymphocyte cooperation for a humoral response to take place ('thymus-dependent' foreign antigens). High responsiveness is dominant over low, and the immune functions influenced by Ir genes involve the development of cell-mediated immunity and production of IgG antibodies against the antigen in question. Both of these responses are due to T lymphocyte activation, and until recently it was believed that the Ir genes were expressed only on T lymphocytes. However, evidence is now accumulating that the Ir gene products are indeed mainly present on B lymphocytes and perhaps even more so on monocytes[29,30]. The picture which seems to emerge[20] parallels that given above for effector cells, differing only in the nature of MHC products and cells involved: some MHC products on monocytes serve a function by binding foreign antigens and presenting them to immunocompetent T-helper lymphocytes (the Lyl-positive subclass in mice[2]) which react not to the simple foreign antigens, but to the complex between antigen and MHC product (Figure 2.4). To do this, the T cells must have receptors on their surface capable of reacting with altered MHC. What then is the nature of the MHC product which presents the antigen to T cells? At the time of writing, the most likely candidates are the Ia antigens (in man the DR antigens) because these antigens are (1) present on monocytes and B lymphocytes, and (2) controlled by genes mapping precisely in the same part of the MHC of mice as the Ir genes. As mentioned above, the DR antigens and D (MLC) antigens may be identical, and the same close genetic relationship between strong MLC determinants and Ia antigens has also been observed in mice[15]. The T-helper lymphocyte receptors must then have specificity for 'altered' D ($\sim$DR) antigens[32]. The nature of these T cell receptors is still an enigma, but there is some evidence that they may be related to immunoglobulins[33]. Activated T helper cells 'help' B lymphocytes to produce IgG antibody and the above T lymphocyte subclass to become killer cells[34]. The cooperation seems to be mediated by soluble factors released from the T helper cells[35].

Space does not allow a detailed discussion of all the evidence upon which the above scheme is based. However, one of the cornerstones in this evidence is the observation that T lymphocytes from a primed (sensitized) individual must 'see' the antigen on the same MHC background as the one being present during the primary immunization if a secondary response is to take place. This has been shown convincingly in guinea pigs[3] and most recently in man[36, 37].

It is a well-known observation that peripheral blood mononuclear cells from humans who have been vaccinated with BCG respond with proliferation of the T lymphocytes when exposed to tuberculin (PPD) *in vitro*. Recently, it has been shown that purified T lymphocytes from such individuals have lost most of their capacity to respond to PPD, but that the response can be restored by the addition of a small number of autologous monocytes[38]. Most recently, it has been observed independently by two different groups[36, 37] that the monocytes added must share HLA-D antigens with the T lymphocytes in order to restore effectively the responsiveness. Moreover, in the experiments of Hansen *et al.*[37], monocytes not sharing any HLA-D antigens with the T cells were totally ineffective in this respect. These findings can be best explained by the assumption that the memory T lymphocytes of the PPD-sensitized individual are primed not solely against PPD but against a complex between PPD and the HLA-D antigens of that individual. Accordingly, a secondary response (e.g. *in vitro* proliferation) only occurs when the T lymphocytes recognize PPD together with the same HLA-D antigens as were originally presenting the antigen. Conceivably, the preferential restriction phenomenon operates also for D antigens (Figure 2.5).

It has always been something of a mystery why as many as about 1 to 2% of the lymphocytes in the peripheral blood were able to respond to allogeneic lymphocytes in the mixed leukocyte culture (MLC) reaction even when the responder individual has not been immunized. In a primary immune response much fewer cells would generally be expected to be present. Now, the 'presentation' mechanism makes it easier to understand the high number of alloreactive cells in unprimed individuals: these cells are predisposed to recognize altered HLA-D antigens, and the foreign HLA-D antigens on the stimulating cells may just as well be regarded as altered HLA-D antigens in relation to the responder's own HLA-D antigens. Moreover, it is conceivable that the HLA-D antigens on the stimulating cells may be combined with many other molecular species normally present on the cell. These combination products may in turn be recognized as further modifications of the original HLA-D antigen, which would amplify the response[39].

The MLC reaction may be considered an *in vitro* model of the *in vivo* transplantation reaction: T lymphocytes react to foreign HLA-D antigens by proliferation and by the formation of both helper cells (specific for HLA-D) and killer cells (and perhaps some suppressor cells[40]) specific for HLA-ABC antigens which is completely in agreement with the 'presentation' theory outlined above. Thus, the biological background for the strong transplantation antigens is their role as presentation factors and this makes it understandable why transplantation across the HLA barrier is met with so strong an immune reaction in untreated recipients.

CONCLUDING REMARKS

Studies of the final products in the humoral immune response, the immunoglobulins, have led to the discovery of three very complex genetic systems (H, κ and λ) which are the basis for antibody production. More recently, it has become clear that another very complex genetic system (MHC, in man HLA) is also of key importance in many immune responses, humoral as well as cell-mediated. Following the above consideration, the HLA-A, B, C, D (and DR) antigens probably have as one of their most important biological properties, a fundamental role in presenting foreign antigens to immunocompetent T lymphocytes. The only difference between the HLA-D antigens on the one side and HLA-ABC antigens on the other would be that the D antigens present foreign antigens to a subset of T lymphocytes (T-helper cells with receptors for altered D) which assist B lymphocytes in their development into IgG antibody producing cells and a subset of T cells to become killer cells, while the ABC antigens present foreign antigen to this latter subset of T cells with receptors for altered ABC.

Although the 'altered self' or 'presentation' theory is gaining more and more support, it would be appropriate at this place to stress that the operation of HLA and related systems in the immune response may not be precisely as discussed above. There are still a number of controversies and many gaps have yet to be filled; in particular, the molecular mechanism of the postulated complex formation between MHC and foreign antigen is difficult to understand. It has been suggested that there are two different receptors on the same T cell, one reacting with foreign antigen and one with MHC[31]. Nevertheless, we believe that the scheme as we have outlined it represents at least roughly the truth. We have deliberately tried to present the situation in the simplest possible way, and Nature is most probably more complicated. Indeed, although the discovery of HLA as an antigen-presenting system has added very significantly to our understanding of the genetics of the immune system, it certainly has not solved the problem of the elusive T cell receptors[41]. Whether or not the genes controlling these receptors are linked to the Ig genes or to MHC, it must be concluded that there are at least four different very complex genetic systems (H, κ, λ, and MHC) involved in the specific immune response towards many antigens. In general, at the cellular level this response would start with the monocytes, in which a certain crude specificity may reside, and continues over T-helper cells and immunocompetent B lymphocytes to end by the formation of antibody-secreting plasma cells. During this sequence of events, an amplification and an increase of specificity takes place. To prevent the reaction running out of control, there must be feedback mechanisms, and as suggested by Jerne[42], the immune system may be considered a very fine network of stimulating and suppressing forces.

Acknowledgements

This study was aided by grants from the Danish Medical Research Council, the Danish Cancer Society, and the Nordic Insulin Foundation. We are grateful to Dr D. Jerne for helpful discussions during preparations of the section on immunoglobulins.

References

1. Edelman, G. M. (1977). Summary: Understanding selective molecular recognition. *Cold Spring Harbor Symposia on Quant. Biol.*, **49**, 891
2. Simonsen, M. (1978). General immunobiology – cell types and effector mechanisms (this volume).
3. Pahwa, R., Pahwa, S., O'Reilly, R., Smithwick, Elizabeth M. and Good, R. A. (1978). Immunodeficiency diseases – a review (p. 3 this volume).
4. Meuwissen, H. J., Parker, K. and Cook, B. (1977). Inborn errors of specific immunity: adenosine deaminase deficiency and purine nucleoside phospherylase deficiencies (p. 89 this volume).
5. Gally, J. A. and Edelman, G. M. (1977). Somatic translocation of antibody genes. *Nature (London)*, **227**, 341
6. Porter, R. R. (1959). The hydrolysis of rabbit-globulin and antibodies with crystalline papain. *Biochem. J.*, **73**, 119
7. Natvig, J. B. and Kunkel, H. (1973). Human immunoglobulins: classes, subclasses, genetic variants and idiotypes. *Adv. Immunol.*, **16**, 1
8. Kindt, T. J. (1975). Rabbit immunoglobulin allotypes: Structure, immunology and genetics. *Adv. Immunol.*, **21**, 35
9. Hood, L., Campbell, J. H. and Elgin, S. C. R. (1975). The organization, expression, and evolution of antibody genes and other multigene families. *Ann. Rev. Genet.*, **19**, 305
10. Roitt, I. (1974). *Essential Immunology*, 2nd Ed. (Oxford: Blackwell Scientific Publications)
11. Wigzell, H. (1973). Antibody diversity: Is it all coded for by the germ line genes? *Scand. J. Immunol.*, **2**, 199
12. Jerne, N. K. (1971). The somatic generation of immune recognition. *Eur. J. Immunol.*, **1**, 1
13. Natvig, J. B., Kunkel, H. G., Yount, W. J. and Nielsen, J. C. (1968). Further

studies of the γG-heavy chain genes complexes, with particular reference to the genetic markers Gm(g) and Gm(h). *J. Exp. Med.*, **128**, 763

14.   McDevitt, H. O. and Benacerraf, B. (1969). Genetic control of specific immune responses. *Adv. Immunol.*, **11**, 31.

15.   Klein, J. (1975). *Biology of the Mouse Histocompatibility-2 Complex* (New York: Springer)

16.   Shreffler, D. C. and Davis, C. S. (1975). The H-2 major histocompatibility complex and the I immune response region: Genetic variation, function and organization. *Adv. Immunol.*, **20**, 125

17.   Snell, G., Dausset, J. and Nathenson, S. (1976). *Histocompatibility*, p. 401. (New York: Academic Press)

18.   Svejgaard, A., Hauge, M., Jersild, C., Platz, P., Ryder, L. P., Staub Nielsen, L. and Thomsen, M. (1975). The HLA system – an introductory survey. In L. Beckman and M. Hauge (eds.). *Monographs in Human Genetics*, 7 (Basel: S. Karger)

19.   *Histocompatibility Testing 1977.* (Copenhagen: Munksgaard) (*In press*)

20.   Miller, J. F. A. P. and Vadas, M. A. (1977). The major histocompatibility complex: Influence on immune reactivity and T-lymphocyte activation. *Scand. J. Immunol.*, **6**, 771

21.   Doherty, P. C. and Zinkernagel, R. M. (1975). A biological role for the major histocompatibility antigens. *Lancet*, **i**, 1406

22.   Shearer, G. M. (1974). Cell-mediated cytotoxicity to trinitrophenyl-modified syngeneic lymphocytes. *Eur. J. Immunol.*, **4**, 527

23.   Zinkernagel, R. M. and Doherty, P. C. (1977). Possible mechanisms of disease susceptibility association with major transplantations antigens. In J. Dausset and A. Svejgaard (eds.). *HLA and Disease*, pp. 256–68. (Copenhagen: Munksgaard)

24.   Goulmy, E., Termijtelen, A., Bradley, B. A. and Rood, J. J. van (1977). Y-Antigen killing by T cells of women is restricted by HLA. *Nature (London)*, **266**, 544

25.   Dickmeiss, E., Soeberg, B. and Svejgaard, A. (1977). Human cell-mediated cytotoxicity against modified target cell is restricted by HLA. *Nature (London)*, **270**, 526

26.   McMichael, A. J., Ting, A., Zweerink, H. J. and Askonas, B. A. (1977). HLA restriction of cell mediated lysis of influenza virus infected human cells. *Nature (London)*, **270**, 524

27.   Shearer, G. M., Rehn, T. G. and Schmitt-Verhulst, A.-M. (1976). Role of the murine major histocompatibility complex in the specificity of *in vivo* T-cell-mediated lympholysis against chemically-modified autologous lymphocytes. *Transpl. Rev.*, **29**, 222

28.   Bubbers, J.-E., Blank, K. J., Freedman, H. A. and Lilly, F. (1977). Mechanism of the H-2 effect on viral leukemogenesis. *Scand. J. Immunol.*, **6**, 533

29.   Rosenthal, A. S. and Svevach, E. M. (1973). Function of macrophages in antigen recognition by guinea-pig T lymphocytes. I. Requirement for histocompatible macrophages and lymphocytes. *J. Exp. Med.*, **138**, 1194

30.   Rosenstreich, D. L. and Oppenheim, J. J. (1976) The role of macrophages in the activation of T and B lymphocytes *in vitro*. In D. S. Nelson (ed.). *Immunobiology of the Macrophages* (London/New York: Academic Press)

31. Thomas, D. W., Yamashita, U. and Shevach, E. M. (1977). The role of Ia antigens in T cell activation. *Immunol. Rev.*, 35, 97

32. Erb, P., Meier, B. and Feldman, M. (1976) Two gene control of T-helper cell induction. *Nature (London)*, 263, 601

33. Janeway, C. A., Wigzell, H. and Binz, H. (1976). Two different V_H gene products make up the T-cell receptors. *Scand. J. Immunol.*, 5, 993

34. Cantor, H. and Boyse, E. A. (1975). Functional subclasses of T lymphocytes bearing different Ly antigens. II Cooperation between subclasses of Ly⁺ cells in the generation of killer activity. *J. Exp. Med.*, 141, 1390

35. Munro, A. J. and Taussig, M. J. (1975). Two genes in the major histocompatibility complex control immune response. *Nature (London)*, 256, 103

36. Bergholtz, B. O. and Thorsby, E. (1977). Macrophage-dependent response of immune human T lymphocytes to PPD *in vitro*. *Scand. J. Immunol.*, 6, 779

37. Hansen, G. S., Rubin, B., Sørensen, S. F. and Svejgaard, A. (1978). Importance of HLA-D antigens for the cooperation between human monocytes and T lymphocytes, *Eur. J. Immunol.*, 7, 520

38. Hansen, G. S., Rubin, B. and Sørensen, S. F. (1977). Human leucocyte response *in vitro*. I. Transformation of purified T lymphocytes with and without addition of partially purified monocytes. *Clin. Exp. Immunol.*, 29 295

39. Matzinger, P. and Bevan, M. J. (1977). Why do so many lymphocytes respond to major histocompatibility antigens? *Cell. Immunol.*, 29, 1

40. Thomson, M., Dickmeiss, E., Jakobsen, B. K., Platz, P., Ryder, L. and Svejgaard, A. (1977). Low responsiveness in MLC induced by certain HLA-A antigens on the stimulator cells. *Tissue Antigens*, 11, 449

41. Crone, M., Koch, C. and Simonsen, M. (1972). The elusive T cell receptor. *Transpl. Rev.*, 10, 36

42. Jerne, N. K. (1974). Towards a network theory of the immune system. *Ann. Immunol. (Institut Pasteur)*, 125c, 373

SECTION TWO

Enzyme Defects and Immunodeficiency

Inborn errors of specific immunity: adenosine deaminase deficiency and purine nucleoside phosphorylase deficiency

H. J. Meuwissen, K. Parker and
B. Cook

INTRODUCTION

Many inborn errors of metabolism are known to occur in immune defence systems. Most of these involve non-specific immunity, particularly the complement and neutrophil granulocyte systems. Inborn errors of specific immunity were not described until recently. In this discussion, we will review the two most important diseases in this latter group, deficiency of adenosine deaminase (ADA) and purine nucleoside phosphorylase (PNP). Lack of transcobalamine II, leading to hypogammaglobulinaemia, may represent a third disorder in this group[1] but we will not consider this entity here.

ADA DEFICIENCY

Lack of ADA activity in children with severe combined immunodeficiency (SCID) was noted almost simultaneously by our group[2] and the Danish investigators Dissing and Knudsen[3], each without knowing about the finding of the other. This association was so unexpected that these cases were not reported until our group happened to come upon the second case, again quite by accident (Dr Flossie Cohen's patient[2]). Our finding was made in the process of searching for a bone marrow donor in a patient withe SCID. SCID refers to a severe disorder of the immune system, in many instances inherited, in which both thymus-dependent (T cells) and cells belonging to the antibody-forming system (B cells) are malfunctioning. ADA is an

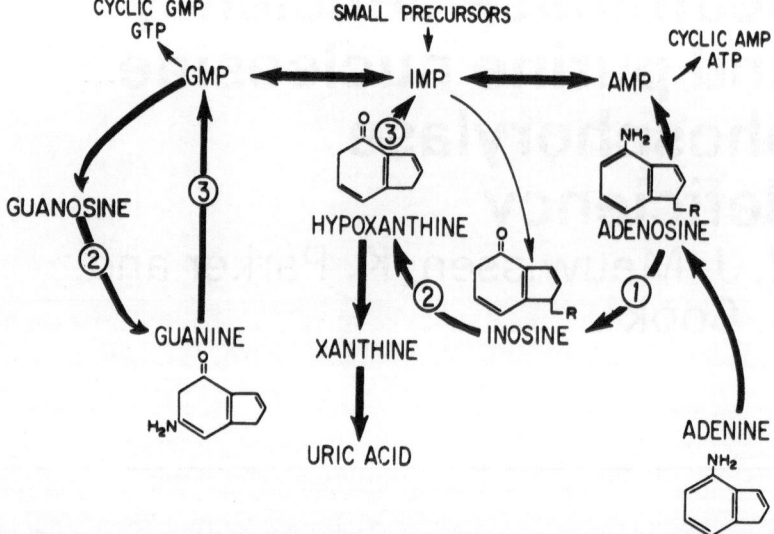

Figure 3.1 A simplified scheme of purine metabolism. 1. Adenosine deaminase. 2. Purine nucleoside phosphorylase. 3. Hypoxanthine guanine phosphoribosyl transferase (deficient in the Lesch–Nyhan syndrome)

enzyme in the purine reutilization pathway, and catabolizes adenosine to inosine by deamination. Inosine is further catabolized to hypoxanthine, and this latter metabolite may be degraded to uric acid or reutilized via the hypoxanthine guanine phosphoribosyl transferase (HGPRT) pathway (Figure 3.1).

Clinical and laboratory data

The first patient with ADA deficiency had many features shared by other patients with SCID and lack of ADA, and therefore we will briefly discuss her case. She was born from healthy but related parents and remained well for the first months of life until pneumonia and chronic *Candida* infection occurred[4]. At 5 months of age, she had considerable evidence of T cell dysfunction but normal levels of immunoglobulins and some antibodies, thus making a diagnosis of SCID unlikely until decay of B cell functions and other signs of immunological attrition occurred in the first year of life. She was nursed in a sterile environment and almost all treatments known at that time were applied in an effort to reconstitute her immune function. Two fetal thymus transplants, then two transplants of fetal thymus and fetal liver, followed by multiple administration of transfer factor and maternal buffy coat, all were without sucess. Finally,

TABLE 3.1   ADA Workshop 1973: Clinical and immunological data in patients with SCID with or without ADA deficiency in red cells*

	RBC ADA absent (12 patients)	RBC ADA normal (9 patients)
Clinical data		
Female	7	3
Alive at time of study	3	7
Failure to thrive	11	4
Candidiasis	9	3
Recurrent pneumonia	8	4
Opportunistic infections	6	3
Immunological data		
Normal to high IgG	4/12	3/9
Normal to high IgM	2/12	2/9
Normal to high IgA	3/12	3/9
Antibodies present	3/6	2/9
Normal PHA	0/12	0/9
Normal MLC	1/9	1/9
Normal T cells	1/5	0/7

* Data modified from Meuwissen, Pollara, Pickering et al. (1975)[6]

a maternal marrow transplant was attempted because the child had inherited the same HLA type from both related parents[4]. The transplant was successful in restoring B cell competence but was followed by flare-up of a dormant cytomegalovirus (CMV) infection and death.

Evidence of a T cell take was inconclusive. ADA was undetectable in her erythrocytes.

A workshop was held in Albany, New York in 1973 to study children suffering from SCID with or without ADA deficiency[5,6]. Data on 55 patients could be evaluated: 38 of the 55 had normal levels of ADA and 17 very low levels, in either red cells, tissues, or serum. Nine patients had normal red cell ADA and 13 had undetectable red cell ADA. A comparison of these two groups revealed that patients with undetectable red cell ADA died earlier and had a greater incidence of complications than patients in the ADA-normal group, while both were comparable in respect to laboratory evidence of B and T cell dysfunction: in both groups, T cell function seemed to be more severely depressed than B cell function (Table 3.1). The comparison between patients with normal and with abnormally low ADA is complicated by the fact that we had tried to include as many ADA-deficient children in the study as possible.

Striking findings were made in two areas. A specific pattern of abnormalities in ribs, pelves and vertebrae was recognized by radiographic examination in a subgroup of ADA-deficient children with SCID[6]. This radiological syndrome is so characteristic that it allows rapid recognition of ADA deficiency. The reason why a number of children lack the bone abnormalities is as yet not clear. A second major finding related to the histological picture of the thymus. Classically in SCID, the thymus is small, often incompletely descended, and lacks corticomedullary differentiation as well as Hassall's corpuscles. These features suggest arrest of development at an embryonic stage. As both B and T cell lines are affected in SCID, a defect of primitive lymphoid stem cells was postulated to explain the combined involvement of the B and T cell systems in these children.

Study of workshop patients whose ADA status was unknown to the participating pathologists showed surprisingly that Hassall's corpuscles and developed germinal epithelium could be found in the thymus of all children with ADA deficiency, while these features were absent in the ADA-normal children with SCID[6]. Thus, on the basis of the histological picture of the thymus, patients with SCID could be differentiated in two distinct groups, one of which (the ADA deficient group) showed evidence not of developmental arrest, but of later occurring thymic involution. This latter feature is in keeping with B cell attrition mentioned above, and with other signs of progressive immunological attrition observed not only in many children with ADA deficiency (Table 3.2)[2,7], but also in patients with PNP deficiency[8], and Wiskott–Aldrich syndrome[9]. We postulate that in ADA deficiency, fetal adenosine may be detoxified by the ADA-rich

TABLE 3.2   Evidence of immunological attrition in patients with SCID and ADA deficiency

1.	Decreasing levels of immunoglobulins
2.	Decreasing number of lymphocytes
3.	Decreasing mitogenic response of lymphocytes
4.	Disappearing thymus shadow on radiology
5.	Histological evidence of thymic involution
6.	Disappearing salivary IgA

placenta during intrauterine life. Postnatally, the immune system becomes progressively more impaired because of failure to deaminate adenosine, while at the same time it is exposed to the onslaught of environmental pathogens.

Strikingly, no evidence of immunodeficiency was found in a healthy 12-year-old boy from the !Kung San population in South Africa[10], whose red cells had low levels of ADA. However, his leukocyte ADA was $\pm 10\%$ of normal, suggesting that residual lymphocyte ADA in this child may have been sufficient for normal function of these cells.

Genetic features

Several families have provided the opportunity to study the pattern of genetic transmission of ADA deficiency[5,11,12]. Most parents studied had levels of ADA activity in red cells more than two standard deviations below the normal mean; the parents of our child had in addition abnormally low levels of lymphocyte and serum ADA (Figure 3.2). In several patients, residual ADA has been found in tissues[5,13], a silent gene has been demonstrated[14], and a mutant form of ADA has been found in cultured fibroblasts from ADA-deficient patients[15]. It appears therefore that the ADA molecule is altered by autosomal recessive mutations leading to decreased enzymatic activity.

Some authors have argued that the fault is not with the ADA molecule itself but with an ADA inhibitor[16]. This hypothesis conflicts with evidence of the silent gene and the data have not yet been confirmed by others.

An extra bonus for genetics derives from the fact that all phenotypically variant forms of ADA are equally affected by the genetic fault. This settles the years-old question of multiple versus single gene control of ADA by demonstrating that only a single locus is involved.

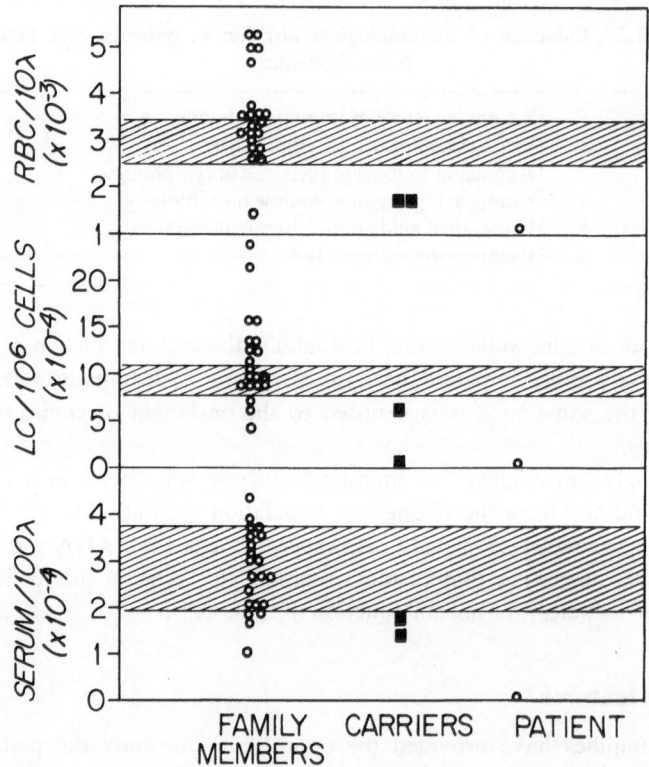

Figure 3.2   ADA levels in H. family. The hatched areas show normal mean ± 2 SD. Square symbols represent ADA values in parents. Some family members other than parents fall below 2 SD of mean, but not consistently so; i.e. none of the relatives is below 2 SD in serum, RBC, and lymphocytes. RBC/10λ: μM adenosine deammated per 10λ packed RBC/min at 37°C. LC/10⁶ cells: μM adenosine deaminated per 10⁶ lymphocytes/min at 37°C. Serum/100λ: μM adenosine deaminated per 100λ serum/min at 37°C. For methods, see caption to Figure 3.3

How does ADA deficiency lead to immune deficiency?

Many years ago, studies of ADA content in tissues showed that spleen and lymph nodes had very high levels of ADA activity in many species[17, 18] (thymus was almost never tested). Similar data have now been obtained for human tissues[19, 20]; in one these studies, thymus was included and had a high ADA content. Recently in our laboratory, Dr Howard Ratech has shown that ADA activity in bursa of embryonic and newly hatched chicks is very high, while it is surprisingly low in thymus[21]. It appears therefore that in general ADA content of lymphoid tissues in most species is high.

Attempts have been made to correlate ADA activity with lymphoid function. After local antigenic stimulation, ADA content of lymph node effluent cells rises significantly in unison with the appearance of plasma cells in the effluent[22]. Recently, production of E rosette binding cells from precursors in peripheral blood and marrow was shown to be impaired by ADA inhibition[23]. Furthermore, administration of ADA inhibitors to experimental animals delays rejection of skin[24] and tumour grafts[25]; graft rejection is a T cell-dependent function.

Several authors have now shown that ADA rises in lymphocytes exposed to plant mitogens[26-28]; protein production and cell proliferation can be diminished or stopped by addition of adenosine in combination with ADA inhibitors coformycin or EHNA[27]. In our laboratory, we have confirmed that ADA activity increases in lymphocyte cultures stimulated with PHA and Con-A but not in cultures stimulated with PWM[29] (Figure 3.3a

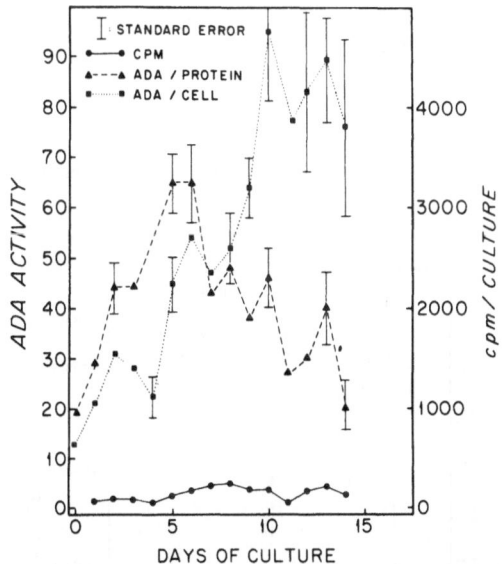

Figure 3.3 (a, b, c)   ADA activity in cultured lymphocytes

Figure 3.3a Human lymphocyte cultures *unstimulated*. ADA/protein: μM adenosine deaminated per min per mg protein. ADA/cell: nM adenosine deaminated per min per 10^7 lymphocytes. Standard errors are not shown for all determinations to prevent crowding, but where not shown are very similar to values shown. Lymphocyte cultures, determination of ADA activity, and protein content were done by methods previously described[58,59,60]. Washed lymphocytes were sonicated in a Branson sonicator. Values similar to those in Con-A stimulated cultures were obtained in PHA stimulated cultures for ADA/protein; in these cultures, ADA/cell could not be measured because of cell aggregation

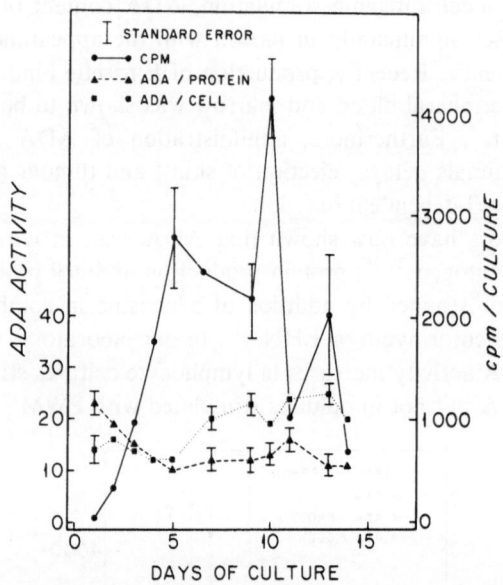

Figure 3.3b   Human lymphocyte cultures stimulated with PWM

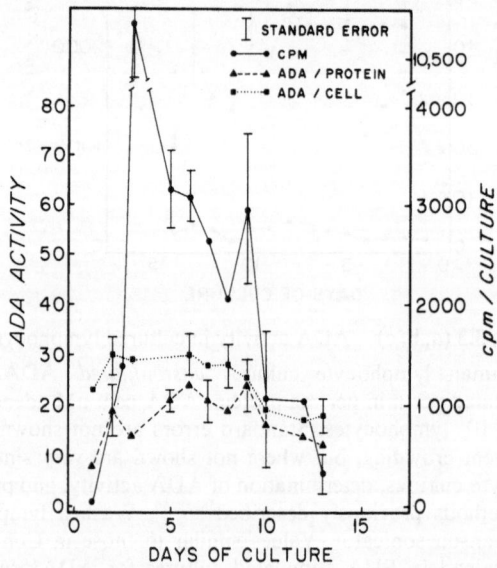

Figure 3.3c   Human lymphocyte cultures stimulated with Con-A

b and c). In unstimulated cultures, a much higher and sustained increase in ADA activity is observed (Figure 3.3a). In parallel experiments, we have shown that in fibroblast cultures, ADA activity remains at a basal level for several days during fibroblast proliferation. Once proliferation ceases and a confluent monolayer is formed, a marked rise in ADA activity occurs (Figure 3.4). These data are in line with recent studies by Fisher and Kelly who showed that maturation of macrophages is associated with increased levels of intracellular ADA[30]. Similarly, Trotta and Balis[31] documented a striking increase of ADA activity in rat gut epithelial cells once the cells had completed the switch from proliferation to differentiation. In regenerating mouse liver, a rise in ADA activity correlates better with increased RNA than DNA synthesis[32]. In differentiated gut epithelial cells, the ADA molecule becomes bound to a 'conversion'[33] or 'stabilizing' molecule, while in lymphocyte cultures, stimulated with PHA or Con-A (but not PWM), the reverse occurs: the amount of ADA bound to the 'stabilizing' factor is much decreased as compared to resting cells[34].

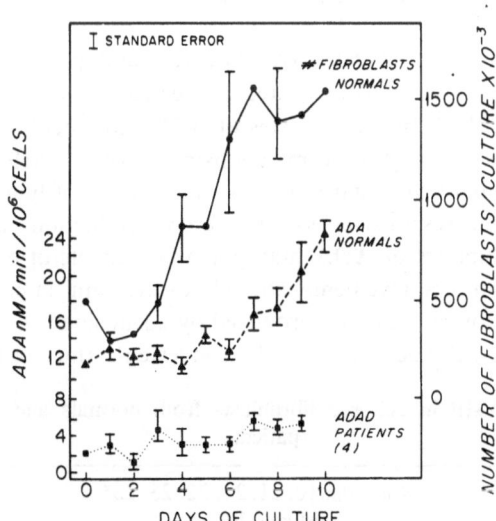

Figure 3.4   ADA activity in cultured fibroblasts. Cell number and ADA content in fibroblast cultures from normal and ADA deficient subjects are shown. Fibroblasts were grown in RPMI 1640 containing penicillin, streptomycin and 15% fetal calf serum. Cells were harvested with 0.05% trypsin. ADA was measured as indicated in caption to Figure 3.3. Two ADA-deficient lines were provided by Dr Arthur Green, Human Genetic Mutant Cell Repository, Camden, NJ (lines GM 469 and 471) and ADA-deficient line IB by Dr N. Goldman, Montreal. ADAD Patients: fibroblast lines from ADA-deficient patients with SCID

Therefore, during the maturation-differentiation phase of cell growth, more ADA activity becomes available to the cell or less ADA is broken down than during the proliferative phase; the hypothesis that absence of ADA blocks lymphoid function simply by impairing cell division obviously needs amplification. The studies cited also suggest an important role for the 'stabilizing' factor in function of the ADA molecule in the cell.

A number of hypotheses have been advanced to explain by which molecular mechanism ADA deficiency leads to immune dysfunction. Green and co-workers were the first to suggest that excess adenosine is toxic for lymphoid cells by decreasing pyrimidine nucleotide synthesis[35]. Many facts however argue against this hypothesis. Uridine therapy has been attempted in children with ADA deficiency and SCID without success[36]. Also, mitogen responsiveness of ADA-deficient lymphocytes and defective growth of ADA-deficient fibroblasts cannot be restored *in vitro* by addition of uridine[37-40]. Furthermore, detailed investigations of cells and plasma from ADA-deficient children with SCID have shown *normal*, not, as was expected on the basis of the hypothesis, *low*, levels of uridine nucleotides[40]. The expected increased levels of orotic acid were also not found[40].

Several studies of red cells, lymphocytes, and plasma from ADA-deficient patients have shown elevated concentrations of ATP, and cyclic AMP (Table 3.3)[40-43]. Increased levels of ATP may interfere with *de novo* purine synthesis[41], and glucose metabolism[44]. Cyclic AMP inhibits lymphocyte functions *in vitro* and *in vivo* by impairment of lymphocyte cytotoxicity, mitogen responsiveness, interferon production, and antibody formation[45]. Inhibitors of ADA may potentiate effects of cAMP[46]. Seegmiller and co-workers have demonstrated however that in cultured human lymphoblasts, growth inhibition produced by adenosine is *not* mediated by nucleotides to which adenosine may be converted[47], thus casting doubt on

TABLE 3.3   cAMP in cultured fibroblasts from normals and ADA-deficient patients

Normals: 10, 21, 21, 22, 23, 25*
Mean: 20
ADA-deficient patient 1: 29
patient 2: 85

* Values represent nM cAMP/μg DNA and were obtained seven days after subculture. Methods used are as described in[46]. All values are means of duplicate determinations except for patient 2 (single determination).
Dr Thomas Zimmerman performed the cAMP determinations.
Fibroblasts from patient 1 were provided by Dr Arthur Green (line GM 469) and those from patient 2 by Dr N. Goldman (line 1B).

the relevance of the studies cited above. Immunosuppressive metabolites such as isopentenyl adenosine[48] may contribute to the immunosuppressive state of ADA-deficient patients. Treatment of ADA deficiency with red cell transfusions and bone marrow transplantation is discussed by Dr Polmar in Chapter 4 of this volume[49].

The frequency of ADA deficiency is unknown at present. In the New York State Newborn Screening Program, more than 700 000 newborns have now been screened[49]. One baby was found to have ADA deficiency; so far, this child is immunologically normal[50]. One child, ADA deficient on newborn screening, was lost to follow-up while four children, negative on newborn screening for ADA, were later found to be normal on testing of whole blood. The incidence of ADA deficiency in the general population in New York State is therefore low.

The proportion of children with SCID who have ADA deficiency is also unknown. A figure for this incidence cannot be deduced from the workshop data as patients were preselected for ADA deficiency. At the most, a figure of 30% (17 patients with ADA deficiency in a total of 55 with SCID) can be taken as a maximum figure.

PNP DEFICIENCY

Four families with PNP deficiency have now been described[8, 51-55]. As in ADA deficiency, a defective mutant gene appears to be transmitted in these families[56]; marked clinical differences between families suggest a number of different gene mutations. The clinical condition of children with PNP

TABLE 3.4   Features of PNP deficiency in four families

Clinical
Progressive generalized vaccinia (two families)
Recurrent severe pyogenic infections (three families)
Red cell aplasia (one family)
Laboratory
T cell abnormalities (in all families studied)
Decreased number of T cells
Absent delayed hypersensitivity
Decreased or absent mitogen response
B cell abnormalities
Decreased number of B cells (three families)
Restricted heterogeneity of immunoglobulins (one family)
Antibody deficiency (mild, in two families)

deficiency differs from those with ADA deficiency (Table 3.4); death in infancy is not as common as in ADA deficiency. B cell dysfunction is mild, but deficient antibody formation and restricted heterogeneity in the presence of normal immunoglobulin levels do occur. In addition to congenital anaemia in the original patient[51], other patients have suffered from chronic, purulent pulmonary infections, purulent otitis media, and mastoiditis. These infections probably are not due to B cell dysfunction, and their cause needs further investigation. It is clear therefore that PNP deficiency is not an example of a 'pure' T cell disease.

Why children with PNP deficiency are immunologically abnormal remains speculative. The enzymatic defect impairs the catabolism of several nucleosides, including inosine and guanosine. The mechanism of immunological impairment may therefore be different from the one seen in ADA deficiency, as also suggested by the clinical and laboratory findings cited above. Some authors have suggested that the increase in guanosine as a result of the PNP defect could have deleterious effects on various aspects of purine metabolism and consequently on immune function[8], but many other possibilities will need to be considered.

CONCLUSION

Since the original description of ADA deficiency, a surprising amount of information has been gathered.

Two new autosomal recessive diseases have been found. It has become clear that both ADA and PNP are controlled by single genes. We now have two specific causes for severe primary immunodeficiencies and have thus gained a new conceptual approach to this group of diseases. A new radiological syndrome has been recognized. Screening for immune deficiency has begun, although in the case of ADA deficiency, with a very low yield. Enzyme replacement in ADA deficiency offers some promise and there are indications that administration of nucleosides or nucleotides to patients with PNP deficiency may be of help.

By investigating patients with defects in purine salvage pathways, the significance of these pathways in nucleic acid metabolism and lymphocyte function may be appreciated. The scope of these studies can be enlarged to include the central nervous system. For instance, the hypothesis that increased levels of hypoxanthine (see Figure 3.1) produce disturbances of the central nervous system in the Lesch–Nyhan syndrome has been strengthened by findings in PNP deficiency, where the blood level of hypoxanthine is low, and where, with one exception[8], no abnormalities of the central nervous system have been found. The metabolic block in the

Lesch–Nyhan syndrome, deficient HGPRT, is only one step removed from that in PNP deficiency (see Figure 3.1).

Finally, new methods for immunosuppression in humans may be developed based on the immunosuppressive effect of drugs inhibiting ADA and PNP; immunosuppression without bone marrow depression might even be possible.

We have begun to think about immunodeficiency disease in new ways. Hopefully this will be the start of new methods for diagnosis and therapy of these and other disorders and lead us into deeper understanding of the complexity of nucleic acid metabolism and lymphocyte function.

Acknowledgements

We thank Mr Andrew Stacey and Mrs R. Null for expert technical and secretarial help, respectively.

References

1. Hitzig, W. H. and Kenny, A. B. (1975). The role of vitamin B_{12} and its transport globulins in the production of antibodies. *Clin. Exp. Immunol.*, **20**, 105

2. Giblett, E. R., Anderson, J. E., Cohen, F. *et al.* (1972). Adenosine deaminase deficiency in two patients with severely impaired cellular immunity. *Lancet*, **ii**, 1067

3. Dissing, J. and Knudsen, B. (1972). Adenosine deaminase deficiency and combined immunodeficiency syndrome. *Lancet*, **ii**, 1316

4. Meuwissen, H. J., Moore, E. C., Pollara, B. *et al.* (1977). Combined immunodeficiency of the ADA deficient type with re-establishment of B cell function after maternal marrow graft. In preparation.

5. Meuwissen, H. J., Pickering, R. J., Pollara, B. and Porter, I. H. (eds.) (1975). *Combined Immunodeficiency Disease and Adenosine Deaminase Deficiency. A molecular defect.* (New York: Academic Press)

6. Meuwissen, H. J., Pollara, B., Pickering, R. J. *et al.* (1975). Combined immunodeficiency disease associated with ADA deficiency. *J. Pediatr.*, **86**, 169

7. Hitzig, W. H., Landolt, R., Müller, G. and Bodmer, P. (1971). Heterogeneity of phenotypic expression in a family with Swiss-type agammaglobulinemia. Observations on the acquisition of agammaglobulinemia. *J. Pediatr.*, **78**, 968

8. Stoop, J. W., Zegers, B. J. M., Hendrickx, G. F. M. *et al.* (1977). Purine nucleoside phosphorylase deficiency associated with selective cellular immunodeficiency. *N. Engl. J. Med.*, **296**, 651

9. Ammann, A. and Hong, R. (1973). Cellular immunodeficiency disorders. In R. Stiehm and V. Fulginiti (eds.). *Immunologic Disorders in Infants and Children*, p. 236. (Philadelphia: Saunders)

10. Jenkins, T., Rabson, A., Nurse, G. *et al.* (1976). Deficiency of adenosine deaminase not associated with severe combined immunodeficiency. *J. Pediatr.*, **89**, 732

11. Scott, C. R., Chen, S. H. and Giblett, E. R. (1974). Detection of the carrier state in combined immunodeficiency disease associated with adenosine deaminase deficiency. *J. Clin. Invest.*, 53, 1194

12. Ackeret, C., Plüss, H. J. and Hitzig, W. H. (1976). Hereditary severe combined immunodeficiency and adenosine deaminase deficiency. *Pediatr. Res.*, 10, 67

13. Van Der Weyden, M., Buckley, R. and Kelley, W. (1974). Molecular form of adenosine deaminase in severe combined immunodeficiency. *Biochem. Biophys. Res. Comm.*, 57, 590

14. Chen, S., Scott, C. and Giblett, E. (1974). Adenosine deaminase: Demonstration of a 'silent' gene associated with combined immunodeficiency disease. *Am. J. Hum. Genet*, 26, 103

15. Hirschhorn, R., Beratis, N. and Rosen, F. S. (1976). Characterization of residual enzyme activity in fibroblasts from patients with adenosine deaminase deficiency and combined immunodeficiency: Evidence for a mutant enzyme. *Proc. Natl. Acad. Sci. USA*, 73, 213

16. Trotta, P. P., Smithwick, E. M. and Balis, M. E. (1976). A normal level of adenosine deaminase activity in the red cell lysates of carriers and patients with severe combined immunodeficiency disease. *Proc. Natl. Acad. Sci. USA*, 73, 104

17. Conway, E. and Cooke, R. (1939). The deaminases of adenosine and adenylic acid in blood and tissues. *Biochem. J.*, 33, 479

18. Brady, T. G. and O'Donovan, C. (1965). A study of the tissue distribution of adenosine deaminase in six mammal species. *Comp. Biochem. Physiol.*, 14, 101

19. Van Der Weyden, M. B. and Kelley, W. N. (1976). Human adenosine deaminase – distribution and properties. *J. Biol. Chem.*, 251, 5448

20. Adams, A. and Harkness, R. A. (1976). Adenosine deaminase activity in thymus and other human tissues. *Clin. Exp. Immunol.*, 26, 647

21. Ratech, H. and Meuwissen, H. J. (1977). Adenosine deaminase in chicken thymus and bursa. (Submitted)

22. Hall, J. G. (1963). Adenosine deaminase activity in lymphoid cells during antibody production. *Aust. J. Exp. Biol.*, 41, 93

23. Ballet, J. J., Insel, R., Merler, E. *et al.* (1976). Inhibition of maturation of human precursor lymphocytes by coformycin, an inhibitor of the enzyme adenosine deaminase. *J. Exp. Med.*, 143, 1271

24. Lum, C. T., Sutherland, D. and Najarian, J. (1977). ADA inhibition and skin graft rejection. ADA inhibition for immunosuppression. *N. Engl. J. Med.*, 296, 819

25. Chassin, M. M., Chirigos, M. A., Johns, D. *et al.* (1977). Adenosine deaminase inhibition for immunosuppression. *N. Engl. J. Med.*, 296, 1232

26. Ochs, H. D. (1975). Combined immunodeficiency and adenosine deaminase deficiency. In H. J. Meuwissen, R. J. Pickering, B. Pollara, I. H. Porter (eds.). *Combined Immunodeficiency Disease and Adenosine Deaminase Deficiency*, p. 190. (New York: Academic Press)

27. Carson, D. and Seegmiller, J. (1976). Effect of adenosine deaminase inhibition upon human lymphocyte blastogenesis. *J. Clin. Invest.*, 57, 274

28. Hovi, T., Smyth, J., Allison, A. *et al.* (1976). Role of adenosine deaminase in lymphocyte proliferation. *Clin. Exp. Immunol.*, 23, 395

29. Meuwissen, H. J., Parker, K., Cook, B. and Pollara, B. (1976). Adenosine deaminase in proliferating lymphocytes and fibroblasts. *Fed. Proc.*, **35**, 821

30. Fischer, D., Van Der Weyden, M. B. *et al.* (1976). A role for adenosine deaminase in human monocyte maturation. *J. Clin. Invest.*, **58**, 399

31. Trotta, P. P. and Balis, M. E. (1977). Structural and kinetic alterations in adenosine deaminase associated with the differentiation of rat intestinal cells. *Cancer Res.*, **37**, 2297

32. Rothman, I., Silber, R. and Klein, K. (1971). Nucleoside deaminase and adenosine deaminase activities in regenerating mouse liver. *Biochim. Biophys. Acta*, **228**, 307

33. Nishihara, H., Satsuki, I., Shinkai, K. *et al.* (1973). Multiple forms of human adenosine deaminase. II. Isolation and properties of a conversion factor from human lung. *Biochim. Biophys. Acta*, **302**, 429

34. Hirschhorn, R. and Levytska, V. (1974). Alterations in isozymes of adenosine deaminase during stimulation of human peripheral blood lymphocytes. *Cell. Immunol.*, **12**, 387

35. Green, H. and Chan, T. S. (1973). Pyrimidine starvation induced by adenosine in fibroblasts and lymphoid cells. Role of adenosine deaminase. *Science*, **182**, 836

36. Pickering, R. J. Personal communication

37. Personal observations

38. Parkman, R., Gelfand, E. W., Rosen, F. *et al.* (1975). Severe combined immunodeficiency and adenosine deaminase deficiency. *N. Engl. J. Med.*, **292**, 714

39. Polmar, S., Wetzler, E., Stern, R. *et al.* (1975). Restoration of *in vitro* lymphocyte responses with exogenous adenosine deaminase in a patient with severe combined immunodeficiency. *Lancet*, ii, 743

40. Schmalstieg, F. C., Nelson, J. A., Mills, G. *et al.* (1977). Increased purine nucleotides in adenosine deaminase-deficient lymphocytes. *J. Pediatr.*, **91**, 48

41. Agarwal, R., Crabtree, G., Parks, R. *et al.* (1976). Purine nucleoside metabolism in the erythrocytes of patients with adenosine deaminase deficiency and severe combined immunodeficiency. *J. Clin. Invest.*, **57**, 1025

42. Mills, G., Schmalstieg, F., Trimmer, K. *et al.* (1976). Purine metabolism in adenosine deaminase deficiency. *Proc. Natl. Acad. Sci. USA*, **73**, 2867

43. Polmar, S., Stern, R., Schwartz, A. *et al.* (1976). Enzyme replacement therapy for adenosine deaminase deficiency and severe combined immunodeficiency. *N. Engl. J. Med.*, **295**, 1337

44. Lardy, H. and Parks, R. (1956). Influence of ATP concentration on rates of some phosphorylation reaction. In O. H. Gaebler (ed.). *Enzymes: Units of Biological Structure and Function*, p. 584. (New York: Academic Press)

45. Bourne, H., Lichtenstein, L., Melmon, K. *et al.* (1974). Modulation of inflammation and immunity by cyclic AMP. *Science*, **184**, 19

46. Wolberg, G., Zimmerman, T. P. and Hiemstra, K. (1975). Adenosine inhibition of lymphocyte-mediated cytolysis. Possible role of cyclic adenosine monophosphate. *Science*, **187**, 957

47. Hershfield, M. S., Snyder, F. F. and Seegmiller, J. E. (1977). Adenine and adenosine are toxic to human lymphoblast mutants defective in purine salvage enzymes. *Science*, **197**, 1284

48. Hacker, B. and Feldbush, T. (1969). N^6-(Δ^2-isopentenyl) adenosine – effects upon nucleic acid synthesis in lymphocytes *in vitro* and the development of immunologic hypersensitivity *in vivo*. *Biochem. Pharmacol.*, **18**, 847

49. Carter, R. Personal communication

50. Hirschhorn, R. Personal communication

51. Giblett, E., Ammann, A., Wara, D. *et al.* (1975). Nucleoside phosphorylase deficiency in a child with severe defective T-cell immunity and normal B-cell immunity. *Lancet*, **i**, 1010

52. Cohen, A., Doyle, D., Martin, D. *et al.* (1976). Abnormal purine metabolism and purine overproduction in a patient deficient in purine nucleoside phosphorylase. *N. Engl. J. Med.*, **295**, 1449

53. Stoop, J. W., Eijsvoogel, V. P., Zegers, B. *et al.* (1976). Selective severe cellular immunodeficiency – effect of thymus transplantation and transfer factor administration. *Clin. Immunol. Immunopathol.*, **6**, 289

54. Griscelli, C., Hauret, M., Ballet, J. *et al.* (1976). Inosine phosphorylase deficiency with fatal vaccinia gangrenosa. Presented at the 3rd International Workshop of the Cooperative Group for Bone Marrow Transplantation in Man, August 19–21, New York.

55. Biggar, W. D. (1977). A new form of nucleoside phosphorylase deficiency in two brothers with defective T cell function. Presented at the National Pediatric Conference Honoring Dr J. Anderson, June 16–18, Minneapolis, Minnesota

56. Fox, I. H., Andres, C. M., Gelfand, E. *et al.* (1977). Purine nucleoside phosphorylase deficiency: Altered kinetic properties of a mutant enzyme. *Science*, **197**, 1084

57. Parker, K., Schreinemachers, D. and Meuwissen, H. J. (1972). Lymphocyte recovery, purification and stimulation: A prospective study. *Transplantation*, **14**, 135

58. Kalckar, H. (1947). Differential spectrophotometry of purine compounds by means of specific enzymes. *J. Biol. Chem.*, **167**, 429

59. Lowry, O. H. and Rosebrough, N. J. (1951). Protein measurement with the folin phenol reagent. *J. Biol. Chem.*, **193**, 265

4

Adenosine deaminase deficiency: enzyme replacement therapy and investigations of the biochemical basis of immunodeficiency
S. H. Polmar

INTRODUCTION

In 1972, Giblett and co-workers[1] and Dissing and Knudsen[2] reported the coexistence of adenosine deaminase (ADA) deficiency and severe combined immunodeficiency disease (SCID). The discovery of an association between deficiency of an enzyme and an immunodeficiency represents a major conceptual landmark in that we now recognize that at least some immunodeficiency diseases, 'experiments of nature' as Dr Robert A. Good so elegantly called them, may indeed be 'inborn errors of metabolism' whose major consequences are manifest in the function of the immune system[3]. Therefore, if some immunodeficiencies are indeed metabolic diseases, the diagnostic and therapeutic approaches to these disorders must be similar to our approach to metabolic diseases, namely biochemical and pharmacological. Rational approaches to therapy presupposes an understanding of the biochemical basis of the immune dysfunction. This paper describes some of our investigations into the adenosine deaminase-deficient form of severe combined immunodeficiency disease, as well as our experience with enzyme replacement therapy for this disorder and some recent studies with pharmacological agents upon adenosine deaminase-deficient lymphocytes.

ADENOSINE DEAMINASE DEFICIENCY

The existence of a causal relationship between deficiency of ADA and severe combined immunodeficiency was first suggested by the finding that ADA deficiency occurs exclusively in patients with an autosomal recessive form of severe combined immunodeficiency and has not been found in normal individuals or patients with other immunodeficiencies such as common variable hypogammaglobulinaemia, sex-linked infantile agamma-globulinaemia, ataxia-telangiectasia, selective IgA deficiency, or Wiskott–Aldrich syndrome[4]. Furthermore, we have observed that adenosine deaminase deficiency is present before the immunological deficiency appears and thus ADA deficiency is not secondary to infection, growth failure or other consequences of immunodeficiency[5].

Patients with ADA deficiency usually manifest marked defects in both cell-mediated, T cell dependent, immunity as well as humoral, B cell dependent, immune functions. There is marked lymphopenia, depression of cutaneous delayed hypersensitivity and diminished or absent *in vitro* lymphocyte responses to mitogens such as phytohaemagglutinin (PHA), Concanavalin-A (Con-A) and pokeweed mitogen (PWM) as well as to antigens such as *Candida* and in mixed leukocyte cultures (MLC). Immunoglobulin levels in the serum are usually depressed and specific antibody production is diminished or absent. There is, however, consider-able heterogeneity in the immunological manifestations of ADA–SCID and some patients show primarily marked defects in cell-mediated immunity and relatively normal B cell function[6]. However, this appears to be related to the stage of the disease; with increasing age both T cell and B cell functions are ultimately lost[7,8].

Approximately 3 years ago we had the opportunity to study a family in which a female child had died with severe combined immunodeficiency. Family studies revealed that both parents had less than one-half normal ADA activity in their erythrocytes and an ADA^0 gene was identified by electrophoretic studies[5]. Aminocentesis and subsequent studies of the ADA activity in amniotic fluid cells revealed only 1% of normal ADA activity. At birth, the enzyme deficiency was confirmed by the finding of no ADA activity in the patient's erythrocytes, but the patient had lymphocytes, relatively normal numbers of T cells and B cells and did manifest *in vitro* lymphocyte response to PHA and Con-A, but these responses were only 25% of normal control responses. During the succeeding 6 weeks the patient became markedly lymphopenic and lost his ability to respond to mitogens *in vitro*. The patient did not have a histocompatible donor suitable for bone marrow transplantation and alternative modes of therapy were sought.

ENZYME REPLACEMENT THERAPY FOR ADENOSINE DEAMINASE DEFICIENCY

If deficiency of ADA resulted in immunodeficiency, then replacement of enzyme might result in restoration of immunological competence. Lymphocyte proliferative responses to mitogens, measured by [³H]thymidine incorporation, are characteristically diminished or absent in patients with SCID and serve as a useful laboratory parameter for study since they require relatively small numbers of cells. Addition of calf-intestine ADA or human erythrocyte ADA was found to markedly increase the ADA–SCID lymphocytes' response to PHA, Con-A and PWM[9] (Table 4.1). These observations suggested that enzyme replacement therapy might be possible for this form of immunodeficiency disease.

Enzyme replacement therapy first requires that sufficient amounts of purified enzyme be available to make therapy feasible and that the infused

TABLE 4.1 Effect of exogenous adenosine deaminase on mitogen-induced lymphocyte proliferation of an adenosine deaminase-deficient patient

ADA[2] source	[³H]Thymidine incorporation (cpm[1])		
	PHA[3]	Con-A[4]	Unstimulated
None	3067 ± 984	6875 ± 386	88 ± 13
Human erythrocyte[5]	$19\,102 \pm 1161$	$14\,029 \pm 557$	115 ± 8
Calf intestine[6]	8636 ± 237	$16\,900 \pm 1465$	98 ± 13

1. cpm = counts per minute ± one standard error of the mean
2. ADA = adenosine deaminase
3. PHA = phytohaemagglutinin
4. Con-A = Concanavalin-A
5. 0.89 international units of human erythrocyte ADA were added to each culture (kindly provided by Dr R. Hirschhorn)
6. 2.0 international units of calf intestine ADA added to each culture (obtained from Sigma, St Louis, Missouri)

enzyme remain biologically active for a sufficient period of time to produce the desired biochemical and immunological effects. Methods for purification of human ADA in quantity have only recently been developed[10, 11]. Furthermore, purified enzymes infused intravenously have been found to have very short half-lives[12]. However, entrapment of enzymes in

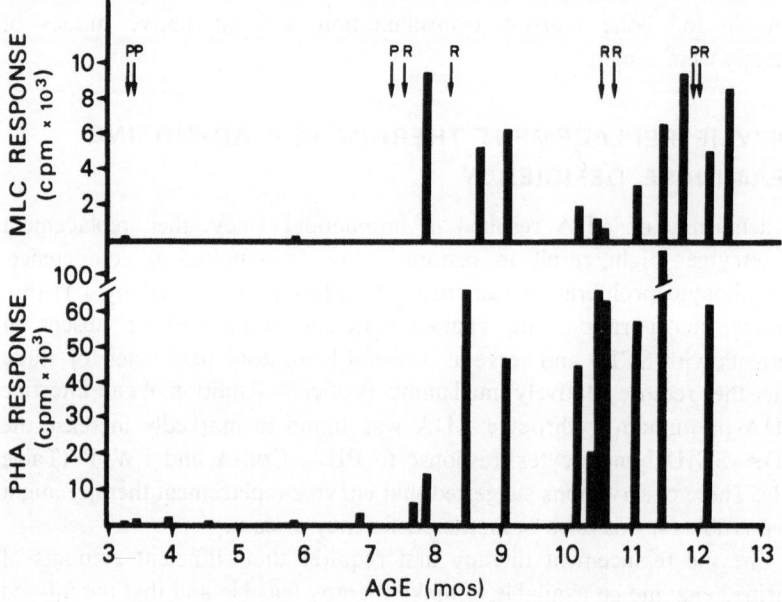

Figure 4.1   Effect of transfusion of frozen irradiated red blood cells (R) or frozen irradiated plasma (P) (or both) on *in vitro* lymphocyte responses to phytohaemagglutinin (PHA) and allogeneic cells in the mixed leukocyte culture (MLC) reaction (reprinted from Polmar *et al.*[8] with permission of the Massachusetts Medical Society)

biodegradable vesicles such as erythrocytes has been shown to prolong the half-life of the infused enzyme[13]. Since ADA is present in the human erythrocyte, this tissue was selected as a source of encapsulated human ADA. The risk of graft-versus-host (GVH) reaction form transfusion of viable donor lymphocytes was minimized by using frozen blood which had been irradiated with 5000 rad.

Enzyme replacement therapy was attempted by transfusing a 7-month-old ADA–SCID patient with 15 ml/kg of frozen, irradiated packed red blood cells[8]. Enzyme levels near the heterozygote range could be achieved by transfusing the child at monthly intervals. The transfused enzyme was found to have a half-life of approximately 30 days. Studies of lymphocyte ADA activity before and during therapy failed to reveal any significant increase in lymphocyte ADA activity; the ADA–SCID lymphocyte remained enzyme-deficient, containing only 6% of normal enzyme activity. Prior to initiation of therapy, the patient's *in vitro* lymphocyte responses to PHA, Con-A, PWM and allogeneic cells were either absent or less than 5% of normal control responses. Improvement in lymphocyte responses was observed within 1 week of initiation of therapy and were within the normal range 3 weeks after therapy was begun (Figure 4.1). If transfusions were withheld for more than 5 weeks, *in vitro* lymphocyte responses decreased significantly, but could be increased approximately 3-fold within 24 h following a transfusion of frozen, irradiated red cells (Table 4.2).

TABLE 4.2 Lymphocyte responses to mitogens and allogeneic cells (MLC reaction) in vitro before and 24 h after transfusion with frozen irradiated red blood cells[1]

		$[^3H]$Thymidine incorporation (cpm^2)			
Time of study	$RBC–ADA^3$	PHA^4	$Con-A^5$	PWM^6	MLC^7
Before transfusion	3.3	8840 ± 351	4100 ± 149	3295 ± 42	3149 ± 99
Twenty-four hours after transfusion	18.8	24 451 ± 1055	10 927 ± 337	6125 ± 148	10 021 ± 1251

1. Reprinted from Polmar *et al.*[8] with permission of the publisher
2. cpm = count per minute $\pm$ one standard error of the mean
3. RBC–ADA = red blood cell adenosine deaminase activity expressed as the nmol of adenosine deaminated/mg of haemoglobin/h at 20 °C
4. PHA = phytohaemagglutinin
5. Con-A = Concanavalin-A
6. PWM = pokeweed mitogen
7. MLC = mixed leukocyte culture

Therapy also resulted in a marked increase in circulating peripheral blood lymphocytes from less than 350/mm^3 to a maximum of 1800/mm^3 (Figure 4.2). Both T lymphocytes (44–48%) and B lymphocytes (18–23%) were identified. Initially, lymphocytosis appeared to be facilitated by infusion of fresh frozen normal plasma. Plasma infusion had no effect upon *in vitro* lymphocyte responses.

Prior to enzyme replacement therapy, a thymic shadow had never been observed on chest roentgenograms of the ADA–SCID patient. A thymus shadow was detected 14 days after initiation of therapy (Figure 4.3). Studies of serum thymic hormone activity performed before and subsequent to therapy showed an increase of thymic hormone activity into the normal range and continued therapy maintained thymic hormone levels within or just slightly below the normal range[14]. However, we have been unable to demonstrate or induce cutaneous delayed hypersensitivity in this patient.

Prior to therapy, the patient was markedly hypogammaglobulinaemic.

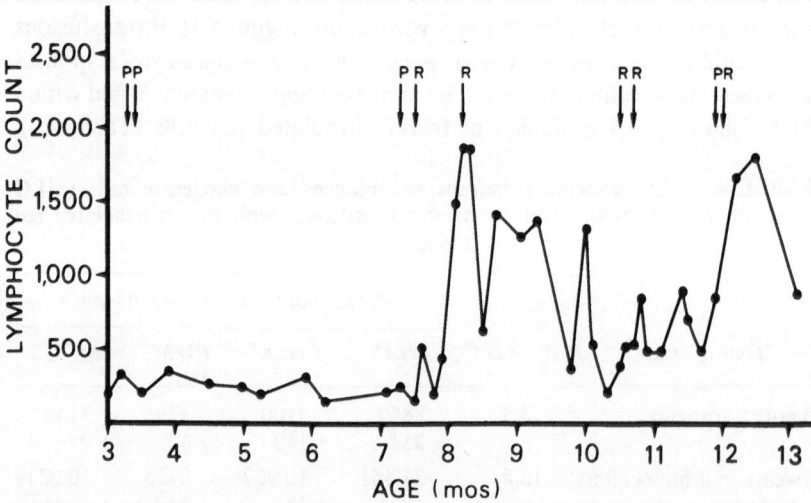

Figure 4.2   Effect of transfusion of frozen irradiated red blood cells (R) or frozen irradiated plasma (P) (or both) on peripheral blood absolute lymphocyte count (cells per mm³) (reprinted from Polmar *et al.*[8] with permission of the Massachusetts Medical Society)

Serum immunoglobulin levels began to rise 5 months after the initiation of therapy and have been within the normal range for the past 18 months. Synthesis of immunoglobulin by peripheral blood lymphocyte *in vitro* could also be demonstrated.

This ADA–SCID patient, now 3 years of age, has been maintained on monthly frozen, irradiated red blood cell transfusions for more than two years. He has had no significant infections and his growth and development, both physically and psychologically, have been normal. Up to the present time there have been no adverse consequences resulting from this form of therapy.

A total of eight ADA–SCID patients have been treated by frozen, irradiated red blood cell. transfusion. Therapy and evaluation of these patients has not been standardized, thus making it difficult to analyse even

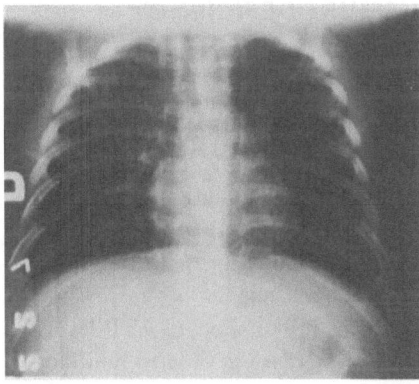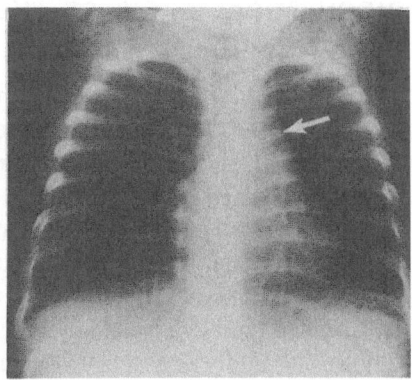

Figure 4.3 Roentgenograms of the chest taken before (left) and 4 months after initiation of transfusion therapy (right). The film taken before therapy shows no thymus shadow in the anterior superior mediastinum, whereas that taken after therapy shows a readily identifiable thymus shadow, indicated by the arrow. A thymus shadow was first detectable 14 days after initiation of transfusion therapy (reprinted from Polmar *et al.*[8] with permission of the Massachusetts Medical Society)

the small amount of available data. In four patients, restoration or improvement of immunological function was observed as well as improvement in general clinical status (i.e. improved growth, decreased infection)[8, 15-17]. In two patients, clinical status improved, but there was no increased immunological competence demonstrated[18]. In three patients there was no improvement in clinical or immunological state[19-21]. Why some patients respond to enzyme replacement therapy while others do not is as yet unclear. There appears to be considerable variability between patients with regard to the severity of their enzyme deficiency as well as their degree of immunodeficiency. It is possible that only patients with less severe enzyme deficiency can respond to enzyme replacement. Alternatively, since the immunodeficiency appears to be acquired, becoming more profound with time, at some point the immunodeficiency may become irreversible. This might occur if the thymus were severely damaged or lymphoid stem cells were lost as a result of metabolic toxicity. In such instances, correction of the metabolic defect could not be expected to restore immunological competence, but the combination of enzyme replacement and thymic epithelial transplantation[22] might be effective.

BIOCHEMICAL BASIS OF THE IMMUNODEFICIENCY IN ADA–SCID

The precise biochemical or pharmacological mechanism(s) by which deficiency of ADA results in immunodeficiency is not entirely understood. When ADA is absent, adenosine cannot be deaminated to inosine and is phosphorylated by adenosine kinase, resulting in accumulation of adenine nucleotides, particularly ATP[23, 24]. We found lymphocyte ATP levels to be 10-fold normal in our ADA-deficient SCID patient prior to therapy[8]. This observation has been confirmed by Schmalsteig *et al.*[25]. Enzyme replacement therapy resulted in a 75% decrease in lymphocyte ATP levels (Figure 4.4) and was associated with a 3-fold increase in *in vitro* lymphocyte responses within 24 hours of erythrocyte transfusion (Table 4.2)[8]. Increased levels of ATP may interfere with lymphocyte function in at least three ways: (1) by inhibiting purine and pyrimidine synthesis, (2) by inhibiting lymphocyte glycolysis, and (3) by increasing cyclic AMP (cAMP) production.

Green and Chan[26] observed inhibition of proliferation of lymphoid cell lines cultured in the presence of adenosine and suggested that this was due to 'pyrimidine starvation' resulting from inhibition of 5-phosphoribosyl-l-pyrophosphate (PRPP) synthesis. However, PRPP-dependent reactions

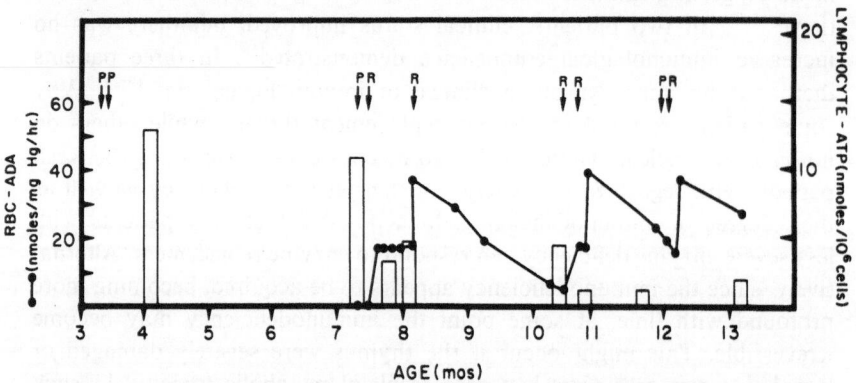

Figure 4.4   Effect of transfusion of frozen irradiated red blood cells (R) or frozen irradiated plasma (P) (or both) on lymphocyte ATP levels and red cell adenosine deaminase activity (RBC–ADA). Lymphocyte ATP levels are indicated by the open bars, and red cell ADA activity by the closed circles; red cell transfusion consistently reduced lymphocyte ATP concentrations. Lymphocyte ATP levels could be maintained near the normal range (1.1 to 1.7 nmol/10⁶ cells) by transfusion of frozen irradiated red blood cells at 4 week intervals (reprinted from Polmar *et al.*[8] with permission of the Massachusetts Medical Society)

occur at normal rates in ADA-deficient lymphocytes indicating no deficiency of PRPP in enzyme-deficient cells[24]. Furthermore, ADA deficient lymphocytes do not show enhanced proliferation in the presence of uridine, which would be expected if there was 'pyrimidine starvation'[9, 27]. In addition, purine and pyrimidine levels have been found to be normal or elevated in ADA-deficient lymphocytes[25].

It is unlikely that ADA deficiency results in significant inhibition of glycolysis in ADA-deficient cells due to ATP accumulation. In ADA-deficient patients, the enzyme deficiency is more extreme in erythrocytes than in lymphocytes[5, 27]. Erythrocytes in which glycolysis is perturbed

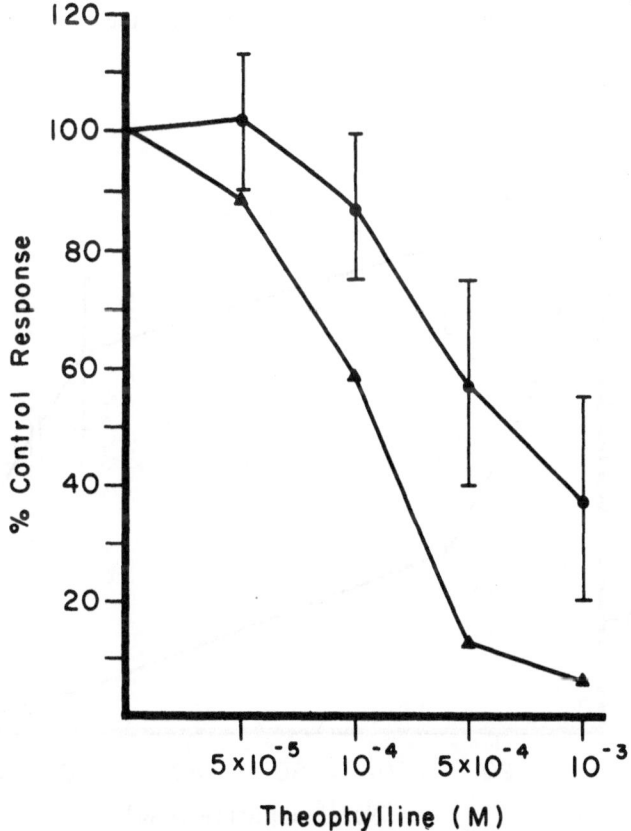

Figure 4.5   Inhibition of *in vitro* lymphocyte responses to phytohaemagglutinin by theophylline. Closed circles (●) represent the mean ± one standard deviation of six normal individuals. Closed triangles (▲) represent the mean response of the ADA-deficient lymphocytes

have shortened half-lives and are usually associated with a haemolytic anaemia which has not been observed in ADA deficiency.

Elevated levels of cAMP have been shown to inhibit many lymphocyte functions including mitogen-induced lymphocyte proliferation[28,29]. Elevated levels of cAMP have been reported in the lymphocytes of one ADA-deficient patient[25] but the functional significance of this observation is difficult to assess in light of the known protein binding and compartmentalization of cAMP within the cell. The availability of ADA-deficient lymphocytes capable of responding to mitogens has permitted us to study the effects of various pharmacological agents on ADA-deficient and normal lymphocytes in order to examine the possible role of cAMP in the causation of the immunodeficiency in ADA–SCID[30,31].

The effects of various pharmacological agents upon the *in vitro* lympho-

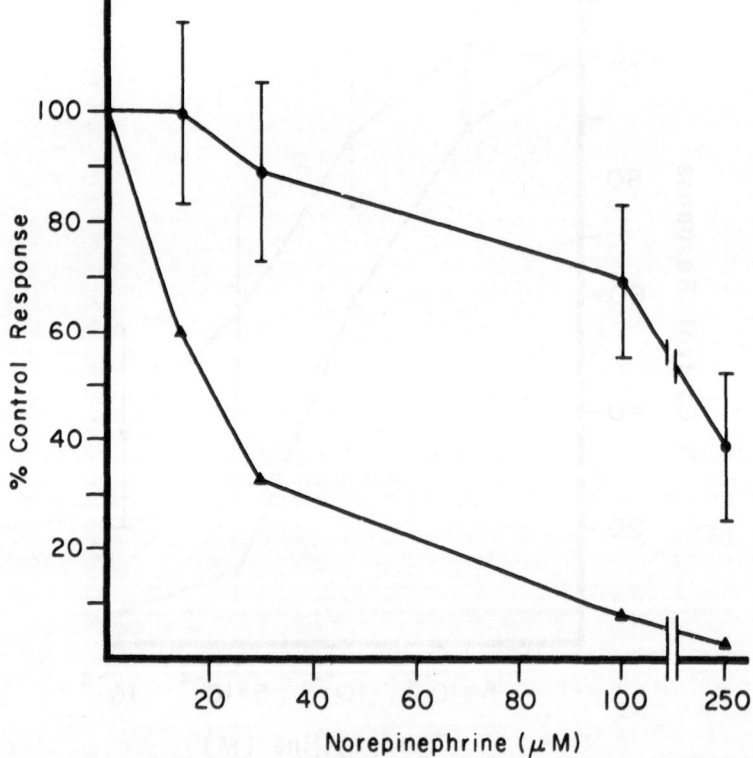

Figure 4.6   Inhibition of *in vitro* lymphocyte responses to phytohaemagglutinin by norepinephrine. Closed circles (●) represent the mean ± one standard deviation of six normal individuals. Closed triangles (▲) represent the mean response of the ADA-deficient lymphocytes

cyte response to PHA was studied by adding the drug to lymphocyte microcultures 5 min prior to the addition of PHA. The lymphocyte proliferative response was measured by [^{3}H]thymidine incorporation after 72 h in culture. The effect of a specific agent was expressed as a percentage of the lymphocyte response in the absence of added pharmacological agents (control response). Percentages less than 100 indicate inhibition while those greater than 100 indicate enhancement of lymphocyte responses.

Theophylline, which elevates cAMP by inhibiting its catabolism by cAMP phosphodiesterase, was found to depress [^{3}H]thymidine incorporation of ADA-deficient lymphocytes to a significantly greater extent than normal lymphocytes at the same theophylline concentration (Figure

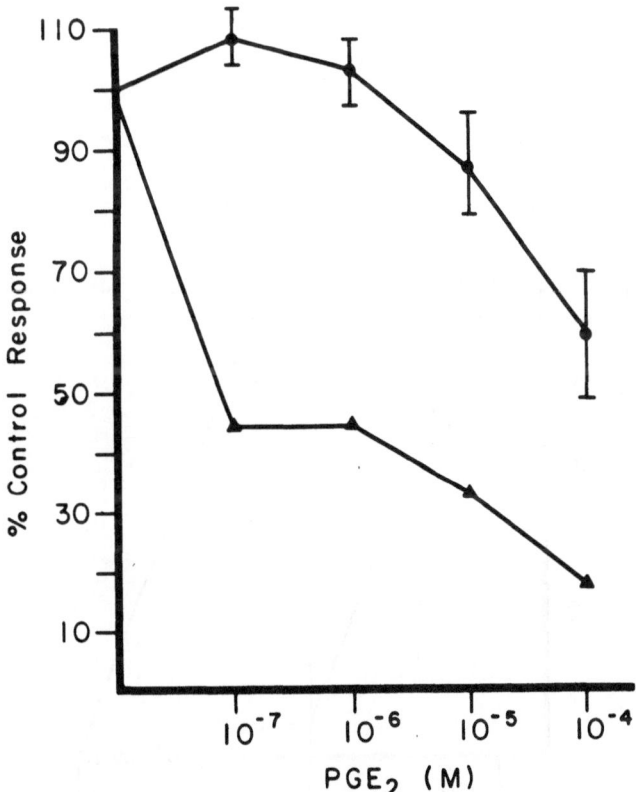

Figure 4.7   Inhibition of *in vitro* lymphocyte responses to phytohaemagglutinin by prostaglandin (PG) E$_2$. Closed circles (●) represent the mean ± one standard deviation of two normal individuals. Closed triangles (▲) represent the mean response of the ADA-deficient lymphocytes

4.5). ADA-deficient lymphocytes were also found to be more sensitive than normal lymphocytes to inhibition by R020-1724, a non-methylxanthine cAMP phosphodiesterase inhibitor.

ADA-deficient lymphocytes were found to be significantly more sensitive than normal lymphocytes to inhibition by norepinephrine, which stimulates adenylate cyclase activity and cAMP synthesis by stimulation of the β-adrenergic receptor (Figure 4.6). However, there was no increased

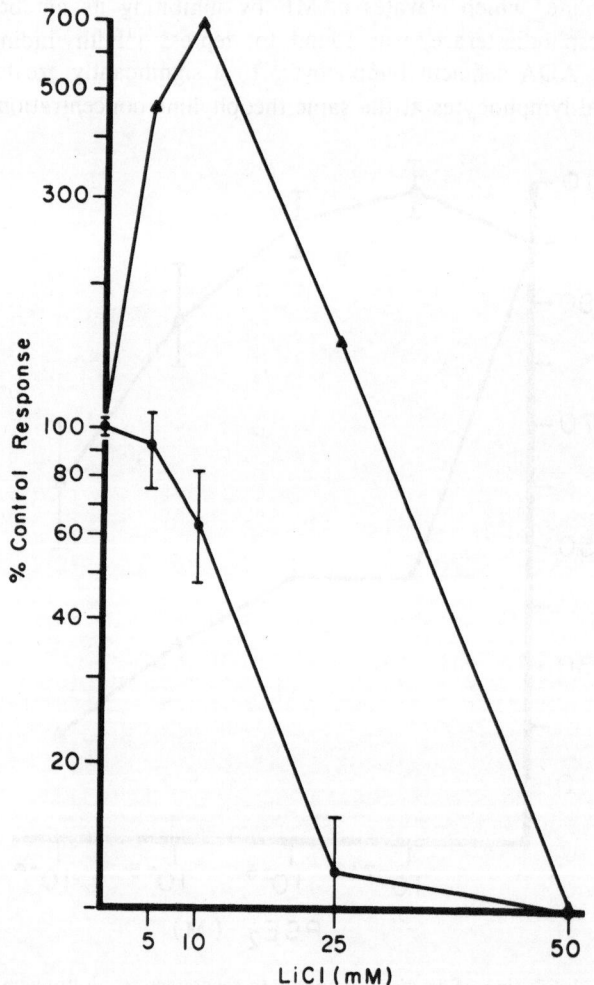

Figure 4.8 Enhancement of *in vitro* lymphocyte response of ADA-deficient lymphocytes (▲) by lithium chloride (LiCl). Responses of normal lymphocytes (●) were either unchanged or inhibited

sensitivity to α-adrenergic or cholinergic drugs, which do not increase cAMP synthesis. Lymphocyte responses of ADA-deficient lymphocytes were exquisitely sensitive to inhibition by prostaglandins (PG) E_1 and E_2 (Figure 4.7), which are potent inducers of cAMP synthesis, but were not unusually sensitive to $PGF_{2\alpha}$, which does not enhance cAMP synthesis. These data indicate that ADA-deficient lymphocytes are uniquely sensitive to inhibition by agents which increase cAMP levels either by increasing its synthesis or inhibiting its catabolism. This sensitivity may result from the increased quantities of ATP available for conversion to cAMP by the action of adenylate cyclase.

One would, therefore, expect that the function of ADA-deficient lymphocytes might be enhanced by agents that inhibited cAMP synthesis. Lithium salts have been shown to inhibit adenylate cyclase in brain[32] and platelets[33]. Lithium chloride was found to markedly enhance the [^{3}H] thymidine incorporation of ADA-deficient lymphocytes at concentrations that either inhibited or had no effect upon normal lymphocytes (Figure 4.8).

The ADA-deficient lymphocyte is not immunologically incompetent merely due to the presence of the enzyme deficiency. Suppression of immunological function may come from extrinsic physiological stimuli' acting upon cellular receptors. The consequences of receptor stimulation may be excessive, namely over production of cAMP. Such stimuli include β-adrenergic catecholamines, prostaglandins of the E type and perhaps adenosine itself, which can also increase adenylate cyclase activity and cAMP synthesis by activation of a lymphocyte adenosine receptor[34]. Restoration or maintenance of immunological competence may, in part, be possible by modulating these physiological stimuli (e.g. decreasing prostaglandin synthesis) or by negating the effects of these stimuli by inhibiting adenylate cyclase.

CONCLUDING REMARKS

Transfusions of frozen, irradiated, normal red blood cells appear to be an efficacious mode of therapy for some patients with the adenosine deaminase deficient form of severe combined immunodeficiency disease. At the present time we do not have sufficient information to predict which patients will respond to replacement therapy and which ones will not respond to this treatment alone. Enzyme replacement therapy using red cell transfusions is a relatively crude and inefficient means to deliver enzyme to the patient and carries with it the potential risks of sensitization to minor blood group antigens, chronic iron overloading and, to a lesser extent, hepatitis. Some of these problems may be overcome by entrapping purified ADA into biodegradable vesicles. However, the major significance of enzyme replacement therapy is that modification of the metabolism of lymphoid cells in certain immunodeficient states can result in the restoration and maintenance of immunological competence. In addition, studies of the effects of pharmacological agents upon mitogen-induced lymphocyte responses indicate that enzyme-deficient lymphocyte function may be enhanced by certain drugs. These observations, although certainly preliminary at this time, suggest that pharmacological approaches to the therapy of immunodeficiency diseases may be possible in the future if enzyme deficiencies can be identified and the biochemical bases of the immunodeficiencies understood.

Acknowledgements

The author wishes to gratefully acknowledge the support of the National Foundation March of Dimes (grant no. 1-424) and the National Institutes of Health (grant nos. HL 06009, HL 13885 and 5 MO 1 RR 000 80).

References

1. Giblett, E. L., Anderson, J. E., Cohen, F., Pollara, B. and Meuwissen, H. J. (1972). Adenosine deaminase deficiency in two patients with severely impaired cellular immunity. *Lancet*, ii, 1067
2. Dissing, J. and Knudsen, B. (1972). Adenosine deaminase deficiency and combined immunodeficiency syndrome. *Lancet*, ii, 1316
3. Polmar, S. H. (1977). Lymphocyte enzyme deficiencies and the metabolic basis of immunodeficiency disease. *Clin. Haematol.*, 6, 423
4. Meuwissen, H. J., Pickering, R. J., Moore, E. C. and Pollara, B. (1975). Impairment of adenosine deaminase activity in combined immunological deficiency disease. In H. J. Meuwissen, R. J. Pickering, B. Pollara and I. H. Porter (eds.). *Combined Immunodeficiency Disease and Adenosine Deaminase Deficiency: A Molecular Defect*, p. 73 (New York: Academic Press)
5. Hirschhorn, R., Beratis, N., Rosen, F. S., Parkman, R., Stern, R. C. and Polmar, S. H. (1975). Adenosine deaminase deficiency in a child diagnosed prenatally. *Lancet*, i, 73
6. Wara, D. W. and Ammann, A. J. (1975). Laboratory data. In H. J. Meuwissen, R. J. Pickering, B. Pollara and I. H. Porter (eds.). *Combined Immunodeficiency Disease and Adenosine Deaminase Deficiency: A Molecular Defect*, p. 247. (New York: Academic Press)
7. Hitzig, W. H., Landolt, R., Muller, G. and Bodmer, P. (1971). Heterogeneity of phenotypic expression in a family with Swiss-type agammaglobulinemia: observations on the acquisition of agammaglobulinemia. *J. Pediatr.*, 78, 968
8. Polmar, S. H., Stern, R. C., Schwartz, A. L., Wetzler, E. M., Chase, P. A. and Hirschhorn, R. (1976). Enzyme replacement therapy for adenosine

deaminase deficiency and severe combined immunodeficiency. *N. Engl. J. Med.*, **295**, 1337

9. Polmar, S. H., Wetzler, E. M., Stern, R. C. and Hirschhorn, R. (1975). Restoration of *in vitro* lymphocyte responses with exogenous adenosine deaminase in a patient with severe combined immunodeficiency. *Lancet*, **ii**, 743

10. Schrader, W. P., Stacy, A. R. and Pollara, B. (1976). Purification of human erythrocyte adenosine deaminase by affinity column chromatograph. *J. Biol. Chem.*, **251**, 4026

11. Daddona, P. E. and Kelley, W. N. (1977). Human adenosine deaminase. Purification and subunit structure. *J. Biol. Chem.*, **252**, 110

12. Brady, R. O., Tallman, J. F., Johnson, W. G., Gal, A. E., Leahy, W. R., Quirk, J. M. and Dekaban, A. S. (1973). Replacement therapy for inherited enzyme deficiency. Use of purified ceramidetrihexosidase in Fabry's disease. *N. Engl. J. Med.*, **289**, 9

13. Thorpe, S. R., Fiddler, M. B. and Desnick, R. J. (1975). Enzyme therapy. V. *In vivo* fate of erythrocyte-entrapped β-glucuronidase in β-glucuronidase-deficient mice. *Ped. Res.*, **9**, 918

14. Lewis, V., Twomey, J., Goldstein, G., O'Reilly, R., Smithwick, E., Pahwa, R., Pahwa, S., Good, R. A., Schulte-Wisserman, H., Horowitz, S., Hong, R., Jones, J., Sieber, O., Kirkpatrick, C., Polmar, S. H. and Bealmear, P. (1977). Circulating thymic hormone activity in congenital immunodeficiency. *Lancet*, **ii**, 471

15. Wolf, J., Reid, R., Anderson, J., Rebuck, J., Lightbody, J., Johnson, R., Uberti, J. and Weiss, L. (1976). Cellular immunodeficiency (Nezelof) associated with ADA deficiency. Treatment with thymosin and ADA enzyme replacement. *J. Reticuloendothelial Soc.*, **20**, 48

16. Lampkin, B. C. and Dauod, A. (1977). Personal communication

17. Rubenstein, A. and Hirschhorn, R. (1977). Personal communication

18. Horowitz, S. and Hong, R. (1977). Personal communication

19. Schmalsteig, F. C., Goldblum, R. M., Mills, G. C., May, L. T. and Goldman, A. S. (1977). The effect of RBC transfusion on adenosine deaminase (ADA) deficient severe-combined immunodeficiency (SCID). *Ped. Res.*, **11**, 493

20. Gelfand, E. W. (1977). Personal communication

21. Ziegler, J. B. (1977). Personal communication

22. Hong, R., Santosham, M., Schulte-Wisserman, H., Horowitz, S., Hsu, S. H. and Winkelstein, J. (1976). Reconstitution of B- and T-lymphocyte function in severe combined immunodeficiency disease after transplantation with thymic epithelium. *Lancet*, **ii**, 1270

23. Agarwal, R. P., Crabtree, G. W., Parks, R. E., Nelson, J. A., Keightley, R., Parkman, R., Rosen, F. S., Stern, R. C. and Polmar, S. H. (1976). Purine metabolism in the erythrocytes of patients with adenosine deaminase deficiency and severe combined immunodeficiency. *J. Clin. Invest.*, **57**, 1025

24. Raivio, K. O., Schwartz, A. L., Stern, R. C. and Polmar, S. H. (1976). Adenine and adenosine metabolism in lymphocytes deficient in adenosine deaminase. In M. M. Müller, E. Kaiser and J. E. Seegmiller (eds.). *Purine Metabolism in Man*, p. 456. (New York: Plenum Press)

25. Schmalsteig, F. C., Nelson, J. A., Mills, G. C., Monahan, T. M., Goldman,

A. S. and Goldblum, R. M. (1977). Increased purine nucleotides in adenosine deaminase deficient lymphocytes. *J. Pediatr.*, 91, 48

26. Green, H. and Chan, T.-S. (1973). Pyrimidine starvation induced by adenosine in fibroblasts and lymphoid cells: role of adenosine deaminase. *Science*, 182, 836

27. Parkman, R., Gelfand, E. W., Rosen, F. S., Sanderson, A. and Hirschhorn, R. (1975). Severe combined immunodeficiency and adenosine deaminase deficiency. *N. Engl. J. Med.*, 292, 714

28. Hirschhorn, R., Grossman, J. and Weismann, G. (1970). Effect of cyclic 3', 5'-adenosine monophosphate and theophylline on lymphocyte transformation. *Proc. Soc. Exp. Biol. Med.*, 133, 1361

29. deRubertis, F. R., Zenser, T. V., Adler, W. H. and Hudson, T. (1974). Role of cyclic adenosine 3', 5'-monophosphate in lymphocyte mitogenesis. *J. Immunol.*, 113, 151

30. Polmar, S. H., Wetzler, E. M. and Stern, R. C. (1977). Immunopharmacologic studies of adenosine deaminase deficient lymphoyctes. *Ped. Res.*, 11, 492

31. Polmar, S. H., Wetzler, E. M. and Stern, R. C. (1977). Studies on adenosine deaminase deficient lymphocytes: I. Differential inhibitory and enhancing effects of various pharmacologic agents upon the *in vitro* lymphocyte responses to phytohemagglutinin. (In preparation)

32. Forn, J. and Valdecasas, F. G. (1971). Effects of lithium on brain adenylate cyclase activity. *Biochem. Pharmacol.*, 20, 2773

33. Wang, Y. C., Pandey, G. N., Mendels, J. and Frazer, A. (1974). Effect of lithium on prostaglandin E_1-stimulated adenylate cyclase activity of human platelets. *Biochem. Pharmacol.*, 23, 845

34. Schwartz, A. L., Stern, R. C. and Polmar, S. H. (1977). Demonstration of an adenosine receptor on human lymphocytes *in vitro* and its possible role in the adenosine deaminase deficient form of severe combined immunodeficiency disease. *Clin. Immunol. Immunopathol.* 99, 499

5

Prenatal diagnosis and heterozygote detection in adenosine deaminase deficiency
Rochelle Hirschhorn

Severe combined immunodeficiency disease (SCID) is a fatal syndrome of infancy characterized by defects of both cellular and humoral immunities[1,2]. Based upon the pattern of inheritance, at least two different forms of the syndrome exist: an X-linked and an autosomal recessive form. In a proportion of families with the autosomal recessive form of SCID, the disorder is due to an inherited deficiency of the purine salvage enzyme, adenosine deaminase (ADA)[3-5].

Once a precise biochemical defect has been defined for a disorder, prenatal diagnosis becomes feasible. We have previously reported successful prenatal diagnosis of a child with ADA deficiency[6]. We would like to report here our cumulative experience to date with seven pregnancies at risk for ADA deficiency in six families.

Our initial prenatal diagnosis was performed in a family which had been ascertained retrospectively because of the earlier death of a child with SCID but with undetermined ADA status. A number of such families exist who are still of childbearing age. We have undertaken to determine the feasibility of retrospective heterozygote detection in such families. We would like to report here some of our experience to date with quantitative and qualitative measures for heterozygote detection.

HETEROZYGOTE DETECTION

We have tested 20 parents and 19 other members of twelve families who have had children with SCID and ADA deficiency. In ten of the families, ADA deficiency was determined by assay of ADA activity in erythrocytes of an affected child. In three families no affected children were alive at the time of testing and the diagnosis of ADA deficiency was based upon the findings of a 'null' gene (see below) segregating in the family. In one of these three families the diagnosis of ADA deficiency was subsequently confirmed by the predicted birth of an affected child[6]. In the analysis of ADA activity of heterozygotes we have included the quantitative RBC–ADA activity of the parents and those relatives who demonstrate inheritance of a 'null' gene for ADA.

Red cell adenosine deaminase activity of 74 normal individuals exhibited a positively skewed distribution, as has been previously reported[7]. The distribution of ADA activity could be partially restored to a normal distribution by a log transformation, but this distribution was still significantly different from a normal distribution (chi-square goodness of fit = 11 429, 4 D.F., 0.02 > p > 0.01). The geometric mean was 83.98 units (nmol uric acid/mg Hb/h at 37 °C)* with 53.8–133.5 representing ± two SD. The red cell ADA activity of 26 heterozygotes showed a similarly positively skewed distribution but a log transformation resulted in a normal distribution of values. The geometric mean of the 26 heterozygotes was 38.26 with 22.2–65.93 representing ± two SD. If a value of two SD below the geometric mean of normals (53.8) is rigidly used as the discriminating value, 11% of heterozygotes will be misclassified as normal. These results

* Normal values for adenosine deaminase activity have been determined in several laboratories by different methods and at different temperatures. I have recalculated these values to a common unit of nmol/mg Hb/h (1 i.u. = 1/60 of this unit). The values obtained are tabulated for the actual temperature of reaction used and after conversion to values for a constant temperature of reaction of 30 °C calculated according to E. Beutler[10]. Values for two SD from the geometric mean are given where available. Values for two SD from the arithmetic mean are not given since these do not take into account the skewed distribution of adenosine deaminase values found in the normal population.

	30 °C
25 °C = 36.1 (± two SD = 22.5–58.1)[7]	55.4
30 °C = 60.0[8]	60.0
37 °C = 62.9[9]	47.2
37 °C = 66.6[10]	50.0
37 °C = 83.8 (± two SD = 58.1–133.5)	62.8

confirm the earlier observations of Scott *et al.*[7] In practice, only one obligate heterozygote of 26 had ADA values well within the normal range and two individuals (both parents of known ADA-deficient SCIDs) had values of 54.9 and 55.3, just slightly above the value of 53.8. Alternatively, if one wanted to ascertain 97.5% of heterozygotes (i.e., + two SD above the mean of heterozygotes) a value of 65.9 could be used. This value would however, misclassify approximately 12% of the normal population as ADA heterozygotes. This is displayed graphically in the probit plot (Figure 5.1) of normals and heterozygotes, from which one can estimate the error involved in classification at any given ADA value. There is therefore no foolproof quantitative value which will discriminate without error between heterozygotes for ADA deficiency and normals. The value one uses will depend upon the purpose for which the study is performed.

Fortunately, there are other methods available for heterozygote detection in this disorder. These methods are based upon demonstration of abnormal transmission of the genetically polymorphic marker of ADA. When applicable (and assuming illegitimacy has been ruled out), this provides definitive evidence for heterozygosity.

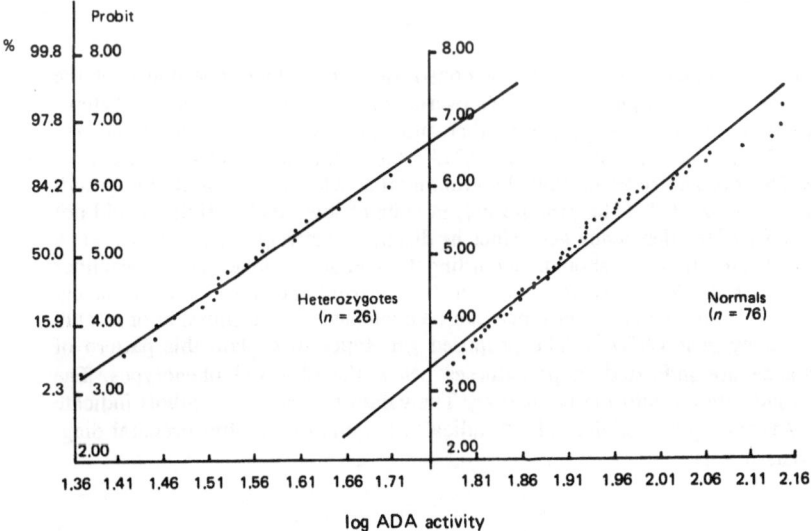

Figure 5.1 Probit plot of ADA activity of normals and individuals heterozygous for ADA deficiency. ADA activity has been transformed to log values to fit more closely a normal distribution. The regression lines have been fitted by least mean squares. The approximate percentage of the population included at each probit point is indicated to allow for easy comparison. To convert to SD, a probit of 5.0 = mean, 6.0 = +one SD, etc. (for additional details see text)

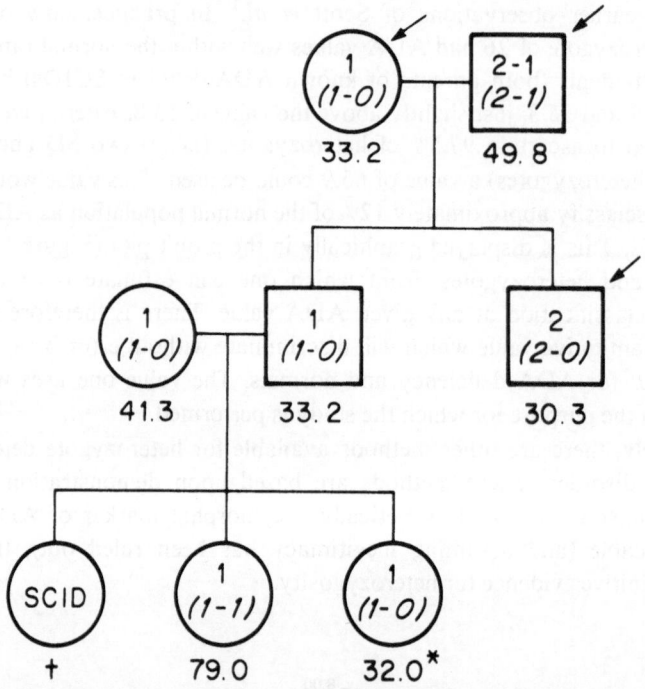

Figure 5.2   Pedigree of a family demonstrating anomalous inheritance of the ADA genetic polymorphism as well as overlap of quantitative normal and heterozygous RBC–ADA activity. The mother and father of the index case (who had died of SCID and was of unknown ADA status) had heterozygous values for ADA. Phenotyping revealed that the grandmother was ADA 1 while the grandfather was ADA 2–1. (The grandfather, in spite of low ADA activity, could not be a carrier of the deficiency gene since he displayed active products of two ADA alleles.) Their offspring should, according to mendelian inheritance, be either ADA 1 or ADA 2–1. Instead, their son (the paternal uncle) was phenotypically ADA 2. This anomalous inheritance can be explained by transmission of a 'null' or deficiency gene (ADA⁰). The proposed genotypes to explain this pattern of inheritance are indicated in parentheses below the observed phenotypes. The arrows indicate the informative mating. The values beneath the symbols indicate RBC–ADA enzyme activity. The * indicates the child born after prenatal diagnosis (case no. 2)

NULL GENE

The red cell enzyme ADA demonstrates a genetic polymorphism in that different individuals in the population inherit different allelic forms of the enzyme[8]. Thus, the three phenotypes, ADA 1, ADA 2 and ADA 2–1, represent the homozygous or heterozygous expression of two allelic genes at the ADA autosomal locus. Anomalous inheritance of the ADA gene has previously been reported fully in four families[6,12-14], including two of the families reported here[6,14]. The inheritance of the null gene in the additional family (family C) is seen in Figure 5.2. In this family, the ADA phenotypes of the mother and father were not informative. The paternal grandparents were respectively phenotypically ADA 2–1 and ADA 1. For normal inheritance, their offspring should be phenotypically ADA 1 or ADA 2–1. However, one of their offspring, the paternal uncle, was ADA 2. The appearance of the ADA 2 phenotype can be explained if his ADA 1 parent is genotypically ADA 1–0. It can be calculated that if two sets of grandparents, the parents and a sib are available for phenotyping as to the genetic polymorphism, approximately one-third of families will have a mating demonstrating a null gene. This percentage increases as additional matings of aunts and uncles and their offspring are considered.

PRENATAL DETECTION

Three of six families studied were known to be at risk for ADA deficiency because of the prior birth of a child with SCID and proven ADA deficiency (cases no. 3, 4, 5 and 6). Three of the families were referred because of an offspring who had died with SCID but prior to the availability of testing for ADA deficiency[1,2,7]. In all three families the parents had values for ADA more than two SD below the normal mean. In one family (case no. 1), other family members were not available for testing and the presence of a null gene could not be tested for. (These parents were not included in the values for heterozygotes.) In the two other families (cases no. 2 and 7), the diagnosis of ADA deficiency was confirmed by the finding of a null gene segregating in the family and in one of these an affected child was subsequently born.

In three pregnancies (Table 5.1) the amniotic fluid fibroblasts exhibited easily detectable enzyme activity which was, however, below the range of simultaneously assayed normal amniotic fluid fibroblasts. A prediction of a normal child who would most probably be heterozygous was made in each of these cases. Two of these children have been born and have indeed had heterozygous levels of ADA activity. In the fourth pregnancy (case no. 3), the ADA activity was in the normal range but was lower than fibroblasts assayed simultaneously. A prediction of a normal child was made as well as a prediction for heterozygosity. This cannot be rigorously supported by the data and, although the child did indeed have heterozygous erythrocyte ADA activity at birth, it must be remembered that the odds are two to three for any normal child to be heterozygous. In the fifth pregnancy,

TABLE 5.1   Prenatal diagnosis for ADA deficiency

	Cases	ADA activity*	Diagnosis‡
(1)	V†	5.56	heterozygote
(2)	C†	5.35	heterozygote
(3)	S	10.7	heterozygote
(4)	S	3.74	[heterozygote]
(5)	R	14.67	[normal]
(6)	D	0.62	affected
(7)	W†	0.2	affected
Normals		13.16 ± 4.82	
		($n = 9$, range 8.8–20.2)§	
		17.2 ± 7.79	
		($n = 17$, range 7.2–31.0)‖	

* nmol/mg prot/min at 37 °C of cultured amniotic fluid fibroblasts
† Family ascertained retrospectively. Family C and W showed a 'null' gene for ADA, as well as heterozygous values for ADA
‡ Diagnosis based upon assay of ADA activity of RBCs, in cases where a child has been born
[ ] Pending outcome of pregnancy
§ Normals assayed simultaneously with diagnoses of cases nos. 1–6
‖ Normals assayed at time of diagnosis of case no. 7

the outcome is still pending but ADA activity well within the normal range was observed. In the last two pregnancies, there was less than 5% of normal ADA activity, and a diagnosis of an affected child was easily made and confirmed at birth. Both mothers elected to bear the child.

In theory, one should have characterized the enzyme deficit in an affected child prior to attempting prenatal diagnosis in any given family. Unfortunately, this is often not feasible. We have, however, begun determining ADA activity both at high and low substrate concentrations so as to at least not misdiagnose a case with a K_m mutation.

In summary, the distinction between affected and non-affected pregnancies has to date been uncomplicated. We feel that heterozygosity cannot be predicted in amniotic fluid fibroblasts with any degree of confidence, even though we have to date been correct in this diagnosis. This inability to reliably discriminate between heterozygotes and normals most probably reflects the great variation in ADA activity of fibroblasts under different growth conditions as well as the overlap between heterozygotes and normals seen in ADA activity of erythrocytes.

Heterozygote detection for adenosine deaminase deficiency is possible by quantitative assay of RBC–ADA activity but with a 10% error. This error can be reduced by study of the genetically polymorphic markers as well as of quantitative RBC–ADA activity in as many relatives as possible.

Acknowledgement

I would like to thank Dr W. Hitzig, Dr M. Ballow, Dr P. Durand, Dr J. L. Simpson, Dr F. Rosen and Dr A. Rubenstein for referral of the patients for prenatal diagnosis and heterozygote detection.

I would like to thank Dr E. Smithwick for allowing me to test parents of one of her patients.

I would like to thank Ms V. Roegner and Mr F. Martiniuk for their technical assistance and Ms J. Handsman for the preparation of this manuscript.

This work was supported by grants (A1 10343) from the National Institutes of Health and (6–4) from the National Foundation March of Dimes.

References

1. Rosen, F. S. (1975). Immunodeficiency. In B. Benacerraf (ed.). *Immunogenetics and Immunodeficiency*, p. 230 (Baltimore University Park Press)
2. Gelfand, E. W., Biggar, W. D. and Orange, R. P. (1974). Immune deficiency: Evaluation, diagnosis, and therapy. *Pediatr. Clin. N. Am.*, 21, 745
3. Giblett, E. R., Anderson, J. E., Cohen, F., Pollara, B. and Meuwissen, H. J. (1972). Adenosine-deaminase deficiency in two patients with severely impaired cellular immunity. *Lancet*, ii, 1067
4. Meuwissen, H. J., Pickering, R. J., Pollara, B. and Porter, I. H., (1975). *Combined Immunodeficiency Disease and Adenosine Deaminase Deficiency: A Molecular Defect.* (New York: Academic Press)
5. Hirschhorn, Rochelle (1977). Defects of purine metabolism in immunodeficiency diseases. In R. S. Schwartz (ed.). *Progress in Clinical Immunology*, Vol. III, p. 67. (New York: Grune and Stratton)
6. Hirschhorn, R., Beratis, N., Rosen, F. S., Parkman, R., Stern, R. and Polmar, S. (1975). Adenosine-deaminase deficiency in a child diagnosed prenatally. *Lancet*, i, 73
7. Scott, C. R., Chen, S.-H. and Giblett, E. R. (1974). Detection of the carrier state in combined immunodeficiency disease associated with adenosine deaminase deficiency. *J. Clin. Invest.*, 53, 1194
8. Agarwal, R. P., Crabtree, G. W., Parks, R. E. Jr., Nelson, J. A., Keightley, R., Parkman, R., Rosen, F. S., Stern, R. C. and Polmar, S. H. (1976). Purine nucleoside metabolism in the erythrocytes of patients with adenosine deaminase deficiency and severe combined immunodeficiency. *J. Clin. Invest.*, 57, 1025

9.   Ackeret, C., Plüss, H. J. and Hitzig, W. H. (1976). Hereditary severe combined immunodeficiency and adenosine deaminase deficiency.*Pediatr. Res.*, **10**, 67

10. Beutler, E. (1975). *Red Cell Metabolism: A Manual of Biochemical Methods*, p. 147. 2nd Ed. (New York: Grune and Stratton)

11. Spencer, N., Hopkinson, D. A. and Harris, H. (1968). Adenosine deaminase polymorphism in man. *Ann. Hum. Genet.*, **32**, 9

12. Chen, S.-H., Scott, C. R. and Giblett, E. R. (1974). Adenosine deaminase: Demonstration of a 'silent' gene associated with combined immunodeficiency disease. *Am. J. Hum. Genet.*, **26**, 103

13. Chen, S.-H., Scott, C. R., Giblett, E. R. and Levin, A. (1977). Adenosine deaminase deficiency: Another family with a 'silent' ADA allele and normal ADA activity in two heterozygotes. *Am. J. Hum. Genet.*, **29**, 642

14. Hirschhorn, R., Vawter, G. F. and Rosch, F. S. (1978). Adenosine deaminase deficiency: Frequency and comparative pathology in autosomally recessive severe combined immunodeficiency. *Pediatr. Res.* (submitted for publication)

6

Pathogenic mechanisms in deficiencies of adenosine deaminase and purine nucleoside phosphorylase

D. A. Carson, J. Kaye and
J. E. Seegmiller

Inherited deficiencies of the enzymes adenosine deaminase (ADA) (E.C.3.5.4.4) and purine nucleoside phosphorylase (PNP) (E.C.2.4.2.1) recently have been associated with human immunodeficiency disease[1,2]. There are two puzzling dilemmas to explain in these conditions. First, why are both enzyme deficiencies associated with similar clinical syndromes? Second, why do *both* diseases preferentially affect lymphoid development while sparing most other organ systems? None of the biochemical mechanisms proposed to explain ADA and PNP deficiency successfully answers both questions posed above[3-5]. Recently we have collected evidence which suggests that lymphospecific toxicity in ADA and PNP deficiency might result from the selective accumulation in lymphoid tissues, particularly the thymus, of toxic deoxyribonucleotides, mediated by deoxyribonucleoside kinase(s).

TABLE 6.1 Enzyme activities in human tissues

	Adenosine kinase		Deoxyadenosine kinase		Deoxyguanosine kinase		Deoxyinosine kinase		Adenosine deaminase	Purine nucleoside phosphorylase
	I	II	I	II	I	II	I	II	II	II
Thymus	0.79	0.86	1.35	0.78	1.92	1.39	0.34	0.31	282.8	23.3
Spleen	Na	0.53	Na	0.20	Na	0.33	Na	0.07	12.4	54.0
Brain	Na	1.01	Na	0.14	Na	0.16	Na	0.05	5.0	10.3
Kidney	Na	1.15	Na	0.07	Na	0.08	Na	0.10	1.8	100.0
Liver	0.81	2.26	0.12	0.07	0.04	0.07	0.05	0.04	1.1	36.2
Lung	1.32	0.81	0.11	0.06	0.03	0.08	0.03	0.02	0.8	38.0
Small intestine	0.41	0.52	0.13	0.08	0.03	0.11	0.09	0.07	14.2	63.9
Heart	0.48	0.51	0.13	0.08	0.03	0.11	0.07	0.06	2.1	32.2
Peripheral lymphocytes	1.00		0.32		0.21		0.09		20.7	114.7
Peripheral granulocytes	0.83		0.05		<0.02		0.03		11.9	121.4

Human tissues were obtained from two babies who died during, or immediately after, parturition. Extracts were prepared by mincing the tissue, freeze thawing five times, and ultracentrifuging the particulate material. Protein concentration in the supernatant was determined by Lowry's method. Kinase activities were determined under the following conditions:

Buffer:	50 mM Tris, pH 8.0
Protein	1 mg/ml
ATP	10 mM
$MgCl_2$	10 mM
NaF	15 mM
Substrate	0.3 mM

Final pH = 7.4

The reaction was initiated by the addition of labelled substrate. After 30 min at 37°C, tubes were boiled for 2 min. insoluble material was sedimented a 4°C, and an aliquot of the reaction mixture was spotted on a PEI cellulose thin-layer chromatography plate to which a paper wick was attached. After overnight chromatography in methanol: water (1 : 1) the nucleotides which remained at the origin were cut out and counted in a liquid scintillation counter. Activities are expressed as nmol/min per mg. protein. No inosine kinase or guanosine kinase activity was detectable in any preparation; Na = not available.

Previous experiments have suggested that in certain instances purines and deoxypurines can be exchanged between tissues at the nucleoside level, and subsequently trapped intracellularly in the form of nucleoside monophosphates, which do not readily traverse cell membranes[6]. Consequently, the rate of phosphorylation of many nucleosides may limit their uptake by cells[7].

With this hypothesis in mind, we measured the ability of human tissues to phosphorylate adenosine and deoxyadenosine, the substrates of ADA, and also inosine, deoxyinosine, guanosine and deoxyguanosine, the substrates of PNP. As shown in Table 6.1, adenosine kinase activity was widespread among the organs examined. Guanosine and inosine kinases were undetectable in any tissue. However, the ability to phosphorylate deoxyadenosine, deoxyinosine and deoxyguanosine was largely confined to lymphoid cells, including both actively dividing thymocytes and resting peripheral blood lymphocytes. A similar tissue distribution has been reported for deoxycytidine kinase[8, 9]. Confirming previous reports, ADA but not PNP also showed a predilection for lymphoid tissues[10].

The approximate Michaelis constant for the phosphorylation of purine deoxyribonucleosides by human thymic extracts was 400 μM, as opposed to a K_m of 7 μM and 50 μM for the alternative metabolic enzymes ADA and PNP[11, 12]. Thus in normal cells purine deoxyribonucleosides at physiological concentrations may not be phosphorylated to a significant degree. In ADA and PNP deficiency, however, either deoxyadenosine, or deoxyinosine and deoxyguanosine, produced by many tissues might be selectively trapped in the thymus by deoxyribonucleoside kinase. Although in

TABLE 6.2 Potentiation of deoxyadenosine toxicity by the ADA inhibitor EHNA

	Per cent control leucine uptake	
Inhibitor	*Without EHNA*	*With EHNA, 5 μM*
EHNA alone	–	82 ± 3
Deoxyadenosine 1 mM	49 ± 10	1 ± 0
Deoxyadenosine 100 μM	97 ± 3	5 ± 1
Deoxyadenosine 10 μM	92 ± 3	25 ± 4
Deoxyadenosine 1 μM	nd	56 ± 3
Deoxyadenosine 0.1 μM	nd	67 ± 4
No phytohaemagglutinin	6 ± 1	

Phytohaemagglutinin-stimulated human peripheral blood lymphocytes were cultured as previously described[13]. After 3 days, they were pulsed with tritiated leucine and the per cent control leucine uptake into protein determined. Each point is the mean $\pm$ SEM of six cultures; nd = not done.

TABLE 6.3 Deoxycytidine reversal of deoxyribonucleoside toxicity during phytohaemagglutinin induced human lymphocyte transformation

Inhibitor	Reversor		Per cent control leucine uptake $\pm$ SEM*	p value†
Deoxyadenosine 1 mM	0		35 ± 1 ($n=6$)‡	
Deoxyadenosine 1 mM	uridine	100 μM	36 ± 2 ($n=6$)	ns
Deoxyadenosine 1 mM	deoxycytidine	100 μM	59 ± 3 ($n=6$)	< 0.05
Deoxyadenosine 10 μM + EHNA 5 μM	0		19 ± 3 ($n=6$)	
Deoxyadenosine 10 μM + EHNA 5 μM	uridine	100 μM	26 ± 2 ($n=6$)	ns
Deoxyadenosine 10 μM + EHNA 5 μM	deoxycytidine	100 μM	70 ± 5 ($n=6$)	< 0.05
Deoxyinosine 2 mM	0		33 ± 6 ($n=6$)	
Deoxyinosine 2 mM	uridine	100 μM	41 ± 5 ($n=6$)	ns
Deoxyinosine 2 mM	deoxycytidine	100 μM	67 ± 7 ($n=6$)	< 0.05
0	uridine	100 μM	96 ± 6 ($n=6$)	
0	deoxycytidine	100 μM	82 ± 4 ($n=6$)	

* human peripheral blood lymphocytes were stimulated with phytohaemagglutinin in the presence or absence of the indicated nucleosides. After three days the per cent control leucine uptake into acid precipitable material $\pm$ SEM was determined

† values compare the means of the cultures with uridine or deoxycytidine with those containing deoxyadenosine alone by Student's t test; ns = not significant

‡ n = number of cultures

theory such a 'phosphate trap' could proceed even at low concentrations, this remains to be confirmed *in vivo*.

If purine deoxyribonucleosides in ADA and PNP deficiency are indeed trapped by lymphocytes, what might be their effects on growth? As shown in Table 6.2, in the presence of the ADA inhibitor EHNA, as little as 0.1 μM deoxyadenosine inhibited the response of normal human peripheral blood lymphocytes to the mitogen phytohaemagglutinin (PHA). Although adenosine toxicity was similarly potentiated by EHNA, the inhibitory effects of deoxyadenosine and adenosine differed. While adenosine toxicity was reversed by adding uridine to the culture medium, the inhibitory effects of deoxyadenosine alone or in combination with EHNA were partially reversed by deoxycytidine but not uridine (Table 6.3). These results are consistent with earlier reports in other systems which suggested that deoxyribonucleotide triphosphates can be inhibitors of ribonucleotide reductase[14, 15].

Since we did not have a PNP inhibitor comparable to the potent ADA inhibitor EHNA, we could not study in isolation the effects of deoxyinosine and deoxyguanosine on human lymphocyte transformation. However deoxyinosine did inhibit the response of lymphocytes to phytohaemagglutinin at concentrations comparable to those of adenosine in the absence of ADA inhibition, while inosine at the same concentration had no effect (results not shown). Deoxyinosine toxicity was reversed by the addition of deoxycytidine but not uridine to the culture medium (Table 6.3).

Not only deoxyguanosine, but also guanosine and guanine at concentrations of 100 μM or greater inhibited human lymphocyte transformation (results not shown). On the other hand, both deoxyinosine and deoxyguanosine, but not their ribonucleoside analogues, inhibited the growth of a human lymphoblastoid cell line deficient in hypoxanthine-guanine phosphoribosyltransferase (HGPRT). This cell line had levels of deoxyinosine kinase and deoxyguanosine kinase equivalent to the wild type, but lacked the ability to phosphorylate inosine and guanosine. However, in this case deoxyinosine and deoxyguanosine toxicity was not circumvented by the addition of deoxycytidine to the culture medium.

SUMMARY

1. Deoxypurine nucleosides and/or their nucleotides are toxic to cells.

2. Under normal conditions, purine deoxyribonucleosides are present in low concentrations, and are rapidly converted to the non-toxic bases via ADA and PNP.

3. In ADA and PNP deficiency, deoxypurines may be selectively trapped in the thymus and other lymphoid cells because of the presence of deoxyribonucleoside kinase(s).

4. The mechanism of deoxypurine toxicity is not fully known, but may involve inhibition of ribonucleotide reductase.

5. Deoxycytidine may partially reverse deoxypurine toxicity by preventing the transport and/or phosphorylation of deoxypurines, as well as providing a source of pyrimidine deoxyribonucleotides. Whether or not deoxycytidine might be of clinical benefit to ADA and PNP-deficient patients remains to be established.

Acknowledgements

This study was supported by NIH grants numbers GM 23200, GM 17702, AM 13622, grants from the Kroc Foundation, National Foundation, and by Special Grant no. 797 from the Californian Division of the American Cancer Society. Dennis Carson is a Special Fellow of the Leukaemia Society of America.

References

1. Giblett, E. R., Anderson, J. E., Cohen, F., Pollara, B. and Meuwissen, H. J. (1972). Adenosine deaminase deficiency in two children with impaired cellular immunity. *Lancet*, ii, 1067

2. Giblett, E. R., Amman, A. J., Sandman, R., Wana, D. W. and Diamond, L. K. (1975). Nucleoside phosphorylase deficiency in a child with severely defective T-cell immunity and normal B-cell immunity. *Lancet*, ii, 1010

3. Green, H. and Chan, T.-S. (1973). Pyrimidine starvation induced by adenosine in fibroblasts and lymphoid cells. Role of adenosine deaminase. *Science*, 182, 367

4. Benke, P. J. and Dittman, D. (1976). Purine dysfunction in cells from patients with adenosine deaminase deficiency. *Pediatr. Res.*, 10, 642

5. Wolberg, G., Zimmerman, T. P., Hiemstra, K., Winston, M. and Chu, L.-C. (1975). Adenosine inhibition of lymphocyte-mediated cytolysis: possible role of cyclic adenosine monophosphate. *Science*, 187, 957

6. Paterson, A. R. P., Kim, S. C., Ora, B. and Cass, C. E. (1975). Transport of nucleosides. *Ann. N.Y. Acad. Sci.*, 255, 402

7. Barlow, S. D. (1976). Deoxycytidine transport and pyrimidine deoxynucleotide metabolism in phytohemagglutinin stimulated pig lymphocytes. *Biochem. J.*, 154, 395

8. Durham, J. P. and Ives, D. H. (1969). Deoxycytidine kinase. 1. Distribution in normal and neoplastic tissues and interrelationships of deoxycytidine and 9-β-D-arabinofuranosylcytosine phosphorylation. *Mol. Pharmacol.*, 5, 358

9. Gray, G. D., Mickelson, M. M., Hall, T. M. and Kessel, D. (1072). Small

lymphocyte phosphorylation of cytarabine – an organ and species survey. *Biochem. Pharmacol.*, **21**, 2227

10. Adams, A. and Harkness, R. A. (1976). Adenosine deaminase activity in thymus and other human tissues. *Clin. Exp. Immunol.*, **26**, 647

11. Agrawal, R. F., Sagar, S. M. and Parks, R. E. Jr. (1975). Adenosine deaminase from human erythrocytes. Purification and effects of adenosine analogs. *Biochem. Pharmacol.*, **24**, 693

12. Kim, B., Cha, S. and Parks, R. E. Jr. (1968). Purine nucleoside phosphorylase from human erythrocytes. Purification and properties. *J. Biol. Chem.*, **243**, 1763

13. Carson, D. A. and Seegmiller, J. E. (1976). Effects of adenosine deaminase inhibition upon human lymphocyte blastogenesis. *J. Clin. Invest.*, **57**, 274

14. Xeros, N. (1962). Deoxyriboside control and synchronization of mitosis. *Nature (London)*, **194**, 682

15. Reichard, P. (1968). The biosynthesis of deoxyribonucleotides. *Eur. J. Biochem.*, **3**, 259

7

Purine nucleoside phosphorylase deficiency associated with cellular immunodeficiency: immunological studies during treatment

B. J. M. Zegers, J. W. Stoop,
G. F. M. Hendrickx, S. K. Wadman
and G. E. J. Staal

INTRODUCTION

The finding of adenosine deaminase (ADA) or purine nucleoside phosphorylase deficiency (PNP) in some immunodeficient patients has opened new perspectives for treatment. The causal relationship between ADA or PNP deficiency and severe combined immunodeficiency (SCID) and selective cellular immunodeficiency respectively is generally accepted. Possible mechanisms leading to the lymphocyte dysfunctions were recently reviewed by Polmar[1].

We were able to study a patient, now $2\frac{1}{2}$ years old, with a PNP deficiency in association with a selective cellular immunodeficiency. The patient was treated by oral substitution with uridine and purines and subsequently with several transfusions of irradiated red cells and plasma. The present study will present part of the immunological follow-up during treatment.

CASE REPORT

The female child was born in January 1975 as the fourth child of healthy unrelated parents. The first child of this family was admitted to our hospital with generalized vaccinia infection as a result of smallpox vaccination. T cell immunodeficiency was documented in the child; she was treated with several fetal thymus transplants resulting in healing of the vaccinia lesions and partial but transient restoration of thymus-dependent immunity. Finally she developed a lymphosarcoma and died. The second child died from a graft-versus-host (GVH) reaction after a blood transfusion. Extensive immunological investigations were not possible; however, the few results obtained as well as the post-mortem findings suggest that this girl also suffered from a T cell immunodeficiency. The third child, a boy, is healthy and is now four years old. Extensive clinical and immunological findings of the first two children of the family have been published[2]. The fourth child was carefully followed after birth. She developed a T cell immunodeficiency in the first months of life, whereas B cell immunity developed normally during the first 15 months of life. She also developed a leukopenia and a granulocytopenia. The blood picture was microcytic with a bone marrow which showed megaloblastosis of erythroid and myeloid cells. A neurological disturbance, spastic tetraparesis, was present. From the first year of life the child occasionally suffered upper respiratory tract infections. A PNP deficiency was found in the child from enzymatic studies on erythrocytes and lymphocytes as well as from the analysis of purines in serum and urine of the patient.

The purine analyses of stored frozen samples of serum and urine of the first two children of the family led to the discovery that these children also had a PNP deficiency. To summarize: we are dealing with a family with PNP deficiency in three members, all of whom had a T cell immunodeficiency. The inheritance pattern is autosomal recessive. Extensive clinical, immunological and metabolic studies have been published[3-5].

METHODS

The immunological studies of the patient were as described earlier[2,3]. The effect of treatment was studied by weekly determinations of the number of leukocytes, granulocytes and lymphocytes; the percentages of sheep red blood rosetting T cells (E_S), immunoglobulin (Ig)-bearing B cells; phytohaemagglutinin (PHA) and one-way allogeneic responsiveness of the lymphocytes and determinations of the Ig levels of the serum. On a few occasions the T lymphocytes were also determined in a direct immunofluorescence test using a well-defined anti-T-cell antiserum[6]. Cyclic AMP levels of the lymphocytes were regularly determined[7]. Bone marrow was examined half yearly.

The metabolic studies during treatment consisted of weekly determinations of serum and urinary purines (Wadman *et al.*, Chapter 8 of this book) and ADA and PNP activity of the erythrocytes. The PNP activity of the lymphocytes was checked regularly.

TREATMENT

Adenine (15 mg/kg bw/d) was given orally for 2 weeks. Subsequently uridine was given (initially 50 mg/kg/d increasing to 150 mg/kg/d) for a period of 4 months. During the last 6 weeks of uridine treatment hypoxanthine 50–100 mg/kg bw/d) was added and then allopurinol for a short period of time. Enzyme replacement therapy by infusion of irradiated erythrocytes and plasma at regular intervals of 4–6 weeks was as described by Polmar *et al.*[8] Initially irradiated erythrocytes and plasma were given on the same day; later erythrocytes and plasma were given separately at intervals of 14 days.

RESULTS OF TREATMENT

Treatment was started at the age of 15 months, when T cell dependent immunity was severely affected and B cell immunity showed deterioration[3]. At that time the granulocyte numbers had decreased to 1600/mm[3].

The rationale for adding purines to the treatment at that time was that there may have existed an intracellular lack of guanine and hypoxanthine. In addition it was found that incubation of PNP-deficient red cells with labelled adenosine resulted in a rapid uptake and conversion to inosine whereas almost no adenosine was incorporated in the adenosine nucleotides[9]. This finding suggested inhibition of adenosine kinase in PNP-deficient red cells, leading to decreased levels of adenosine nucleotides.

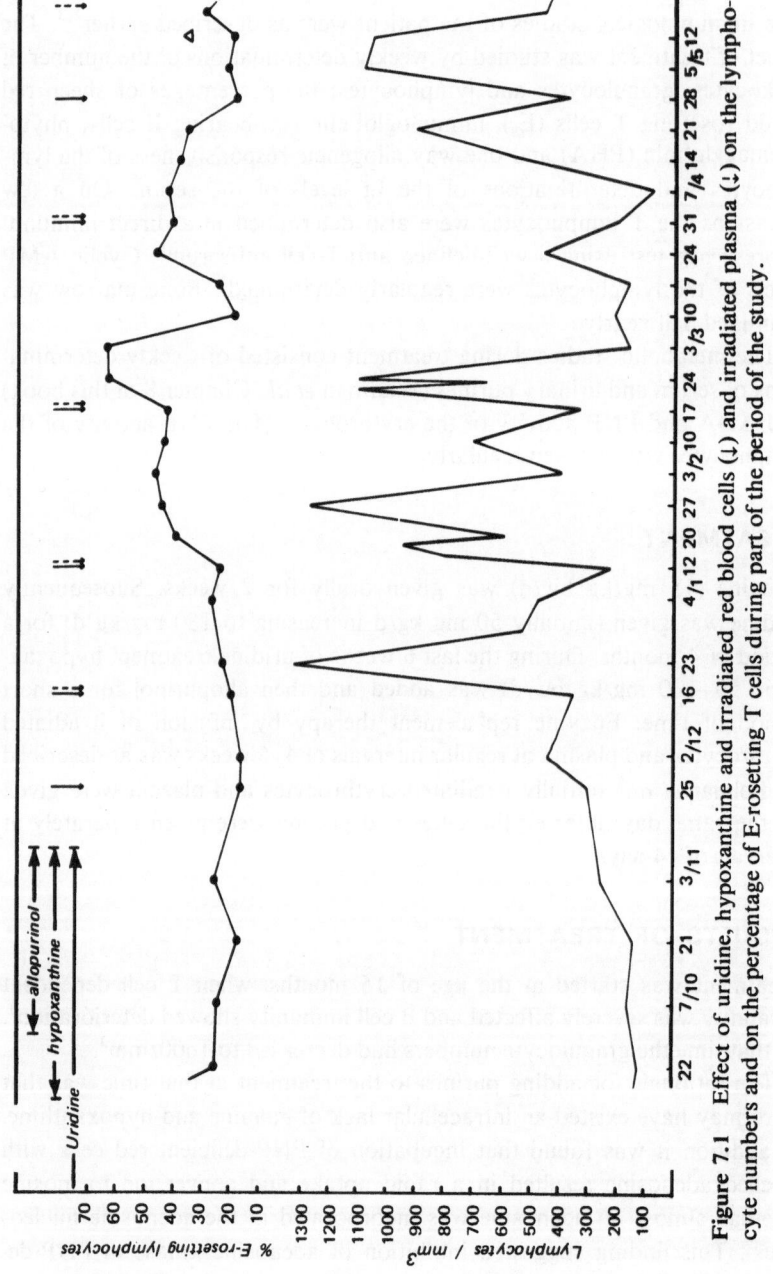

Figure 7.1 Effect of uridine, hypoxanthine and irradiated red blood cells (↓) and irradiated plasma (↓) on the lymphocyte numbers and on the percentage of E-rosetting T cells during part of the period of the study.

Later it was found that the cyclic AMP concentration in the lymphocytes was in the lower part of the range, which agrees with the conclusions from incubation experiments with red cells. For the above reasons adenine was also considered to be a good supplement for the patient.

The rationale for the addition of pyrimidines to the treatment was the presence of megaloblastic changes in the bone marrow suggesting a pyrimidine starvation as seen in orotic aciduria[10]. Moreover, it has been suggested that inosine, being produced in high levels, induces a secondary ADA deficiency[11] from which pyrimidine starvation may result[12]. Before starting the oral supplements, adenine, hypoxanthine and uridine were added to PHA-stimulated lymphocyte cultures of the patient. Adenine and uridine had no effect, whereas hypoxanthine addition resulted in a slight increase of [^{14}C]thymidine uptake of the PHA-stimulated lymphocytes. Uridine addition to ADA-deficient lymphocytes cultured with PHA did not restore proliferative responses[1]. The effects of the oral supplementation with uridine and hypoxanthine on the various parameters are partly shown in Fugure 7.1. During the period of supplementation with either purines or uridine the absolute lymphocyte and granulocyte numbers remained consistently low. Uridine and adenine treatment resulted in some increase in the percentage of E-rosetting T cells but no definite conclusion was possible on the effect of adenine and uridine supplementation on lymphocyte function.

In view of the diminished lymphocyte functions it was decided to try enzyme replacement by infusion of irradiated erythrocytes and plasma. Addition of PNP containing erythrocytes or purified enzyme preparations to in vitro lymphocyte cultures of the patient stimulated with PHA did not lead to an increase in the proliferative response of the lymphocytes. This was interpreted as being the result of either a toxic effect on lymphocytes of some of the enzyme preparations used or reflecting a severe intracellular metabolic disturbance of the lymphocytes. This observation was in contrast with the finding in an ADA-deficient patient in whom restoration of in vitro proliferative mitogenic responses was achieved by addition of ADA to the cultures[1].

Part of the effects of the enzyme replacement during the first months of treatment are given in Figure 7.1. After the second transfusion there was, following each treatment, an increase in the lymphocytes up to about 1000 per mm^3. However, this was transient. Also, the number of granulocytes, initially below 1600 per mm^3, increased after the third transfusion and remained normal thereafter. The percentage of E-rosetting T cells gradually increased from a low value of 20% to 60% and then fell (Figure 7.1). PHA-responsiveness of the lymphocytes increases after the later transfusions showed levels up to 50% of the responsiveness of age-matched controls were attained. The bone marrow showed less megaloblasts in the last months of treatment with enzyme replacement.

During treatment the NP activity of the red cells increased to low–normal levels after the third transfusion, simply as a result of admixture with donor erythrocytes[13]. However, the lymphocytes of the patient did not have any NP activity on several occasions. This result is in agreement with observations on a transfused ADA-deficient patient[5] and a three-times transfused NP-deficient patient[14]. It must be concluded that NP does not enter the lymphocyte and that changes in the serum concentration and urinary excretion of purines indicate that the infused red cells metabolize inosine and guanosine (Wadman et al., Chapter 8 in this book).

During the immunological follow-up a discrepancy was observed between the percentages of T cells as determined by immunofluorescence with a specific T cell antiserum and by the E rosette test. Table 7.1 shows the results of some of the investigations throughout the enzyme treatment period. On the day the transfusions started the discrepancy was rather high, 67% versus 16%. Throughout the treatment period the discrepancy diminished. Since the functioning of the receptor of human T lymphocytes for sheep erythrocytes is modulated by intracellular cyclic AMP[15] the discrepancies observed may simply reflect the degree of metabolic disturbance of the lymphocytes on different days. The immunofluorescence studies with anti-T antiserum should not be influenced by the metabolic state of the patient's lymphocytes. Alternatively the increase in E-rosetting T cells may be related to maturation processes of immature T cells induced by the enzyme replacement. Thymosin administration in a NP-deficient child has

TABLE 7.1   Lymphocytes populations during treatment (%)

Date	E_s	Anti-T	sig[+]
25–11	16	67	14
3–2	46	nt	15
5–5	21	76.5	17
18–8	53	nt	5
1–9	47	78.5	9
mean normal values*	62	80†	13
range	(49–73)	(73–85)	(5–22)

nt: not tested
* F. Gmelig Meyling et al.[19]
† G. Asma et al.[6]

resulted in an increase of the percentage of E-rosetting lymphocytes[16]. This phenomenon has been ascribed to maturation of precursor T cells. Our patient gained IgM-binding T lymphocytes[17] during treatment, which supports the supposition that maturation of T cell-dependent immunity does occur as a result of enzyme replacement therapy[18]. Moreover, these maturation processes may concurrently give rise to a change in the metabolic state of the lymphocytes.

CONCLUSIONS

1. Erythrocyte transfusions in our patient increased the number of lymphocytes and granulocytes. The effect on the lymphocytes was transient and normal levels were never attained; in contrast the effect on the granulocytes was permanent.

2.   Some immunological reconstitution can be attained in NP-deficient patients by erythrocyte and plasma transfusions. Complete immunological reconstitution however, is not achieved. Whether or not additional supplementations of uridine and purine are necessary remains to be answered.

Acknowledgements

Thanks are due to Dr J. M. Vossen and Mrs R. Langlois van de Berg, Academic Hospital, Leiden, to Dr A. Astaldi, Central Laboratory of the Netherlands Red Cross, Amsterdam and to Dr Ch. M. M. de Bruijn, Department of Anthropogenetics, University of Nijmegen, for the analysis of the T lymphocytes with anti-T cell antiserum, the determination of cyclic AMP in the lymphocytes and the enzymological investigations of the lymphocytes respectively.

References

1.   Polmar, S. H. (1977). Lymphocyte enzyme deficiencies and the metabolic basis of immunodeficiency disease. In H. H. Fudenberg (ed.). *Clin. Hematol.*, 6, p. 423. London: Saunders.
2.   Stoop, J. W., Eysvoogel, V. P., Zegers, B. J. M., Blok-Schut, B., van Bekkum, D. W. and Ballieux, R. E. (1976). Selective cellular immunodeficiency: effect of thymus transplantation and transfer factor administration. *Clin. Immunol. Immunopathol.*, 6, 289
3.   Stoop, J. W., Zegers, B. J. M., Hendrickx, G. F. M., Siegenbeek van Heukelom, L. H., Staal, G. E. J., de Bree, P. K., Wadman, S. K. and

Ballieux, R. E. (1977). Purine nucleoside phosphorylase deficiency associated with selective cellular immunodeficiency. *N. Engl. J. Med.*, **296**, 651

4. Siegenbeek van Heukelom, L. H., Staal, G. E. J., Stoop, J. W. and Zegers, B. J. M. (1976). An abnormal form of purine nucleoside phosphorylase in a family with a child with severe defective T-cell and normal B-cell immunity. *Clin. Chim. Acta*, **72**, 117

5. Wadman, S. K., de Bree, P. K., van Gennip, A. H., Stoop, J. W., Zegers, B. J. M., Staal, G. E. J. and Siegenbeek van Heukelom, L. H. (1977). Urinary purines in a patient with a severely defective T-cell immunity and a purine nucleoside phosphorylase deficiency. *Adv. Exp. Med. Biol.*, **76A**, 471

6. Asma, G., Schuit, H. R. E. and Hijmans, W. (1977). The determination of numbers of T and B lymphocytes in the blood of children and adults by the direct immunofluorescence technique. *Clin. Exp. Immunol.*, **29**, 286

7. Astaldi, A., Astaldi, G. C. B., Schellekens, P. Th. A. and Eysvoogel, V. P. (1976). Thymic factor in human sera demonstrable by a cyclic AMP assay. *Nature (London)*, **260**, 713

8. Polmar, S. H., Stern, R. C., Schwartz, A. L., Wetzler, E. M., Chase, P. A. and Hirschhorn, R. (1976). Enzyme replacement therapy for adenosine deaminase deficiency and severe combined immunodeficiency. *N. Engl. J. Med.*, **295**, 1337

9. Siegenbeek van Heukelom, L. H., Akkerman, J. W. N., Staal, G. E. J., de Bruyn, Ch. M. M., Stoop, J. W., Zegers, B. J. M., de Bree, P. K. and Wadman, S. K. (1977). A patient with purine nucleoside phosphorylase deficiency: enzymological and metabolic aspects. *Clin. Chim. Acta*, **74**, 271

10. Smith, L. H., Jr., Huguley, C. M., Jr. and Bain, J. A. (1972). Hereditary orotic aciduria. In J. B. Stanbury, J. B. Wijngaarden and D. S. Frederickson (eds.). *The Metabolic Basis of Inherited Disease*, p. 1003. (New York: McGraw-Hill)

11. Cohen, A., Doyle, D., Martin D. W. Jr., and Ammann, A. J. (1976). Abnormal purine metabolism and purine overproduction in a patient deficient in purine nucleoside phosphorylase. *N. Engl. J. Med.*, **295**, 1449

12. Green, S. H. and Chan, T. S. (1973). Pyrimidine starvation induced by adenosine in fibroblasts and lymphoid cells: role of adenosine deaminase. *Science*, **182**, 836

13. Staal, G. E. J., Stoop, J. W., Zegers, B. J. M., de Bruyn, Ch. M. M. and Wadman, S. K. (1977). Red cell metabolism in purine nucleoside phosphorylase deficiency after enzyme replacement therapy, *Hum. Hered.*, **27**, 215

14. Sandman, R., Ammann, A. J., Grose, Ch. and Wara, D. W. (1977). Cellular immunodeficiency associated with nucleoside phosphorylase deficiency: immunologic and biochemical studies. *Clin. Immunol. Immunopathol.*, **8**, 247

15. Chisari, F. V. and Edgington, Th. S. (1974). Human T lymphocyte E rosette function. I. A process modulated by intracellular cyclic AMP. *J. Exp. Med.*, **140**, 1122

16. Wara, D. W., Goldstein, A. L., Doyle, N. E. and Ammann, A. J. (1975). Thymosin activity in patients with cellular immunodeficiency, *N. Engl. J. Med.*, **292**, 70

17. Gmelig Meyling F., van der Ham, M. and Ballieux, R. E. (1976). Binding of IgM by human T lymphocytes. *Scand. J. Immunol.*, **5**, 487

18. Stoop, J. W., Hendrickx, G. F. M., Zegers, B. J. M., Wadman, S. K. and Staal, G. E. J. (1978). Immunological and metabolic follow-up of treatment of a NP deficient patient with cellular immunodeficiency. In preparation
19. Gmelig Meyling, F., Dollekamp, I., Zegers, B. J. M. and Ballieux, R. E. (1978). Lymphocyte subpopulations in neonates, children and adults. (In press)

8

Purine nucleoside phosphorylase deficiency associated with cellular immunodeficiency: metabolic studies during treatment

S. K. Wadman, P. K. de Bree,
G. F. M. Hendrickx, B. J. M.
Zegers and J. W. Stoop

INTRODUCTION

Until now only a few patients with purine nucleoside phosphorylase (PNP) deficiency have been described and knowledge about quantitative aspects of purine metabolism in this disease is limited[1, 2]. The data available suggest that PNP deficiency brings about major metabolic disturbances. A massive urinary excretion of inosine, guanosine and the corresponding deoxynucleosides was observed. Presumably these metabolites replace uric acid as the principal end product of purine metabolism as do xanthine and hypoxanthine in xanthine oxidase deficiency. We had the opportunity to study purine excretion in our patient during purine supplement therapy and enzyme replacement with irradiated erythrocytes containing PNP. Daily oral supplements of adenine and hypoxanthine were tried in order to compensate for the lack of purine salvage. Uridine was given at the instigation of American workers, who thought that inosine may induce a secondary adenosine deaminase deficiency state[1], from which pyrimidine starvation may result[3, 4]. Enzyme replacement therapy was inspired by the success of this approach in a patient with adenosine deaminase deficiency and severe combined immunodeficiency[5].

Previously, purine analyses were performed by cation exchange column chromatography. This technique is rather cumbersome for deoxynucleosides, which partly decompose[6]. Meanwhile high pressure liquid chroma-

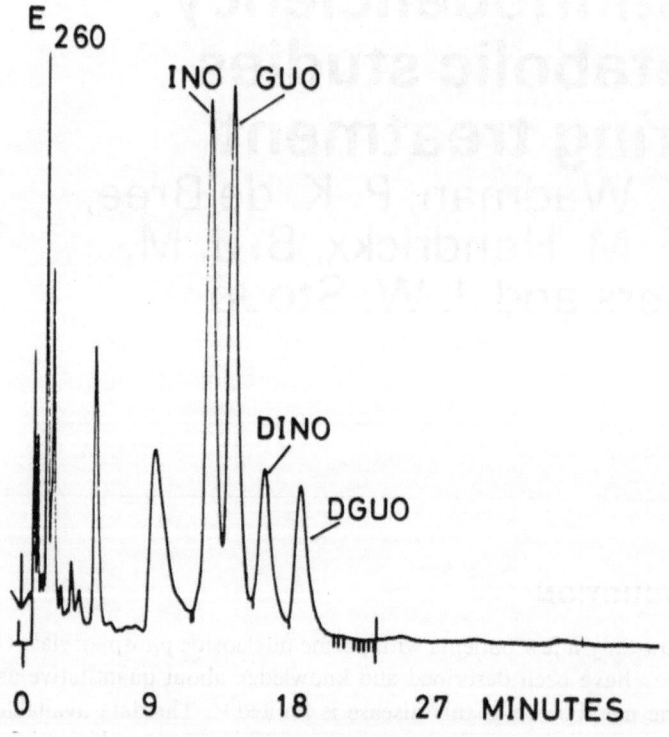

Figure 8.1 A high pressure liquid chromatogram of urinary inosine (Ino), deoxyinosine (dIno), guanosine (Guo) and deoxyguanosine (dGuo)

tography became available, making detailed analyses of nucleosides and deoxynucleosides possible.

METHODS

Urinary ribonucleosides and deoxyribonucleosides

Instrument: Waters Associates solvent delivery system 6000 A with universal liquid chromatograph injector U6K and a Schoeffel Instr. Corp. Spectroflow monitor SF 770. Column: Li Chromosorb 10 RP 18, 30 cm × 4.6 mm ID (Chrompack). Injected: 4–10 μl urine. Buffer 0.01 M KH_2PO_4 adjusted to pH 5.7 with KOH. Flow rate 3.0 ml/min. Monitoring of the effluent at 260 nm. Regeneration of the column: 4 min with buffer pH 5.7:methanol (1:1) followed by buffer pH 5.7 for 6 min. A chromatogram is shown in Figure 8.1.

Pyrimidines and uric acid

These were determined by cation exchange chromatography as described previously[6,7]. If uric acid was low it was determined enzymatically with uricase. Serum uric acid was also determined with uricase.

For the case report and treatment, see Chapter 7 in this book.

RESULTS AND DISCUSSION

The excretory patterns obtained confirmed our previous hypothesis concerning the presence of deoxyribonucleosides. The results (Table 8.1) show that uric acid was low and inosine (Ino), deoxyinosine (dIno), guanosine (Guo) and deoxyguanosine (dGuo) were very high. Previously evidence was obtained for an increased *de novo* synthesis of purines, possibly due to a lack of salvage resulting in diminished feedback inhibition at the level of amidophosphoribosyltransferase[6,7]. There was no accumulation of adenosine and no xanthosine was detected, indicating that the xanthosine pathway was practically inoperative in our patient. Little influence was seen from dietary purine restriction, indicating that the amount of endogenously produced purines is large compared to the influx from the intestine.

Addition of 1.35 mmol adenine to the meals for 2 weeks did not alter the pattern (see Table 8.2). Uridine (6.15 mmol per day) did not increase uric acid excretion and nucleosides remained at the same level. Uracil and uridine increased. When hypoxanthine also was added, uric acid increased

TABLE 8.1   Urinary excretion of purines, pyrimidines and their nucleosides in R.V. with nucleoside phosphorylase deficiency (mmol/g creatinine)

	Free diet			*Purine restricted*		
Cation exchange						
Pseudouridine	0.3	0.2	0.2	0.2	—	0.4
Uridine	—	—	—	—	—	—
Uracil	0.3	0.1	0.1	0.2	—	0.2
Enzymatic						
Uric acid	0.2	0.4	0.2	0.07	0.13	0.04
HPLC						
Inosine	10.5	11.8	10.0	12.1	10.6	13.1
Deoxyinosine	3.8	4.5	4.6	5.4	8.4	5.6
Guanosine	7.8	6.2	5.7	7.2	6.2	7.0
Deoxyguanosine	3.7	3.0	3.0	4.3	3.0	4.1

strikingly, which could be expected as a result of xanthine oxidase activity. Nucleosides, however, remained high.

In Table 8.3 we see the dramatic metabolic changes when transfusions of irradiated erythrocytes are given (for details see Chapter 7 in this book). Serum uric acid increased to normal levels. After each transfusion uric acid excretion rose sharply and nucleosides decreased. These phenomena are shown in Figure 8.2 and detailed data about the individual nucleosides

TABLE 8.2   Urinary purine, pyrimidine and their nucleoside excretion (mmol/g creatinine) in R.V. on a purine-restricted diet; effects of oral supplements

	Adenine 1.35 mmol/d	*Uridine* 6.15 mmol/d			*Uridine* 4.1 mmol/d *HYP* 3.8 mmol
Sample date	22/23–6	16/17–7	30/31–7	13/14–8	9/10–9
Cation exchange compounds					
Pseudouridine	0.2	0.3	0.2	0.8	0.5
Uridine	0.1	0.5	0.9	3.1	1.1
Uracil	0.3	2.3	2.6	3.2	1.3
Enzymatic					
Uric acid	0.3	0.10	0.13	0.35	5.9
HPLC					
Inosine	16.7	12.3	11.2	10.4	17.8
Deoxyinosine	5.6	5.5	3.9	4.4	8.6
Guanosine	7.0	6.4	6.5	4.6	8.0
Deoxyguanosine	3.7	3.4	2.8	2.9	4.3

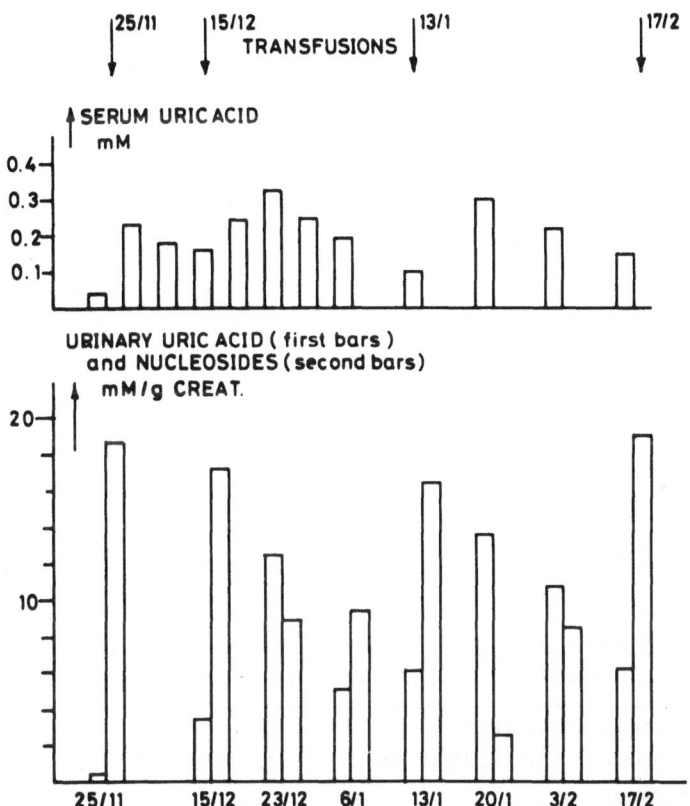

Figure 8.2   Effects of 'enzyme substitution' in R.V.: urinary uric acid and sum of nucleosides (Ino, dIno, Guo, dGuo) as mmol/g creatinine and serum uric acid as mmol/l

can be seen in Table 8.4. We have seen this tendency after each of the ten transfusions which have been given so far. There was a favourable effect on the number of lymphocytes and granulocytes, the percentage of E-rosetting T cells and their PHA-responsiveness of the lymphocytes, although complete restoration of thymus-dependent immunity has not yet been achieved. It is tempting to presume that the clearing of the accumulated nucleosides by the circulating PNP-containing foreign red cells, leads to the removal of the hindrance of lymphocyte proliferation. These data are consistent with inhibition of an essential mechanism by accumulated nucleosides, rather than purine starvation due to insufficient salvage.

In Table 8.5 the ratios of urinary ribonucleosides and deoxyribonucleosides are presented. The excretion of the latter was much higher than we would expect if we consider the ratio RNA/(DNA + mRNA), which is > 2.

TABLE 8.3   Effects of 'enzyme substitution' by transfusion in R.V. urinary uric acid and sum of nucleosides (Ino, dIno, Guo, dGuo) as mmol/g creatinine and serum uric acid as mmol/l.

Date of transf.	25/11			15/12				13/1
Sample date	25/11	30/11	13/12	15/12	20/12	23/12	30/12	6/1
Serum uric acid Normal 0.12–0.33 mM	0.04	0.23	0.18	0.16	0.24	0.32	0.24	0.19
Urine								
Uric acid	0.41			3.5		12.2	7.6	5.1
Nucleosides	(18.6)			17.2		8.8	<8.9	9.4

Date of transf.			13/1				17/2	
Sample date	6/1	12–13/1	13/1	20/1	3/2	10/2	16–17/2	17/2
Serum uric acid Normal 0.12–0.33 mM	0.19			0.10	0.30	0.22	0.24	0.15
Urine								
Uric acid	5.1	6.1		13.6	10.7	8.6	6.2	6.2
Nucleosides	9.4	16.4		2.5	8.5	19.4	19.4	19.0

TABLE 8.4   Urinary purine, pyrimidine and their nucleoside excretion (mmol/g creatinine) in R.V. effects of 'enzyme substitution' by transfusion

Date of transf.	16/12					13/1			
Sample date	15/12	23/12	30/12	6/1	12–13/1	20/1	3/2	10/2	16–17/2
Compounds									
Pseudouridine	0.5	0.3	0.3	0.3	0.4	0.3	0.4	0.4	0.3
Uridine	—	—	—	—	—	—	—	—	—
Uracil	0.2	0.2	0.2	0.2	0.3	0.1	0.2	0.2	0.2
Uric acid	3.5	12.2	7.6	5.1	6.1	13.6	10.7	8.6	6.2
Ino	6.4	3.7	3.5	3.8	6.5	1.5	3.1	6.8	6.6
dIno	3.6	2.1	<2.0	1.8	3.6	n.d	1.4	3.8	4.9
Guo	5.4	2.4	2.7	2.9	4.8	0.7	2.5	5.9	4.8
dGuo	1.8	0.6	<0.7	0.9	1.5	0.3	1.5	2.9	3.1

TABLE 8.5   Ratios of urinary nucleosides and deoxynucleosides

	$\overline{X}$	SD	SD/$\sqrt{n}$
Inosine/deoxyinosine ($n=19$)	2.14	0.48	0.11
Guanosine/deoxyguanosine ($n=20$)	2.30	0.76	0.17
Inosine/guanosine ($n=20$)	1.71	0.38	0.09
Deoxyinosine/deoxyguanosine ($n=19$)	1.84	0.67	0.16

The ratios Ino/dIno and Guo/dGuo were approximately equal (≈ 2), which may indicate that dIMP was a common precursor of dIno and dGuo. Ino predominated over Guo and dIno over dGuo. It is interesting to compare the excretory pattern of PNP deficiency with that of adenosine deaminase (ADA) deficiency, a disease which manifests itself also by severe immunodeficiency. In the latter uric excretion is normal and only a small amount of adenine was reported[8]. We could not detect adenine in a urine sample of such a patient although a trace of adenosine may have been present.

SUMMARY

Our patient with PNP deficiency showed continuous overproduction and loss of Ino, dIno, Guo and dGuo and a decreased formation of uric acid. After transfusions with irradiated red cells transient reversal of the abnormalities was observed, while white cells increased and lymphocytic functions improved. The immunological aberrations may be connected with accumulation of nucleosides.

References

1. Cohen, A., Doyle, D., Martin, D. W. Jr. and Ammann, A. J. (1976). Abnormal purine metabolism and purine overproduction in a patient deficient in purine nucleoside phosphorylase. *N. Engl. J. Med.*, **295**, 1449
2. Stoop, J. W., Zegers, B. J. M., Hendrickx, G. F. M., Siegenbeek van Heukelom, L. H., Staal, G. E. J., de Bree, P. K., Wadman, S. K. and Ballieux, R. E. (1977). Purine nucleoside phosphorylase deficiency associated with selective cellular immunodeficiency. *N. Engl. J. Med.*, **296**, 651
3. Ullman, B., Cohen, A. and Martin, D. W. Jr. (1976). Characterization of a cell culture model for the study of adenosine deaminase and purine nucleoside phosphorylase deficient immunologic disease. *Cell*, **9**, 205
4. Green, H. and Chan, T. S. (1973). Pyrimidine starvation induced by adenosine in fibroblasts and lymphoid cells: role of adenosine deaminase. *Science*, **182**, 836
5. Polmar, S. H., Stern, R. C., Schwartz, A. L., Wetzler, E. M., Chase, P. A. and Hirschhorn, R. (1976). Enzyme replacement therapy for adenosine deaminase deficiency and severe combined immunodeficiency. *N. Engl. J. Med.*, **295**, 1337
6. Wadman, S. K., de Bree, P. K., van Gennip, A. H., Stoop, J. W., Zegers, B. J. M., Staal, G. E. J. and Siegenbeek van Heukelom, L. H. (1976). Urinary purines in a patient with a severely defective T cell immunity and a purine nucleoside phosphorylase deficiency. 2nd International Symposium on Purine Metabolism in Man, Baden near Vienna, Austria. In M. M. Müller, E. Kaiser and J. E. Seegmiller (eds.) (1977). *Purine Metabolism in Man–II: Regulation of Pathways and Enzyme Defects.*

7. Siegenbeek van Heukelom, L. H., Akkerman, J. W., Staal, G. E. J., de Bruyn, C. H. M. M., Stoop, J. W., Zegers, B. J. M., de Bree, P. K. and Wadman, S. K. (1977). A patient with purine nucleoside phosphorylase deficiency: enzymological and metabolic aspects. *Clin. Chim. Acta*, **74**, 271

8. Mills, G. C., Schalstieg, F. C., Trimmer, K. B., Goldman, A. S. and Gold-blum, R. M. (1976). Purine metabolism in adenosine deaminase deficiency. *Proc. Natl. Acad. Sci. USA*, **73**, 2867

9

Severe combined immunodeficiency with B lymphocytes: a selective defect of precursor T cells

C. Griscelli, A. Durandy and
F. Daguillard

Severe combined immunodeficiency (SCID) is a rare disorder character-ized by profound abnormalities of both cellular (T) and humoral (B) func-tions and a fatal outcome during the first year of life.

The first patients described had lymphopenia associated with agamma-globulinaemia; the syndrome was attributed to a defect of bone marrow lymphoid stem cells[1,2]. Several observations have indicated, however, that the immunological parameters varied from one patient to another and that SCID was a heterogeneous disease[3].

Recently, an enzymatic defect of adenosine deaminase (ADA)[4] or nucleoside phosphorylase (PNP)[5-7] activities was found to be associated with immunodeficiency and several studies indicated a relationship be-tween ADA deficiency and abnormal differentiation of the lymphoid precursor cells[8].

TABLE 9.1 SCID with normal ADA and NP activities: heterogeneity of the B cell defect

Number of patients	Circulating lymphocytes	E-RFC %	Anti-HBLA	B cell markers (%)						Serum Ig (mg%)			Antibody formation
				μ	δ	μ+δ	L chains	C3	Fc	IgM	IgA	IgD	
4	≤400	≤1	nt	≤2	0	0	≤2	nt	nt	≤10	≤10	0	no
1	1500	≤1	90	5	3	2	4	6	8	<10	<10	0	no
9	900–3500	≤1	70–93	49–76	75–97	50–70	82–95	45–96	57–83	3–162*	≤10	0	no†

* 19S IgM in three patients

† Two patients had some anti-A and/or anti-B allohaemagglutinins

nt = not tested

We have observed nine SCID patients without marked lymphopenia and without enzymatic defect (Table 9.1). They had no T lymphocytes and carried an increased number of B lymphocytes bearing μ or $\mu + \delta$ Ig determinants. This situation suggested that the humoral defect was secondary to an absence of helper T cells.

Two of these SCID patients with B lymphocytes were transplanted with HLA compatible bone marrow which was presumably able to repopulate an existing thymus gland because this became visible on X-ray and gave rise to mature T cells bearing donor's markers and capable of full co-operation with host B cells in immunoglobulin and antibody production. This suggests that these patients had a selective defect of a precursor T cell.

MATERIAL AND METHODS

Case reports

The first patient (SA) was a girl born on 24 April 1972 from parents who were cousins. Three of her brothers had died before the age of one, two of them being well defined as SCID. *Post mortem* examination confirmed the diagnosis of SCID. The family history suggested an autosomal recessive transmission. The patient was placed in a Trexler isolator one week after birth and kept for 6 months. No attempt was made to decontaminate the

TABLE 9.2 Cellular immunity before and after bone marrow transplantation (BMT)

	Before transplantation		After transplantation	
	patient 1 (SA)	patient 2 (NG)	patient 1 (SA) 4 years*	patient 2 (NG) 10 months*
Lymphocytes/mm³	1000–2000	900–3500	3000	2500
E-RFC (%)	NT†	≤1	71	52
Skin tests‡	−	−	+	+
Polyclonal mitogens§	−	−	+	+
MLR‖	+	−	+	+
Thymic shadow	−	−	+	+
Thymic factor¶	NT	1:16	1:64	NT

* Time after transplantation
† First E-RFC determination was performed one month after B transplantation. At that time, 8% of E-RFC were present
‡ Skin tests were performed with *Candida*, SK–SD, diphtheria, KLH, DNCB, PHA
§ Phytohaemagglutinin, Concanavalin-A and pokeweed mitogen
‖ One way mixed leukocyte reaction with mitomicin C inactivated cells
¶ Performed by M. Dardenne and J. F. Bach. Normal values 1:16 to 1:64[16]

TABLE 9.3   Humoral immunity before and after bone marrow transplantation (BMT)

	Before transplantation		After transplantation	
	patient 1 (SA)	patient 2 (NG)	patient 1 (SA) 4 years B.M.*	patient 2 (NG) 10 months B.M.*
Ig-bearing cells				
μ	62	60	8	6
δ	NT	97	1	12
$\mu + \delta$	NT	58	NT	NT
L chains	94	95	18	NT
IgM (mg%)	≤10	≤10	220	27
IgA	≤5	≤5	120	11
IgD	0	0	0.1	0
Isohaemagglutinins A		0		1:32
B	0	0	1:256	1:16
Antibody formation†	−	−	+	+

* Time after transplantation

† The first patient was immunized against diphtheria and pertussis several times before and after transplantation. Polioviruses were given shortly after transplantation and tetanus toxoid 2 years later. The second patient was immunized with tetanus and blood group substances A and B before and after transplantation. Pertussis, polio and diphtheria were administered after transplantation

child with oral antibiotics. No lymph nodes were palpable. Tonsils were absent. Routine immunological studies showed a normal postnatal level of serum immunoglobulin but an increased number of B cells and a mild lymphopenia − 1300/mm³ (Tables 9.2 and 9.3). No antibody activity could be detected after immunization with diphtheria and tetanus toxoids, *H. pertussis* and killed polio virus. Delayed skin-reaction remained absent following sensitization with DNCB. At day 37, the patient was transplanted with a 12 weeks' gestation female fetal thymus. In the absence of any clinical and biological improvement a transplant of 10⁸ bone marrow lymphoid cells (BMT) from an histocompatible brother was performed on day 58. HL-A antigens (1-W17/192, 12) blood group substances and immunoglobulin allotypes were identical in both donor and recipient. A mild graft-versus-host (GVH) reaction was observed by day 22 after BMT characterized by a transient skin rash and a neutropenia. A thymus shadow, not previously observed, became apparent 5 months after the marrow graft.

The second patient (NG) was a boy born on 3 November 1976 from unrelated parents. Two brothers had died before the age of 8 months from a graft-versus-host reaction following bone marrow transplantation or blood transfusion. Five maternally related boys had died within the first year of life from infections, progressive vaccinia or BCG sepsis. This family history suggested a sex-linked transmission. In three of the seven cases autopsy (performed by Dr C. Nezelof) had confirmed the diagnosis of SCID. The patient was placed in a Trexler isolator immediately after a sterile delivery; 42 days later, the recovery of three different bacteria in the stools prompted decontamination with oral antibiotic therapy for the remaining 6 months of isolation. No lymph nodes were palpable and tonsils were absent. Routine immunological studies showed the same picture as that seen in the first patient, i.e., mild lymphopenia (Tables 9.2 and 9.3) (900–3500/mm^3), an increase of circulating B cells, the presence of maternal IgG, low levels of the other immunoglobulin classes, absence of isohaemagglutinins and antibodies after various immunizations. Skin tests to phytohaemagglutinin (PHA), and haemocyanin (KHL) remained negative. The patient was transplanted on day 47 with 1.5×10^8 bone marrow cells/kg from a maternal aunt who was HLA, ABO identical (HLA: 1, 8/W29, 12 blood group O) but mixed leukocyte reaction (MLR) slightly positive (cpm/min=2800, proliferative index=1.8). Evidence for a graft-versus-host reaction was obtained 10 days after the graft with a recurrent skin rash following by a persisting eosinophilia. A thymic shadow, absent on the first X-rays, became apparent 5 months after marrow graft. The patient has left the hospital, fully reconstituted, in good health and has never received gammaglobulin therapy.

Methods

Blood lymphocytes were isolated on Ficoll-Hypaque gradients. E rosettes with sheep erythrocytes[9], with E sensitized with antibody and complement (EAC)[10] and membrane immunofluorescence studies with rabbit aggregated immunoglobulins and antibodies specific for human μ, α, γ and δ chains (before and after trypsinization) were performed as described[11,12]. A double-staining technique was used for the simultaneous detection of μ and δ chains[13]. T and B cells were also identified using an anti-T serum (Institut Mérieux, Lyon, France) and a locally prepared anti-B serum[11]. Serum antibodies were assessed using routine haemagglutination or infectivity neutralization techniques.

Lymphocytes were cultured in RPMI 1640 medium supplemented with 20% inactivated human serum (from AB + donors) and antibiotics. Mitogen-induced proliferations were tested at various times. Mixed lymphocyte cultures were performed using X-irradiated stimulator cells. Cell stimulation was also obtained using activated supernatants from mixed leukocyte cultures. In each case, the proliferative response was estimated by measuring the 18 h incorporation of [^{3}H]thymidine.

In vitro T–B cooperation was performed using a culture technique modified from Wu *et al.*[14] Normal T cells were isolated by sedimentation of E rosettes. B cells were concentrated by depleting of E rosettes. The T cell : B cell ratio was 4 : 1 and intracellular immunoglobulin synthesis was studied on the 7th day of culture.

Chimerism studies were performed by karyotyping patients' dividing lymphocytes in the presence of PHA, PWM (pokeweed mitogen) or allogeneic cells detected by a chromosomal translocation. Fluorescence quinacrine of the Y chromosome[15] was used in order to detect the donor cells in the first patient or recipient cells in the second. This technique was also coupled with membrane or intracytoplasmic immunofluorescence with specific antisera directed against IgM, IgG, IgA and IgD.

IMMUNOLOGICAL STUDIES

Before transplantation

The majority of lymphocytes from the two patients carried surface Ig determinants. In the second case, membrane staining with antibodies specific for the various Ig classes revealed that almost the whole of these cells carried μ and/or δ chains (see Table 9.3). These B cells also carried receptors for complement and were stained by an antiserum specific for B cells. Besides IgG of maternal origin, immunoglobulins or antibodies were undetectable after various antigenic stimulations including, in the second patient, blood group substances and pneumococcal polysaccharide antigens (SIII). The number of E-RFC was not assessed in the first case (Table 9.2). It was below 1% in the second patient, as was the number of cells reacting with an antiserum specific for T lymphocytes. There was no *in vitro* response to polyclonal mitogens but the lymphocytes of patient 1 were able to respond *in vitro* to allogeneic leukocytes in a one-way stimulation test. This ability to respond in MLR has been previously described[12]. Serum thymic factor was within the normal ranges in the second patient[16]. Lymphocytes from the second patient, a boy, unable to proliferate and to mature *in vitro* in the presence of PWM alone, were co-cultured with normal female T cells and PWM. This study showed that, under these conditions, patient lymphocytes matured into IgM- and IgD-containing cells.

After transplantation

The two patients had a complete immunological reconstitution and are now 5 years and 11 months old respectively and free from infections. Immunoglobulins and antibodies to blood group substances and various specific antigens rose to normal or very high levels in patients 1 and 2. At the same time, their lymphocytes bearing μ and δ chains decreased slowly, reaching normal values within 5 months after transplantation. The number of E-RFC rose in the two cases in the months following transplantation. All two patients became rapidly capable of responding to polyclonal mitogens. Their skin tests also became positive to various antigens, DNCB or PHA. A thymic shadow, not previously present, appeared in patients 1 and 2, 5 months after the BM transplantation.

Chimerism

Chimerism was established by identification of grafted cells. In patients 1 and 2, karyotype studies indicated that dividing cells in the presence of PHA and PWM were of donor origin (XY in patient 1, XX in patient 2) when the cultures were terminated at day 3. On the other hand, both donor and recipient cells were detectable in 5-day culture of lymphocytes from patient 1 stimulated with allogeneic cells or PWM. These results suggested that mainly donor T cells were stimulated at the beginning of culture but that a small percentage of recipient B cells could be subsequently involved in the proliferative process.

Fluorescent staining of Y chromosome by quinacrine coupled with membrane immunofluorescence studies indicated that B cells of patients 1 and 2 were of recipient origin. Intracytoplasmic Ig-containing cells, obtained in a 7-day culture of lymphocytes from patient 1 in the presence of PWM, were also of recipient origin. The isohaemagglutinins of the second patient contained a Gm(1+) allotype not present on the immunoglobulins of the donor. Indeed, blood group A red blood cells (RBC) sensitized with the immune isohaemagglutinins present in the serum of the second patient after immunization with blood group substances were agglutinated with two antiGm(1+) antisera.

DISCUSSION

Studies of two SCID patients demonstrated that, after bone marrow transplantation, an existing thymus gland can be repopulated, becomes visible on X-rays, and gives rise to T cells capable of manifesting cell-mediated immunity and of cooperating with recipient's B cells in humoral functions. In these patients, the newly arising T cells carried chromosomal markers showing that they originated from marrow precursors which presumably matured in the recipient thymus. Although it cannot completely be ruled out that a few mature T cells contaminating our marrow suspension contributed directly to the restoration of immune functions, it is more probable that the continuing supply of T cells originated from the thymus. On the other hand, *in vitro* studies demonstrated that donor's B cells were not the ones bearing and secreting immunoglobulins, and, finally, allotype studies in patient 2 showed that the isoagglutinins produced were of host origin.

It is generally assumed that, following bone marrow transplantation, the grafted precursor cells provide both T and B lineages. T cell chimerism has been amply demonstrated by karyotype studies in several marrow transplantations[1, 17-21]. Some studies based on allotype analysis indicate also that immunoglobulins are produced by donor cells[19, 22-24]. However, in one patient, immunoglobulins carrying recipient's Gm markers were found following a marrow transplant[21, 25]. There was no information on the characteristics of the B cells, but it is most likely that in this patient as in our first case, donor T cells induced the terminal differentiation of the recipient's Ig-bearing cells.

The heterogeneous nature of the deficits observed in the humoral functions of SCID patients must be due to various defects of either T or B lineages and their complex interactions. Immunoglobulin levels are known to vary greatly from one case to another[3]. The same is true for the number of B cells[26-28]. Nine of the 14 cases of non-ADA or NP-deficient SCID patients which we have studied had normal or increased levels of B cells. These B cells bore only μ and δ membrane determinants. Little is known about the functional capacities of these cells. In the presence of normal T cells, the B cells of our second patient matured into μ- and δ-containing cells. In a recent study B cells from a SCID patient were induced to secrete IgG *in vitro* by normal T cells[27], but it was not mentioned which specific Ig determinants were carried by these B lymphocytes. Moreover, this patient had a small percentage (8–10%) of T cells in his peripheral blood. Various studies show that SCID with residual T cells as well as partial DiGeorge and Nezelof syndromes may secrete IgG[3, 29-31]. The heterogeneity of humoral functions seen in these patients may well be attributable to the degree of T cell maturation rather than to anomalies of the B cell line. Our observations could indicate that in the complete absence of T cells, B lymphocyte maturation remains blocked at the level of μ and δ chain expression and that T cell help may be required at this stage in the ontogeny of the B cell.

The complete absence of T cell functions is a rare pathological finding. Our study shows that besides thymic aplasia, a pre-thymic defect (selective defect of bone marrow precursor T cells) can be responsible for this anomaly. It helps also to define the scheme of lymphocyte differentiation. Based on the study of immunodeficiencies it was assumed that both cell lineages derive from a common precursor. SCID resulted from an absence of this precursor whereas Bruton disease and DiGeorge syndrome were caused by a defect of central lymphoid organs (bursa equivalent or thymus gland) which favour the development of this stem cell[2]. In our patients, only precursors of T cells were absent, indicating that, early in the differentiation of the common stem cell, separate precursors of the T and B cell lines appear. In the same vein, Bruton type agammaglobulinaemia might well represent a selective defect of the B cell precursor rather than the anomaly of an elusive equivalent of the bursa of Fabricius.

References

1. Rosen, F. S. (1975). Immunodeficiency. In B. Benacerraf (ed.). *Immunogenetics and Immunodeficiency*, p. 229 (Lancaster: MTP)

2. Cooper, M. D., Faulk, W. P., Fudenberg, H. H., Good, R. A., Hitzig, W. H., Rosen, F. S., Seligmann, M., Soothill, J. and Wedgwood, R. J. (1973). Classification of primary immunodeficiencies. *N. Engl. J. Med.*, **288**, 966

3. Hitzig, W. H., Landolt, R., Müller, G. and Bodmer, P. (1971). Heterogeneity of phenotype expression in a family with Swiss type agammaglobulinemia: observations on the acquisition of agammaglobulinemia. *J. Pediatr.*, **78**, 968

4. Meuwissen, H. J., Pollara, B. and Pickering, R. J. (1975). Combined immunodeficiency disease associated with adenosine deaminase deficiency. *J. Pediatr.*, **86**, 169

5. Giblett, E. R., Ammann, A. J., Wara, D. W., Sandman, R. and Diamond, L. K. (1975). Nucleoside phosphorylase deficiency in a child with severely defective T-cell immunity and normal B-cell immunity. *Lancet*, **ii**, 1010

6. Griscelli, C., Hamet, M., Ballet, J. J., Nezelof, C., De Bruyn, C. H. M. M., Hosli, P. and Cartier, P. (1977). Severe T-cell immunodeficiency associated with inosine phosphorylase (IP) deficiency: A new case with fatal vaccinia gangrenosa. *Third Workshop on Bone Marrow Transplantation in Immunodeficiency*. J. Finstad and R. A. Good (ed.) (in press)

7. Stopp, J. W., Zegers, B. J. M., Hendrickx, G. F. M., Siegenbeek van Heukelom, L. H., Staal, G. E. J., de Bree, P. K., Wadman, S. K. and Ballieux, R. E. (1977). Purine nucleoside phosphorylase deficiency associated with selective cellular immunodeficiency. *N. Engl. J. Med.*, **296**, 651

8. Ballet, J. J., Insel, R., Merler, E. and Rosen, F. S. (1976). Inhibition of maturation of human precursor lymphocytes by Coformycin, an inhibitor of the enzyme adenosine deaminase. *J. Exp. Med.*, **143**, 1271

9. Stjernwärd, J., Jondal, M., Vancky, F., Wigzell, H. and Sealy, R. (1972). Lymphopenia and change in distribution of human T and B lymphocytes in peripheral blood induced by irradiation of mammary carcinoma. *Lancet*, i, 1352

10. Bianco, D., Patrick, R. and Nussenczweig, V. (1970). A population of lymphocytes bearing a membrane receptor for antigen–antibody complement complexes. *J. Exp. Med.*, 132, 702

11. Durandy, A., Wioland, M., Sabolovic, D. and Griscelli, C. (1975). Electrophoretic characteristics and membrane receptors of lymphocytes in primary immunodeficiency diseases. *Clin. Immunol. Immunopathol.*, 4, 440

12. Seligmann, M., Griscelli, C., Preud'Homme, J. L., Sasportes, M., Herzog, C. and Brouet, J. C. (1974). A variant of severe combined immunodeficiency with normal *in vitro* response to allogeneic cells and an increase in circulating B lymphocytes persisting several months after successful bone marrow graft. *Clin. Exp. Immunol.*, 17, 245

13. Preud'Homme, J. L., and Labaume, S. (1977). Detection of surface immunoglobulins on human cells by direct immunofluorescence. In B. R. Bloom and J. R. David (eds.). In vitro *Methods in Cell Mediated Immunity* (New York: Academic Press) (in press)

14. Wu, L. Y., Lawton, A. R. and Cooper, M. D. (1973). Differentiation capacity of cultured B lymphocyte from immunodeficient patients. *J. Clin. Invest.*, 52, 3180

15. Capersson, T., Zech, L., Johansson, C. and Modest, E. J. (1970). Identification of human chromosomes by DNA-binding fluorescent agents. *Chromosoma (Berlin)*, 30, 215

16. Dardenne, M. and Bach, J. F. (1975). The circulating thymic factor (TF). Biochemistry, physiology, biological activity and thymic application. A summary. In D. W. Van Bekkum (ed.). *Biological Activity of Thymic Hormones*, p. 145. (New York: Academic Press).

17. Gatti, R. A., Allen, H. D., Meuwissen, H. J., Hong, R. and Good, R. A. (1968). Immunological reconstitution of sex-linked lymphopenic immunological deficiency. *Lancet*, ii, 1366

18. De Koning, J., van Bekkum, D. W., Dicke, K. A., Dooren, L. J., van Rood, J. J. and Radl, J. (1969). Transplantation of bone marrow cells and fetal thymus in an infant with lymphopenic immunological deficiency. *Lancet*, i, 1223

19. Stiehm, E. R., Lawlor, G. J., Kaplan, M. S., Greenwald, H. L., Neerhout, R. C., Sengar, D. P. S. and Terasaki, P. I. (1972). Immunologic reconstitution in severe combined immunodeficiency without bone marrow chromosomal chimerism. *N. Engl. J. Med.*, 286, 797

20. Yamamura, M., Newton, R. C. F., James, D. C. O., Humbie, J. G., Buttler, L. J. and Hobbs, J. R. (1972). Umcomplicated HL-A matched sibling bone marrow graft for combined immune deficiency. *Br. Med. J.*, 2, 265

21. Vossen, J. M. J. J. (1975). *The Development of the B Immune System in Man* (Rotterdam: Bronder-Offset B.V.)

22. Levey, R. H., Gelfand, E. W., Batchelor, J. R., Klemperer, M. R., Sanderson, A. R., Berkel, A. I. and Rosen, F. S. (1971). Bone marrow transplantation in severe combined immunodeficiency syndrome. *Lancet*, ii, 571

23. Rubinstein, A., Speck, B. and Jeannet, M. (1971). Successful bone marrow transplantation in a lymphopenic immunologic deficiency syndrome. *N. Engl. J. Med.*, **285**, 1399

24. Yount, W. J., Utsinger, P. D., Gatti, R. A. and Good, R. A. (1974). Immunoglobulin classes, IgG subclasses, Gm genetic markers, and C1q following bone marrow transplantation in X-linked combined immunodeficiency. *J. Pediatr.*, **84**, 193

25. Vossen, J. M., de Koning, J., van Bekkum, D. W., Dicke, K. A., Eysvoogel, V. P., Hijmans, W., van Loghem, E., Radl, J., van Rood, J. J., van der Waay, D. and Dooren, L. J. (1973). Successful treatment of an infant with severe combined immunodeficiency by transplantation of bone marrow cells from an uncle. *Clin. Exp. Immunol.*, **13**, 9

26. Griscelli, C. (1975). T and B markers in immunodeficiencies. *Birth Defects*, p. 45. (New York: National Foundation March of Dimes)

27. Seeger, R. C., Robins, R. A., Stevens, R. H., Klein, R. B., Waldman, D. J., Zeltze, P. M. and Kessler, S. W. (1976). Severe combined immunodeficiency with B lymphocytes: *in vitro* correction of defective immunoglobulin production by addition of normal T lymphocytes. *Clin. Exp. Immunol.*, **26**, 1

28. Geha, R. S. (1976). Is the B-cell abnormality secondary to T-cell abnormality in severe combined immunodeficiency? *Clin. Immunol. Immunopathol.*, **6**, 102

29. Pabst, H. F., Wright, W. C., Le Riche, J. and Stiehm, E. R. (1976). Partial DiGeorge syndrome with substantial cell-mediated immunity. *Am. J. Dis. Child.*, **130**, 316

30. Griscelli, C. and Diebold, N. (1976). Le syndrome de DiGeorge. A propos de 4 nouvelles observations. In *Journées Parisiennes de Pédiatrie*, p. 171. (Paris: Flammarion)

31. Nezelof, C., Jammet, M. L., Lortholary, P., Labrune, B. and Lamy, M. (1964). L'hypoplasie héréditaire du thymus; sa place et sa responsabilité dans une observation d'aplasie lymphocytaire normoplasmocytaire et normoglobulinémique du nourrisson. *Arch. Franç. Pédiatr.*, **21**, 897

10

Purine metabolism and the control of lymphocyte proliferation. Effects of exogenous adenosine on normal human lymphocytes
T. Hovi

Proliferation of antigen-sensitized lymphocytes is one of the basic phenomena in the immune response. Several lines of evidence suggest that proliferation of lymphocytes is relatively sensitive to changes in purine metabolism[1,2]. Hereditary deficiencies in either adenosine deaminase (ADA) or purine nucleoside phosphorylase (PNP), enzymes of the pathways responsible for the degradation of purine nucleotides and nucleosides, result in severe immunodeficiency diseases leaving the functions of most other tissues almost unaffected[3,4]. The failure of the immune system in ADA deficiency seems to be based on the accumulation of adenosine, the substrate of ADA, or its metabolic products in the tissues[3,5,6]. This hypothesis is supported by the findings that exposure of normal mitogen-stimulated lymphocyte cultures to exogenous adenosine can inhibit proliferation of the

167

cells[7-9]. Molecular mechanisms of this inhibition are not known, but several alternatives have been suggested, all of which can be approached experimentally[9-11].

In this paper I shall describe some experiments that were designed to answer mainly two questions. First, is the inhibition of phytohaemagglutinin-induced lymphocyte proliferation due to a direct action of the added adenosine on the T lymphocytes themselves, or does it require the presence of some other cell types such as monocytes or macrophages[11]? Secondly, is it possible to prevent the adenosine-induced inhibition of lymphocyte proliferation by adding to the cell culture pyrimidine nucleosides[10]?

MATERIALS AND METHODS

T lymphocyte-enriched normal human peripheral blood leukocytes (more then 85% sheep erythrocyte-rosetting cells) were prepared as described in detail recently[12]. Cultures of 1×10^6 living cells in 1 ml of the RPMI–1640 medium supplemented with 10% dialysed horse serum, antibiotics and the indicated additions were incubated at 37 °C in flat-bottomed tubes (diameter 8 mm).

A quantitative estimate of the mitogen-induced proliferation was obtained by measuring the incorporation of [^{3}H]thymidine or [^{14}C]hypoxanthine into acid-insoluble material in the cultures (standard acid-precipitation and scintillation counting).

RESULTS AND DISCUSSION

The earlier studies on the effects of exogenous adenosine, or of a combination of adenosine and an inhibitor of ADA on mitogen-induced lymphocyte proliferation, have been carried out using lymphocyte–monocyte mixtures[7-9]. Therefore, it was necessary to repeat the experiments with cultures depleted of monocytes. It was observed in these studies that the minimal initial concentrations of extracellular adenosine, resulting in 50% or 90% inhibition of the PHA-induced [^{3}H]thymidine incorporation in the 'T lymphocytes', were of the same order (Table 10.1) as previously found for the unfractionated mononuclear leukocyte cultures under identical conditions[9]. Coformycin, a specific inhibitor of ADA, also synergistically potentiated the effects of adenosine (Table 10.1) on the cells[9].

Though our cultures of the T lymphocyte-enriched leukocytes never were completely free of monocytes[12], it is obvious from these studies that exogenous adenosine can inhibit the proliferation of lymphocytes by a direct action on the stimulated lymphocytes.

TABLE 10.1   Synergistic inhibition of phytohaemagglutinin (PHA) induced thymidine incorporation in human T lymphocytes by adenosine (rA) and coformycin (Cfm)

Compounds added	Thymidine incorporation (cpm/culture)	Ratio to PHA control
None	900 ± 300	0.01
PHA	75500 ± 8300	1.00
10^{-4}M rA + PHA	19700 ± 3500	0.26
10^{-5}M rA + PHA	118500 ± 6300	1.57
10^{-6}M rA + PHA	76400 ± 9200	1.01
10^{-7}M Cfm + PHA	88300 ± 5500	1.17
10^{-5}M rA + 10^{-7}M Cfm + PHA	13900 ± 1100	0.18
10^{-6}M rA + 10^{-7}M Cfm + PHA	87100 ± 1500	1.15

T lymphocyte-enriched human peripheral blood leukocytes were distributed into plastic tubes at 1×10^6 cells/ml of RPMI-1640 medium supplemented with 10% dialysed horse serum. 0.5 μg/ml PHA type HA16 (Wellcome Research Laboratories, Kent, UK), adenosine and coformycin were added to the indicated final concentrations. DNA synthesis was assayed after 38 h incubation at 37 °C by labelling the cultures with 1 μCi [³H]thymidine (sp. act. 5 Ci/mmol, Radiochemical Centre, Amersham, UK for the subsequent 4 h. Means and ranges of duplicate cultures of a representative experiment are shown

Unlike our previous observations in the less purified lymphocyte cultures[9] I now found a reproducible and strong potentiation of the PHA-induced DNA synthesis at a relatively narrow range of subinhibitory concentrations of exogenous adenosine (Figure 10.1). It is interesting to note that the switch from potentiation to the inhibitory action took place at or slightly below the level of the nucleoside resulting in saturation of nucleotide synthesis[13]. These findings support the views that a delicately regulated supply of purine nucleotides is an important part of the cellular mechanisms controlling lymphocyte proliferation[1, 2], and suggest that the inhibition of lymphocyte proliferation by adenosine might be due to an oversaturation of the adenine nucleotide pools.

It has been reported that inhibition of [³H]thymidine incorporation by adenosine in mitogen-stimulated lymphocytes can be almost completely reversed by exogenous uridine or other pyrimidine nucleosides[8, 14]. However, other workers have not succeeded in achieving this reversion[1]. In the present series of experiments the adenosine-induced inhibition of [³H] thymidine incorporation was reduced by micromolar concentrations of uridine to a variable extent. Figures shown in Table 10.2 represent the greatest degree of reversion; in most experiments much less reversion was

TABLE 10.2   Effect of uridine on the adenosine-induced inhibition of nucleic acid synthesis in phytohaemagglutinin (PHA)-stimulated human T lymphocytes

Compounds added	Label incorporated into nucleic acids (stimulation index)	
	[³H]thymidine	[¹⁴C]hypoxanthine
A. PHA alone	25	86
B. 10^{-4}M adenosine + PHA	2.0	2
C. B + 10^{-4}M uridine	5.0	5
D. B + 10^{-5}M uridine	21	8
E. B + 10^{-6}M uridine	18	3
F. 3×10^{-5}M adenosine + 10^{-8}M coformycin + PHA	2.5	2
G. F + 10^{-4}M uridine	3.2	3
H. F + 10^{-5}M uridine	2.9	4
I. F + 10^{-6}M uridine	nt	4

For experimental details see Table 10.1. Cultures were labelled from 38 to 42 h of incubation either with 1 μCi of [³H]thymidine (see Table 10.1) or 1 μCi of [¹⁴C]hypoxanthine (56 mCi/mmol). Means of duplicate cultures form the basis of the calculated indices. Effect of 10^{-4}M adenosine, or the combination of adenosine + coformycin, on nucleic acid synthesis in the unstimulated cells was negligible under these conditions

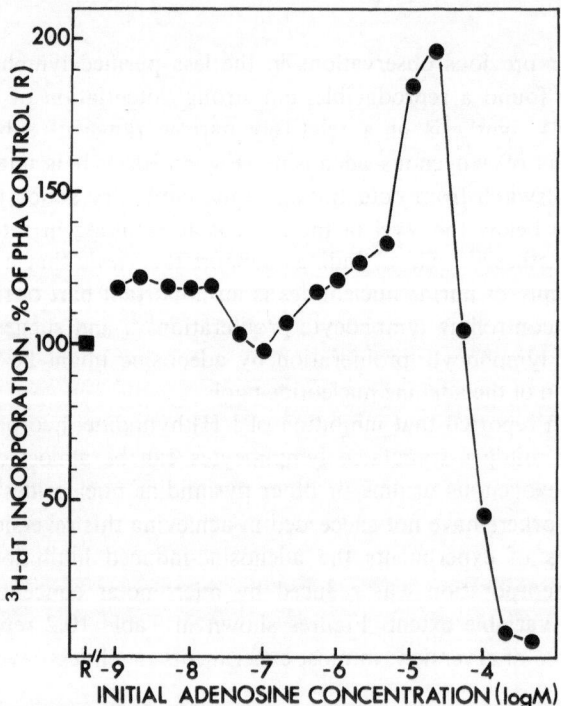

Figure 10.1   Dose–response curve of the effects of exogenous adenosine on phytohaemagglutinin-induced proliferation of T lymphocyte-enriched leukocytes from normal human peripheral blood. For experimental details see Table 10.1

obtained. If the cultures were incubated with a combination of adenosine and coformycin – which may better mimic the deficiency of ADA – practically no reduction in the inhibition of nucleic acid synthesis was obtained by exogenous uridine (Table 10.2) or cytidine (not shown). Furthermore, if the mitogenic response was quantitated by labelling the cells with [14C] hypoxanthine or [14C]guanine (not shown), very little if any reduction of the inhibition induced even by adenosine alone was achieved by adding uridine to the culture medium (Table 10.2).

In conclusion, these results do not support the view[8, 10, 14] that adenosine inhibits lymphocyte proliferation mainly by specifically depleting the cells of pyrimidine nucleotides. Instead, I would like to suggest that increased levels of exogenous adenosine may result in oversaturation of the adenine nucleotide pools in lymphocytes. Consequently, phosphoribosyl pyrophosphate synthetase is inhibited[15] resulting in disturbances in the *de novo* synthesis of not only pyrimidine but also purine nucleotides, as well as in the salvage reactions utilizing nucleobases[9]. Alternatively, an even more widespread perturbation of nucleotide-dependent metabolism may exist in the cells, and inhibit the normal cellular responses to mitogenic stimuli.

Acknowledgements

This work was supported by the State Medical Research Council, Finnish Academy, and by the Cancer Research Foundation, Helsinki. Technical assistance by Mrs Anneli Virtanen, Miss Helena Kainulainen and Mrs Virpi Tiilikainen is gratefully acknowledged.

References

1. Allison, A. C., Hovi, T., Watts, R. W. E. and Webster, A. D. B. (1977). The role of *de novo* purine synthesis in lymphocyte responses to antigenic and mitogenic stimulation. In *Purine and Pyrimidine Metabolism*. Ciba Foundation Symposium 48, p. 207. (Amsterdam: Elsevier/Excerpta Medica/ North-Holland and Elsevier North-Holland Inc.)

2. Hovi, T., Allison, A. C., Raivio, K. O. and Vaheri, A. (1977). Purine metabolism and control of cell proliferation. In *Purine and Pyrimidine Metabolism*, Ciba Foundation Symposium 48, p. 225. (Amsterdam: Elsevier/ Excerpta Medica/North-Holland and Elsevier North-Holland Inc.)

3. Giblett, E. R., Anderson, J. E., Cohen, F. *et al.* (1972). Adenosine-deaminase deficiency in two patients with severely impaired cellular immunity. *Lancet*, ii, 1067

4. Giblett, E. R., Ammann, A. J., Wara, D. W., *et al.* (1975). Nucleoside-phosphorylase deficiency in a child with severely defective T-cell immunity and normal B-cell immunity. *Lancet*, i, 1010

5. Wara, D. W. and Ammann, A. J. (1975). Laboratory data. In H. J. Meuwissen, R. J. Pickering, B. Pollara, and I. H. Porter (eds.). *Combined Immunodeficiency Disease and Adenosine Deaminase Deficiency. A Molecular Defect.* p. 247. (New York: Academic Press)

6. Polmar, J. H., Stern, R. C., Schwartz, A. L., Wetzler, E. M., Chase, P. A. and Hirschhorn, R. (1976). Enzyme replacement therapy for adenosine deaminase deficiency and severe combined immunodeficiency disease. *N. Engl. J. Med.*, **295**, 1337

7. Fox, I. H., Keystone, E. C., Gladman, D. D., Moore, M. and Cane, D. (1975). Inhibition of mitogen-mediated lymphocyte blastogenesis by adenosine. *Immunol. Commun.*, **4**, 419

8. Carson, D. A. and Seegmiller, J. E. (1976). Effect of adenosine deaminase inhibition upon human lymphocyte blastogenesis. *J. Clin. Invest.*, **57**, 274

9. Hovi, T., Smyth, J. F., Allison, A. C. and Williams, S. C. (1976). Role of adenosine deaminase in lymphocyte proliferation. *Clin. Exp. Immunol.*, **23**, 395

10. Green, H. (1975). Pyrimidine starvation induced by adenosine in cultured cells and its bearing on the lymphocyte deficiency disease associated with absence of adenosine deaminase. In H. J. Meuwissen, R. J. Pickering, B. Pollara, and I. H. Porter (eds.). *Combined Immunodeficiency Disease and Adenosine Deaminase Deficiency. A Molecular Defect.*, p. 141. (New York: Academic Press)

11. Kelley, W. N., Paddona, P. E. and van der Weyden, M. B. (1977). Characterization of human adenosine deaminase. In *Purine and Pyrimidine Metabolism*, Ciba Foundation Symposium 48, p. 277. (Amsterdam: Elsevier/ Excerpta Medica/North-Holland and Elsevier North-Holland Inc.)

12. Hovi, T., Mosher, D. and Vaheri, A. (1977). Cultured human monocytes synthesize and secrete α_2-macroglobulin. *J. Exp. Med.*, **145**, 1580

13. Raivio, K. O. and Hovi, T. (1977) Adenine and adenosine metabolism in phytohaemagglutinin (PHA) – stimulated and unstimulated normal human lymphocytes. In M. M. Müller, E. Kaisch and J. E. Seegmiller (eds.). *Purine Metabolism in Man – II: Regulation of Pathways and Enzyme Defects.* (New York: Plenum Publishing Corp.)

14. Seegmiller, J. E., Watanabe, T. and Schreier, M. H. (1977). The effect of adenosine on lymphoid cell proliferation and antibody formation. In *Purine and Pyrimidine Metabolism*, Ciba Foundation Symposium 48, p. 249. (Amsterdam: Elsevier/Excerpta Medica/North-Holland and Elsevier North-Holland Inc.)

15. Fox, I. and Kelley, W. N. (1972). Human phosphoribosyl pyrophosphate synthetase. Kinetic mechanism and end-product inhibition. *J. Biol. Chem.*, **247**, 2126

11

Activity of adenosine deaminase and purine nucleoside phosphorylase in lymphocytes of man, horse and cattle

W. J. M. Tax and J. H. Veerkamp

INTRODUCTION

Deficiency of adenosine deaminase (ADA) or purine nucleoside phosphorylase (PNP) in man is associated with defects of cell-mediated immunity. In horse and cattle ADA activity is virtually absent from erythrocytes[1, 2]. A low activity of PNP was reported for bovine erythrocytes[3]. If ADA and PNP activities in lymphocytes from horse and cattle are also low, these cells might provide suitable animal models for studying the metabolic disturbances caused by deficiency of ADA or PNP. Therefore we measured the activities of ADA and PNP in erythrocytes and lymphocytes of horse, cattle and man. Previously we reported large differences between erythrocytes of ten mammalian species in activities of several other enzymes of purine and pyrimidine metabolism[4, 5]. We have now found large variations between man, horse and cattle in ADA and PNP activities of erythrocytes and lymphocytes. The ADA activity in horse lymphocytes is low and comparable to that in lymphocytes of patients with severe combined immunodeficiency. Since several lines of evidence[6-9] suggest that ADA and PNP deficiency lead to interference with pyrimidine metabolism, we tried to evaluate the relative contributions of *de novo* synthesis and the salvage pathway to the synthesis of pyrimidine nucleotides in lymphocytes of man and horse. The ratio of activities of orotidylate decarboxylase and uridine kinase in lymphocytes showed a large difference between these two species.

MATERIALS AND METHODS

Enzyme preparation

Heparinized blood samples were obtained from adult human volunteers, from healthy adult horses, and from cattle at the local slaughterhouse. Erythrocytes were isolated by centrifugation, washed twice with Tris-buffered saline (pH 7.4) and lysed by adding 3 vol 10 mM Tris (pH 7.4). Lymphocytes were isolated from peripheral blood using Ficoll-Isopaque according to Böyum[10]. Cells were counted with a haemocytometer and lysed by sonication (Branson sonifier, eight periods of 5 s at maximal output). Intact or sonicated lymphocytes as indicated were used for all enzyme assays except for uridine kinase which was measured in the 20 000 g (30 min) supernatant of sonicated extracts. All enzyme assays with lymphocytes were performed immediately upon preparation. Freshly prepared haemolysates were used for ADA assays.

Enzyme assays

All enzymes were assayed at 37 °C by radiochemical methods. Enzyme activities are expressed as nmol/h per 10^6 lymphocytes or for erythrocytes as nmol/h per mg protein. Protein was measured according to Lowry *et al.*[11] Isotonic conditions were maintained during incubations with intact lymphocytes.

Adenosine deaminase assay

The reaction mixture (60 μl) of lymphocytes contained 40 mM phosphate buffer (pH 7.4), 110 mM NaCl, 0.16 mM [8-^{14}C]adenosine (49 mCi/mmol) and the equivalent of $0.025–0.25 \times 10^6$ cells. Haemolysates were assayed by incubating haemolysate protein (60–3000 μg) with 50 mM Tris-HCl buffer (pH 7.4), 1 mM EDTA and 0.16 mM [8-^{14}C]adenosine in a final volume of 60 μl. After 30 min reaction was terminated by boiling for 2 min and addition of excess carrier adenosine, inosine and hypoxanthine. Separation was achieved by high voltage electrophoresis using 40 mM sodium borate (pH 8.65) containing 1 mM EDTA (1 h at 70 V/cm). Spots were localized under ultraviolet light and eluted with 5 ml of 0.1 M NaOH. Radioactivity was determined in 10 ml of Aquasol.

Purine nucleoside phosphorylase assay

Assay conditions in lymphocytes were the same as for ADA except that 0.35 mM [8-^{14}C]inosine (9 mCi/mmol) replaced adenosine and total volume was 50 μl. Incubation mixture for measuring PNP in haemolysates contained 30 mM Tris-HCl (pH 7.4), 1 mM EDTA, 100 mM phosphate (pH 7.4) and 0.35 mM [8-^{14}C]inosine in a volume of 50 μl. Incubations were terminated after 10 min by boiling for 2 min and adding of carrier inosine and hypoxanthine. Substrate and product were separated by thin-layer chromatography on polyethyleneimine-cellulose using distilled water as developer and eluted with 1 ml 0.1 M HCl/0.2 M KCl. Radioactivity was determined after addition of 10 ml of Aquasol.

Uridine kinase assay

The system (100 μl) contained 25 mM Tris (pH 7.4), 50 mM NaCl, 5 mM ATP, 5 mM MgCl$_2$, 0.15 mM [2-^{14}C]uridine (57 mCi/mmol) and the supernatant of $0.5–2 \times 10^6$ cells. Reaction was terminated after 60 min by boiling the reaction mixture for 2 min. After addition of carrier uridine and uracil samples were analysed as described for PNP assay.

Orotidylate decarboxylase assay

The incubation mixture (525 μl) contained 50 mM tris buffer (pH 7.4), 100 mM NaCl, 0.1 mM [carboxyl-^{14}C]orotidine-5′-monophosphate (1 mCi/mmol) and the sonicated suspension of $2–20 \times 10^6$ lymphocytes. Reaction was terminated after 60 min by injection of 0.2 ml 5 M perchloric acid. Production of $^{14}CO_2$ was measured as described before[12].

RESULTS

With all enzyme assays, product formation was linear with time and protein concentration. In ADA assays, both inosine and hypoxanthine were formed due to the presence of PNP activity. No AMP was formed from adenosine by lymphocytes, and the addition of EDTA prevented the production of AMP in haemolysates. Hypoxanthine was the only product formed from inosine in PNP assays. When uridine kinase was assayed, no significant radioactivity was associated with uracil due to the absence of phosphate in the incubation mixture.

ADA activity in cattle haemolysate was low when compared with the activity in human haemolysate and was below detection limit in horse haemolysate (Table 11.1). Cattle haemolysate also showed a low PNP

TABLE 11.1 ADA and PNP activities in haemolysates of man, cattle and horse

Species	ADA	PNP
Man	59 ± 18	1249 ± 222
Cattle	0.7 ± 0.7	39 ± 17
Horse	< 0.2	1.0 ± 0.5

Enzyme activities in nmol/h per mg protein. Values are the means $\pm$ SD of three to five determinations

activity. PNP activity was still lower in haemolysate of horse. Species differences in PNP activity were much smaller in lymphocytes (Table 11.2). PNP and ADA activities were consistently lower (about 50%) in intact lymphocytes than in sonicated lymphocytes. ADA activity in horse lymphocytes was only a few per cent of the value found in human lymphocytes, while cattle lymphocytes had an intermediate value.

The activity of orotidylate decarboxylase was lower in horse lympho-

TABLE 11.2 ADA and PNP activities in lymphocytes of man, cattle and horse

	ADA		PNP	
Species	Intact cells	Lysate	Intact cells	Lysate
Man	44 ± 15	102 ± 30	177 ± 48	385 ± 154
Cattle	21 ± 7	50 ± 18	48 ± 18	96 ± 12
Horse	4 ± 2	7 ± 2	42 ± 3	74 ± 22

Enzyme activities in nmol/h per 10^6 cells
Values are the means $\pm$ SD of four determinations

TABLE 11.3   Activities of uridine kinase and orotidylate decarboxylase in lymphocytes of man and horse

Species	Uridine kinase	Orotidylate decarboxylase	Ratio ODC/ Uridine kinase
Man	0.38 ± 0.20 (5)	0.67 ± 0.24 (7)	1.76
Horse	1.08 ± 0.49 (5)	0.11 ± 0.02 (3)	0.10

Enzyme activities in nmol/h per 10^6 cells. Values are the means ± SD. Numbers in parentheses refer to the number of individuals. Orotidylate decarboxylase was measured in sonic extracts of lymphocytes. Uridine kinase was measured in 20 000 g (30 min) supernatant of sonic extracts

cytes than in human lymphocytes (Table 11.3), but uridine kinase activity was higher. The ratio of ODC activity over uridine kinase activity differs markedly between the two species.

DISCUSSION

Activities of ADA and PNP in human haemolysate (Table 11.1) are comparable to those reported by other investigators[13-19]. The low value of PNP activity in horse haemolysate has not been reported before. ADA activity in lysed human lymphocytes (Table 11.2) is similar to values measured by others in total lysate from lymphocytes[13] or in 20 000 g supernatant of sonic extracts[18]. However, PNP activity in total lysate (Table 11.2) seems to be much higher than the values reported for 20 000 g supernatants[18,19]. This finding suggests that part of the lymphocyte PNP activity is membrane-associated, as is proposed for fibroblasts[20]. Both ADA and PNP activities are lower in intact lymphocytes than in sonicated lymphocytes (Table 11.2) probably because the uptake of nucleosides is rate-limiting[18].

Deficiency of ADA in man is associated with immunodeficiency. Horses have a normal immune response despite low ADA activity in their lymphocytes (Table 11.2). This discrepancy may be related to major differences in lymphocyte purine and/or pyrimidine metabolism between man and horse. Adenosine is involved in the salvage pathway of purines (Figure 11.1). The consecutive action of ADA and PNP on adenosine produces ribose-1-P which may serve as a precursor of PRPP. In this way adenosine metabolism may be involved in *de novo* synthesis of both purine nucleotides (Figure 11.1) and pyrimidine nucleotides (Figure 11.2). Accumulation of adenosine may also cause increased concentrations of adenine nucleotides, which may inhibit either PRPP synthetase or enzymes of

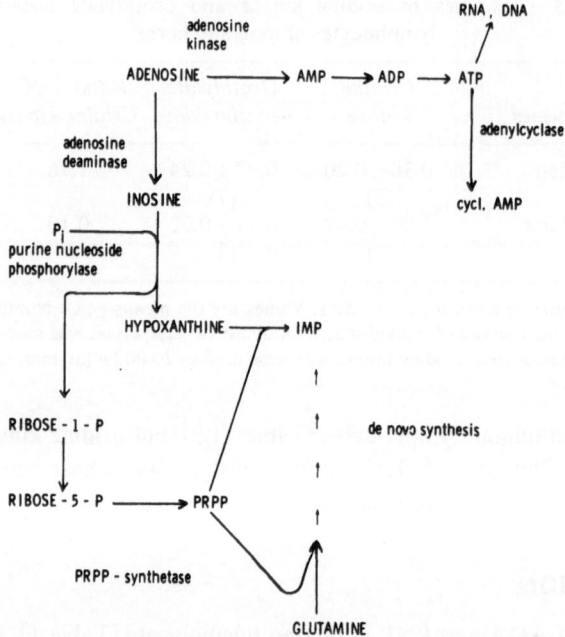

Figure 11.1   Salvage pathway and *de novo* synthesis of purine nucleotides

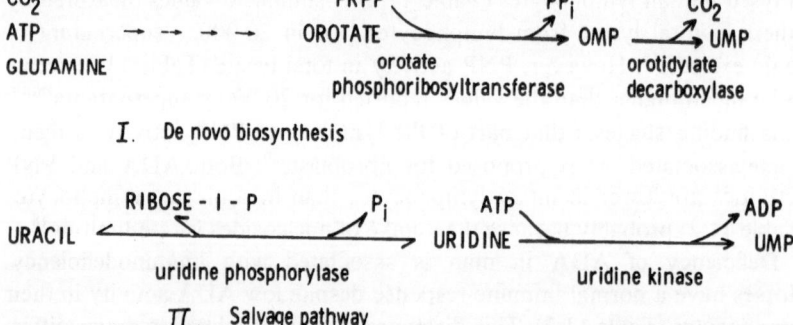

Figure 11.2   Salvage pathway and *de novo* synthesis of pyrimidine nucleotides

pyrimidine nucleotide synthesis *de novo*. When ADA and PNP deficiency lead to interference with pyrimidine synthesis *de novo* (and there is ample evidence[6-9] that they do) then such an interference could be bypassed if pyrimidine nucleotides are formed by the salvage pathway. The activity of human lymphocyte orotidylate decarboxylase (Table 11.3), an enzyme of *de novo* synthesis, is comparable to its activity in human leukocytes[12].

Uridine kinase activity is similar to the value reported by others[21]. The ratio of orotidylate decarboxylase and uridine kinase activities in horse lymphocytes appeared to be much lower than in human lymphocytes. This may indicate a preference for the salvage pathway in horse lymphocytes. The presence of cell-mediated immunity of horse despite ADA deficiency in lymphocytes might also be related to a low plasma concentration of adenosine, a low uptake rate of adenosine and/or low adenosine kinase activity in lymphocytes of horse in comparison to man and/or by an adequate synthesis in horse lymphocytes of PRPP from ribose-5-P obtained from the hexose monophosphate shunt.

Acknowledgements

We like to thank Miss M. Jaminon, Mr A. Oosterhof and Mr F. Peters for technical assistance. This investigation was supported by the Dutch Foundation for Medical Scientific Research (Z.W.O.–FUNGO).

References

1. Moore, E. C. and Meuwissen, H. J. (1974). Screening for ADA deficiency. *J. Pediatr.*, **85**, 802
2. Van Belle, H. (1969). Uptake and deamination of adenosine by blood. Species differences, effect of pH, ions, temperature and metabolic inhibitors. *Biochim. Biophys. Acta*, **192**, 124
3. Duhm, J. (1974). Inosine permeability and purine nucleoside phosphorylase activity as limiting factors for the synthesis of 2,3-diphosphoglycerate from inosine, pyruvate, and inorganic phosphate in erythrocytes of various mammalian species. *Biochim. Biophys. Acta*, **343**, 89
4. Tax, W. J. M., Veerkamp, J. H. and Trijbels, J. M. F. (1976). Activity of purine phosphoribosyltransferases and of two enzymes of pyrimidine biosynthesis in erythrocytes of ten mammalian species. *Comp. Biochem. Physiol.*, **54B**, 209
5. Tax, W. J. M. and Veerkamp, J. H. (1978). Phosphoribosylpyrophosphate in erythrocytes of ten mammalian species: concentration, synthesis and degradation. *Comp. Biochem. Physiol.* **59B**, 219
6. Green, H. (1975). Pyrimidine starvation induced by adenosine in cultured cells and its bearing on the lymphocyte deficiency disease associated with absence of adenosine deaminase. In H. J. Meuwissen, B. Pollara and R. J. Pickering (eds.). *Combined Immunodeficiency Disease and Adenosine Deaminase Deficiency: A Molecular Defect.* p. 141. (New York: Academic Press)
7. Snyder, F. F. and Seegmiller, J. E. (1976). The adenosine-like effect of exogenous cyclic AMP upon nucleotide and PP-ribose-P concentrations of cultured human lymphoblasts. *FEBS Lett.*, **66**, 102
8. Cohen, A., Staal, G. E., Ammann, A. J. and Martin, D. W. (1977). Orotic

aciduria in two unrelated patients with inherited deficiencies of purine nucleoside phosphorylase. *J. Clin. Invest.*, **60**, 491

9. Ullman, B., Cohen, A. and Martin, D. W. (1976). Characterization of a cell culture model for the study of adenosine deaminase and purine nucleoside phosphorylase deficient immunologic disease. *Cell*. **9**, 205

10. Böyum, A. (1968). Isolation of mononuclear cells and granulocytes from human blood. Isolation of mononuclear cells by one centrifugation, and of granulocytes by combining centrifugation and sedimentation at 1 *g. Scand. J. Clin. Lab. Invest.*, **21 (Suppl. 97)**, 77

11. Lowry, O. H., Rosebrough, N. J., Farr, A. L. and Randall, R. J. (1951). Protein measurement with the Folin phenol reagent. *J. Biol. Chem.*, **193**, 265

12. Tax, W. J. M., Veerkamp, J. H., Trijbels, J. M. F. and Schretlen, E. D. A. M. (1976). Mechanism of allopurinol-mediated inhibition and stabilization of human orotate phosphoribosyltransferase and orotidine phosphate decarboxylase. *Biochem. Pharmacol.*, **25**, 2025

13. Cartier, P. and Hamet. M. (1976). Dosage de l'activité adénosine désaminasique dans les érythrocytes et les lymphocytes humains. *Clin. Chim. Acta*, **71**, 429

14. Polmar, S. H., Stern, R. C., Schwartz, A. L., Wetzler, E. M., Chase, P. A. and Hirschhorn, R. (1976). Enzyme replacement therapy for adenosine deaminase deficiency and severe combined immunodeficiency. *N. Engl. J. Med.*, **295**, 1337

15. Parkman, R., Gelfand, E. W., Rosen, F. S., Sanderson, A. and Hirschhorn, R. (1975). Combined immuno- and adenosine deaminase deficiency. *N. Engl. J. Med.*, **292**, 714

16. Coleman, M. S. and Hutton, J. J. (1975). Micromethod for quantitation of adenosine deaminase activity in cells from human peripheral blood. *Biochem. Medicine*, **13**, 46

17. Tung, R., Silber, R., Quagliata, F., Conklyn, M., Gottesman, J. and Hirschhorn, R. (1977). Adenosine deaminase activity in chronic lymphocytic leukemia. Relationship to B- and T-cell subpopulations. *J Clin. Invest.*, **57**, 756

18. Snyder, F. F., Mendelsohn, J. and Seegmiller, J. F. (1976). Adenosine metabolism in phytohemagglutinin-stimulated human lymphocytes. *J. Clin. Invest.*, **58**, 654

19. Scholar, E. M. and Calabresi, P. (1973). Identification of the enzymatic pathways of nucleotide metabolism in human lymphocytes and leukemia cells. *Cancer Res.*, **33**, 94

20. Cohen, A. and Martin, D. W. (1977). Inosine uptake by cultured fibroblasts from normal and purine nucleoside phosphorylase-deficient humans. *J. Biol. Chem.*, **252**, 4428

21. Ito, K. and Uchino, H. (1976). Control of pyrimidine biosynthesis in human lymphocytes. Inhibitory effect of guanine and guanosine on induction of enzymes for pyrimidine biosynthesis *de novo* in phytohemagglutinin-stimulated lymphocytes. *J. Biol. Chem.*, **251**, 1427

12

Ageing and activities of purine metabolizing enzymes in leukocytes
J. Mejer and P. Nygaard

Purine metabolizing enzymes refer to a series of enzymes which synthesize, transform and catabolize purine compounds. The salvage of purines and purine nucleosides provides the cells with nucleotides in addition to those derived from the biosynthesis *de novo*; purine salvage may be the only or major pathway by which leukocytes synthesize their purine nucleotides.

The enzymatic reactions involved in the reutilization of purines and purine nucleosides have attracted great interest as a result of their relevance to a number of diseases.

Thus the occurrence of a deficiency of adenosine deaminase in some patients with severe combined immunodeficiency[1], and a deficiency of purine nucleoside phosphorylase activity associated with impaired T lymphocyte function[2], suggested a relationship between purine metabolism and the functioning of the immune system. Studies with synthetic inhibitors of adenosine deaminase also led to the conclusion that inhibition of adenosine deaminase in lymphocyte cultures resulted in an inhibition of cellular proliferation and function[3].

Purine metabolism also includes enzymes which are not known to be directly involved in the function of the immunocompetent cells. However, changes in the activity of some of these enzymes might be compensated for by variations in other enzymes of this group.

The purpose of the present investigation was to determine whether there was an age-related change in the activities of purine metabolizing enzymes in leukocytes, in order to evaluate the hypothesis that altered patterns of purine metabolizing enzymes might be associated with a reduced immune response during ageing.

Our interest in purine salvage pathways in relation to ageing was primarily stimulated by the finding of large variations in adenosine deaminase activities in leukocytes from patients with malignancies.

The enzymes whose activities were measured were the basic enzymes in the salvage pathways (Figure 12.1) and include: (1) adenosine deaminase,

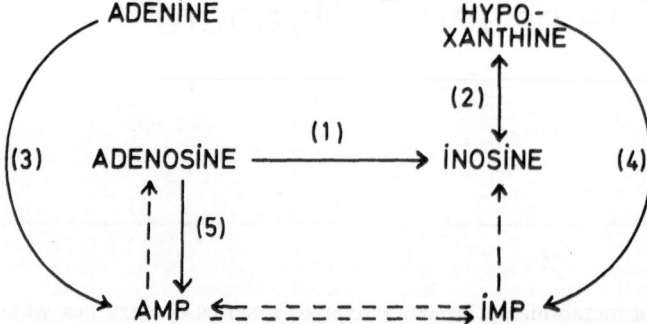

Figure 12.1 Purine metabolizing enzymes in leukocytes: ⎯⎯ enzymes studied; ⎯ ⎯ ⎯ other enzymes where presence or function is not well established. Reactions including deoxynucleosides, guanine and xanthine compounds are not depicted. The enzymes studied here are (1) adenosine deaminase, (2) purine nucleoside phosphorylase, (3) adenine phosphoribosyltransferase, (4) hypoxanthine phosphoribosyltransferase and (5) adenosine kinase. These pathways are required for the utilization and catabolism of purine bases and nucleosides from nucleic acid and nucleotide breakdown, derived from the diet or released from other tissues into blood circulation

which deaminates adenosine to inosine; (2) purine nucleoside phosphorylase, which phosphorolyzes inosine and guanosine to ribose-1-phosphate and hypoxanthine or guanine; (3) adenine phosphoribosyltransferase, which catalyses AMP synthesis from adenine and phosphoribosylpyrophosphate; (4) hypoxanthine phosphoribosyltransferase, which catalyses the synthesis of IMP and GMP from phosphoribosylpyrophosphate and hypoxanthine and guanine respectively; and (5) adenosine kinase, which catalyses the synthesis of AMP from adenosine.

METHODS

Leukocytes were obtained from heparinized peripheral blood by sedimentation of erythrocytes in 6% dextran[4]. From the leukocyte-rich plasma a granulocyte-rich fraction and a fraction of mononuclear cells, predominantly composed of lymphocytes, were isolated by isopycnic separation[4]. The isolated cells were frozen at -20 °C, and were thawed by resuspension in 0.1 M Tris-Cl pH 8.1 at 0–4 °C. Homogenization was performed with an ultrasonic probe for 1 min. The homogenate was centrifuged for 5 min at 8000 g. Enzyme assays were performed at 37 °C and activities are expressed as nmol substrate converted per mg protein in 1 h. Protein was determined according to Lowry et al.[5]

Purine nucleoside phosphorylase activity was determined spectrophotometrically with inosine as substrate[6]. Adenosine deaminase activity was performed by spectrophotometric measurement of the conversion of adenosine to inosine[7]. Adenine and hypoxanthine phosphoribosyltransferase activities were assayed chromatographically by measuring the conversion of ^{14}C-labelled adenine or hypoxanthine into their corresponding mononucleotides[7].

For adenosine kinase the assay mixture consisted of 50 mM Tris-Cl pH 7.6; 30 μM [8-^{14}C]adenosine (10 μCi/μmol); 1.5 mM ATP; 2.5 mM phosphoenolpyruvate; 25 units of pyruvate kinase; 0.3 mM dithiothreitol; 5 μM coformycin; 1.5 mM $MgCl_2$; 25 mM KCl; 1 mM KF and 25 μl of enzyme solution (2–6 mg protein/ml) in a total volume of 100 μl. At 2, 4 and 8 min 10 μl samples were removed and mixed with 5 μl 5 mM AMP and chromatographed on polyethyleneimine-impregnated cellulose plates. Quantitative determinations were performed as described for other purine enzymes[6].

RESULTS AND DISCUSSION

Table 12.1 presents the activities of adenosine deaminase and purine nucleoside phosphorylase obtained from different separated cell groups including leukocytes, mononuclear cells and granulocytes. Sixteen donors from 20 to 57 years were investigated, all had a normal leukocyte and differential count and haemoglobin. No differences were observed in activities per mg protein of adenosine deaminase and purine nucleoside phosphorylase between any of the different cell groups. From these findings, it was decided to assay on leukocytes rather than on separate types of leukocytes.

In malignancies (Table 12.2) it was observed that in acute myeloblastic

TABLE 12.1 Adenosine deaminase and purine nucleoside phosphorylase levels in white blood cells

	No	Adenosine deaminase nmol/h/mg protein		Purine nucleoside phosphorylase nmol/h/mg protein	
		mean	range	mean	range
Leukocytes	16	526	368–768	5426	3888–7640
Mononuclear cells	16	587	178–906	5223	2670–8876
Granulocytes	16	482	252–1035	5712	3293–8192

TABLE 12.2 Adenosine deaminase and purine nucleoside phosphorylase levels in leukocytes from patients with malignancies

Diagnosis	No	Adenosine deaminase nmol/h/mg protein range	Purine nucleoside phosphorylase nmol/h/mg protein range
Bronchogenic carcinoma	4	130–207	4729–4892
Lymphosarcoma	2	207–424	2346–5094
Chronic lymphocytic leukaemia	4	282–1120	1440–4441
Chronic myelocytic leukaemia	4	330–3384	5011–11085
Acute myeloblastic leukaemia	4	896–6125	2636–5114
Acute lymphoblastic leukaemia	2	207–478	4800–5094
Controls	16	368–786	3888–7640

leukaemia patients high activities of adenosine deaminase were present, whereas the opposite was found in leukocytes from patients with bronchogenic carcinoma. Low activities were also found in acute lymphoblastic leukaemia, whereas in chronic myelocytic leukaemia, chronic lymphocytic leukaemia and lymphosarcoma varying levels of activities were present.

Variations in enzyme activities in leukocytes from patients with malignancies were apparently unaffected by age. No differences in purine nucleoside phosphorylase activity were found between controls and patients with malignancies, except one patient with chronic lymphocytic leukaemia with low activity.

If age-dependent variations in purine metabolism were present, one might find minor variations in adenosine deaminase or purine nucleoside phosphorylase. Other enzymes in the salvage pathways might compensate for such minor variations. For example one patient with chronic lymphocytic leukaemia had a high level of adenosine deaminase activity (1120 nmol/mg/h). At the same time, adenine phosphoribosyltransferase and

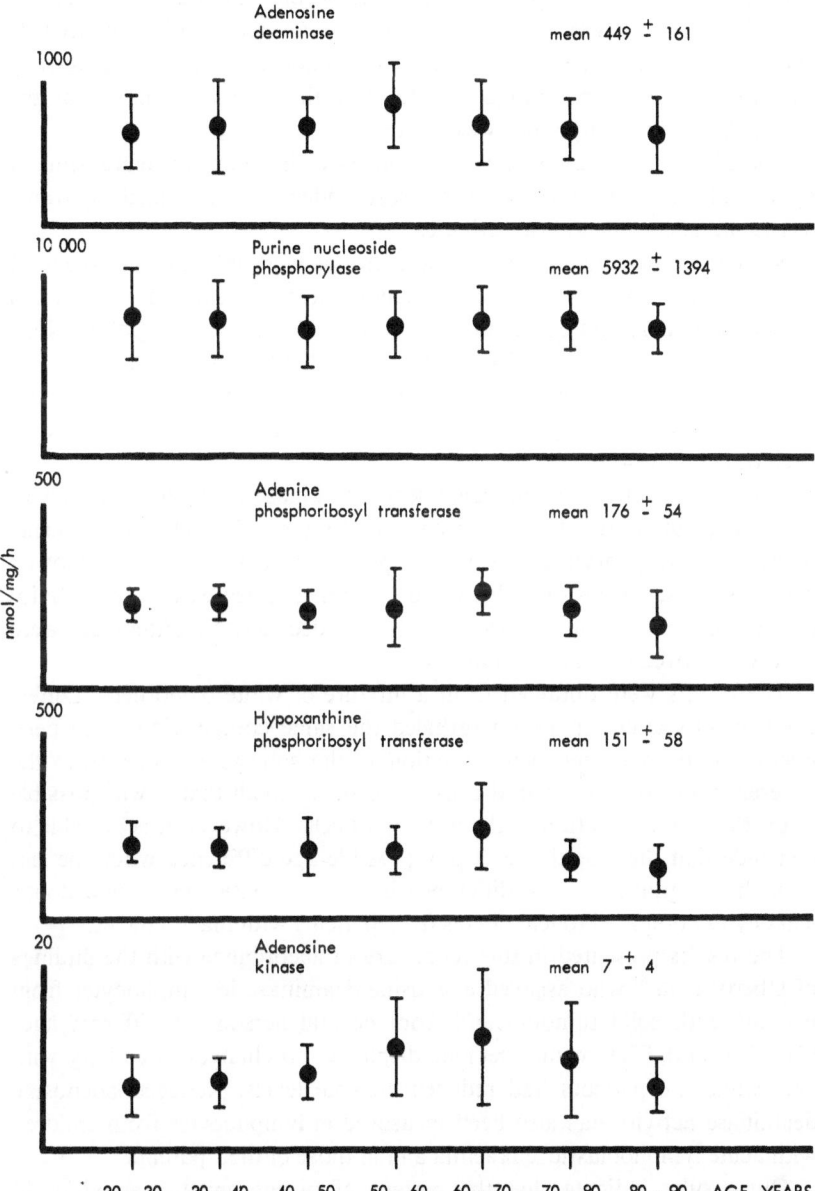

Figure 12.2   Levels of purine metabolizing enzymes in leukocytes of healthy persons from 20 to 90 years. Mean values ± standard deviation from the different age groups are included. Enzymes activities are expressed as (nmol/h per mg protein)

adenosine kinase activities were elevated 4-fold and purine nucleoside phosphorylase activity (1440 nmol/mg/h) was decreased compared to activities from controls; hypoxanthine phosphoribosyltransferase activity was within the normal range. In this way the enzymatic basis for the salvage of purine compounds was present.

Therefore, the present investigation also includes measurement of hypoxanthine phosphoribosyltransferase, adenine phosphoribosyltransferase and adenosine kinase activities.

Sixty-three persons of different age groups were investigated. None of the 63 persons had any malignant diagnosis at the time of study; each had normal leukocyte and differential count and a normal haemoglobin. None of the persons had had any disease in the month preceding the study.

Nine persons were investigated in each decade from 20 to 90 years. Of the 63 studied, 32 were females and 31 males. The female:male ratio in each decade was 4 to 5.

The activity of adenosine deaminase and kinase at different age levels from 20 to 90 years showed no changes (Figure 12.2). Assay of purine nucleoside phosphorylase and the two phosphoribosyltransferases showed similar results, except for a slight and insignificant decrease in the activity of the phosphoribosyltransferases in the last decades. No differences were observed between females and males.

The results were obtained from a mixture of white blood cells. Differential counts after separation revealed the same composition as in peripheral blood. Age-dependent variation in the salvage enzymes from the different types of white blood cells could be so small that it was possible to overlook this variation in the mixture of cells. However, it is possible to conclude that the magnitude of any possible age difference would be less than the magnitude of the difference between activities in normal donor leukocytes compared to leukocytes from patients with malignancies.

The results presented in this report are in accordance with the findings of Uberty et al.[8], who assayed adenosine deaminase in lymphocytes from patients with solid tumours and from normal persons of different ages (21–62 years). The normal persons displayed no changes in activity with age, while the patients had reduced enzyme levels. Reduced adenosine deaminase activity has also been measured in lymphocytes from children with acute lymphoblastic leukaemia and in those of their parents[9].

Our results indicate that the pattern of purine enzyme activities in leukocytes is apparently unaffected by age. However, it cannot be excluded that the impaired function and the increased incidence of neoplastic disease with age are influenced by variations in the functioning of purine salvage pathways.

Acknowledgements

This study was supported by grants from Danish Cancer Society and The Danish Medical Research Council.

References

1. Giblett, E. R., Anderson, J. E., Cohen, F., Pollara, B. and Meuwissen, H. J. (1972). Adenosine deaminase deficiency in two patients with severely impaired cellular immunity. *Lancet*, **ii**, 1067
2. Giblett, E. R., Ammann, A. J., Wara, D. W., Sandman, R. and Diamand, L. K. (1975). Nucleoside phosphorylase deficiency in a child with severely defective T-cell immunity and normal B-cell immunity. *Lancet*, **i**, 1010
3. Carson, D. A. and Seegmiller J. E. (1976). Effect of adenosine deaminase inhibition upon human lymphocyte blastogenesis. *J. Clin. Invest.*, **57**, 274
4. Bøyum, A. (1974). Separation of blood leukocytes, granulocytes and lymphocytes. *Tissue Antigens*, **4**, 269
5. Lowry, O. H., Rosebrough, N. J., Farr, A. L. and Randall, R. J. (1951). Protein measurement with folin phenol reagent. *J. Biol. Chem.*, **193**, 256
6. Jensen, K. F. and Nygaard, P. (1975). Purine nucleoside phosphorylase from *Escherichia coli* and *Salmonella typhimurium*. Purification and some properties. *Eur. J. Biochem.*, **51**, 253
7. Jochimsen, B., Nygaard, P. and Vestergaard, T. (1975). Location on the chromosome of *Escherichia coli* of genes governing purine metabolism. *Mol. Gen. Genet.*, **143**, 85
8. Uberti, J., Johnson, R. M., Talley, R. and Lightbody, J. J. (1976). Decreased lymphocyte adenosine deaminase activity in tumor patients. *Cancer Res.*, **36**, 2046
9. Zimmer, J., Khalifa, S. A. and Lightbody, J. J. (1975). Decreased lymphocyte adenosine deaminase activity in acute lymphocytic leukaemic children and their parents. *Cancer Res.*, **35**, 68

13

Immune function in Down's syndrome

B. Björkstén, O. Bäck, B. Hägglöf and A. Tärnvik

Children with Down's syndrome (DS) suffer from frequent infections and show an increased mortality in infectious diseases compared to a normal population[1]. There is an association between DS and acute leukaemia[2]. Several recent studies have demonstrated abnormalities in cell-mediated and humoral immunity[3-5], and in phagocyte function[6-8].

We have studied the host response including cell-mediated and humoral immunity, neutrophil granulocyte function and complement levels in a group of patients with DS in relation to frequency and severity of infections. We found depressed T cell function and neutrophil chemotactic responsiveness and low levels of IgM in the patients but we were not able to correlate the degree of immune deficiency with frequency and severity of infections.

MATERIALS AND METHODS

All patients between 6 and 20 years of age with DS living in Umeå were selected from a recent comprehensive investigation of severe mental deficiency in the county of Västerbotten, Sweden[9]. The records of these 38 patients were analysed with regard to frequency and type of infections and the patients were divided into three groups: Group I, patients with osteo-myelitis, septicaemia, bacterial meningitis, pneumonia on at least two occasions or recurrent fungal or severe viral infections, e.g. encephalitis or hepatitis. Group II were patients with chronic otitis or sinusitis. Patients without a history of increased number of infections belonged to group III.

A total of 16 patients were selected randomly for laboratory studies of host defence mechanisms, five from each groups I and III and six from group II. An informed consent was obtained from the parents of all these patients.

The patients were also sensitized to DNCB (1-chloro-2,4-dinitrobenzene) by the application of 25 μl of a 2% solution of DNCB in acetone to a skin area of 3 cm^2. The skin was then covered with a plastic film for 72 h. Three to four weeks later the patients were tested epicutaneously with graded amounts of DNCB. A normal patch test response provided redness and infiltration with 5 or 10 μg of DNCB after 72 h. Redness with 20 μg was considered as a weak response. Path tests with more than 20 μg DNCB applied to the circular test area (diameter 10 mm) regularly gave toxic reactions. Proportion of T lymphocytes in blood was determined by means of E-rosettes[10].

For lymphocyte stimulation defibrinated blood was separated on Ficoll-Isopaque[11]. Lymphocytes were suspended in a culture medium consisting of RPMI-HEPES (Gibco, Madison, Wisc.) supplemented with 15% pooled inactivated (56 °C, 30 min) human serum and antibiotics. To each well of a Microtest II tissue culture plate (Falcon Plastics, Los Angeles, Cal.) was added 100 μl of lymphocyte suspension and 100μl of phytohaemagglutinin (PHA, leukoagglutinin, Pharmacia AB, Uppsala, Sweden) appropriately diluted in culture medium. The final lymphocyte density was 10^6 per ml. Each microplate was closed with a film (Falcon Plastics) and incubated at 37 °C for 3 days. DNA synthesis of the lymphocytes was assayed as previously described[12].

Immunoglobulin IgG, IgM, IgA and complement factors (3 and 4) were determined by the radial immunodiffusion of Mancini et al.[13], using Partigen plates (Behringewerke AG, Marburg, W. Germany).

Total haemolytic activity of serum was tested according to routine techniques[14].

Neutrophil chemotaxis was measured by the leading front technique in modified Boyden chambers as described by Wilkinson[15], using 5% zymosan-activated pooled human serum as cytotaxin.

For the chemiluminescence assay[16], whole blood was drawn into heparinized tubes (20–30 IU heparin/ml) mixed with Dextran 4% (Pharmacia AB, Uppsala, Sweden) in proportion 2:1 and allowed to sediment in room temperature for 45–75 min. The leukocyte-rich supernatant was collected with great care taken to minimize erythrocyte contamination and centrifuged at $150 \times g$ for 5 min. The cell button was resuspended in 0.87% NH_4Cl for 5 min to lyse remaining red cells and then washed twice in RPMI (Flow Laboratories) to a final concentration of 10^7 polymorphonuclear leukocytes (PMN) per ml.

Zymosan (Sigma Co, St Louis, Mo) 50 mg/ml was suspended in saline. To opsonize the zymosan one volume of the suspension was incubated with three volumes pooled human serum at 37 °C for 30 min and then centrifuged at $2000 \times g$ at 4 °C for 30 min. The supernatant was used in a 5% dilution as 'activated serum' in the chemotaxis assays. The preopsonized zymosan particles were resuspended in RPMI to a final concentration of 12.5 mg/ml and used in the chemiluminescence assay within 2 h. One ml of the leukocyte suspension and 4.1 ml of RPMI were added into glass vials (Beckman Instruments). Chemiluminescence was measured in a liquid scintillation counter (Beckman LS 3100) operated in the out-of-coincidence mode at an ambient temperature of 23 °C. When constant background counts were recorded 0.4 ml of the preopsonized zymosan suspension was added to the vials. The mixture was then shaken vigorously for 30 sec. Chemiluminescence for the various mixtures was expressed as the peak values from which background counts were subtracted. Vials containing zymosan without PMN and PMN without zymosan served as controls.

RESULTS

Of the 38 patients with DS, nine (24%) belonged to group I, eleven (30%) to group II and 18 (46%) to group III (Table 13.1).

TABLE 13.1 Susceptibility to infections in DS and number of patients studied immunologically in each group

Group	Number boys	girls	%	Number studied immunologically
I. Recurrent severe infections	8	1	24	5
II. Recurrent respiratory tract infections	3	8	30	6
III. No increased incidence of infections	10	8	46	5
Total	21	17	100	16

TABLE 13.2   Results of certain laboratory studies of defence mechanisms against infections in DS

	DS	Normal values
Erythrocyte rosette-binding lymphocytes (%, mean ± SEM)	70 ± 3	71 ± 3
Reactivity to DNCB (no. of patients)		
normal	2	—
weak	4	—
absent	3	—
IgE units (± two SD)	18 ± 26	25 (−300)*
C3 g/l (mean ± two SD)	1.00 ± 0.48	0.95 ± 0.45
C4 g/l (mean ± two SD)	0.44 ± 0.50	0.26 ± 0.12
Neutrophil chemiluminescence (c.p.m. × 10³, mean ± SEM)	25.4 ± 2.8	24.6 ± 2.8

* Values represent geometric mean and + two SD

Studies on T cells were done in 12 patients, three from groups I, five from group II and four from group III. The proportion of E rosette binding lymphocytes was 70 ± 3%, i.e. normal in the patients (Table 13.2). However, lymphocytes from the patients showed significantly depressed

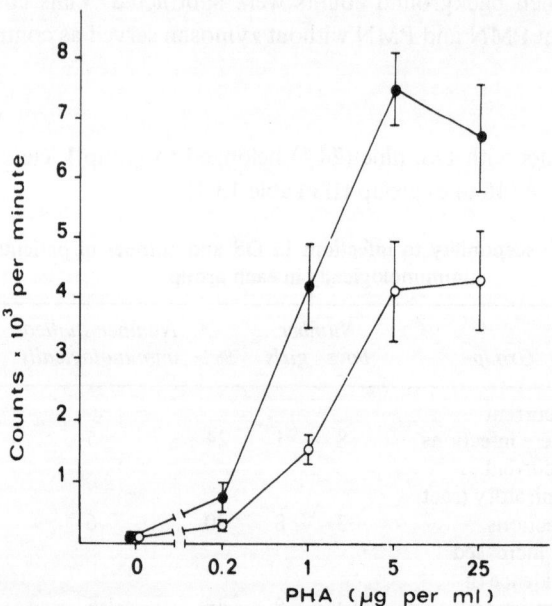

Figure 13.1   Dose–response curve to PHA by lymphocytes from patients with DS (open circles) and healthy persons (closed circles)

responsiveness to various concentrations of PHA (Figure 13.1). Skin tests revealed depressed delayed hypersensitivity in seven out of nine tested patients (Table 13.2). The results of these tests did not differ between the three groups of DS patients.

As shown in Figure 13.2 the serum levels of IgM were low, or in the low part of the normal range, while the levels of IgA were elevated in most patients. Similar results were obtained in all the three groups of patients.

The serum levels of IgG, IgE and C3 did not differ from normal. Elevated C4 levels (>0.5 g per 1) was seen in two patients. Total complement haemolytic activity, number and proportion of the various types of blood

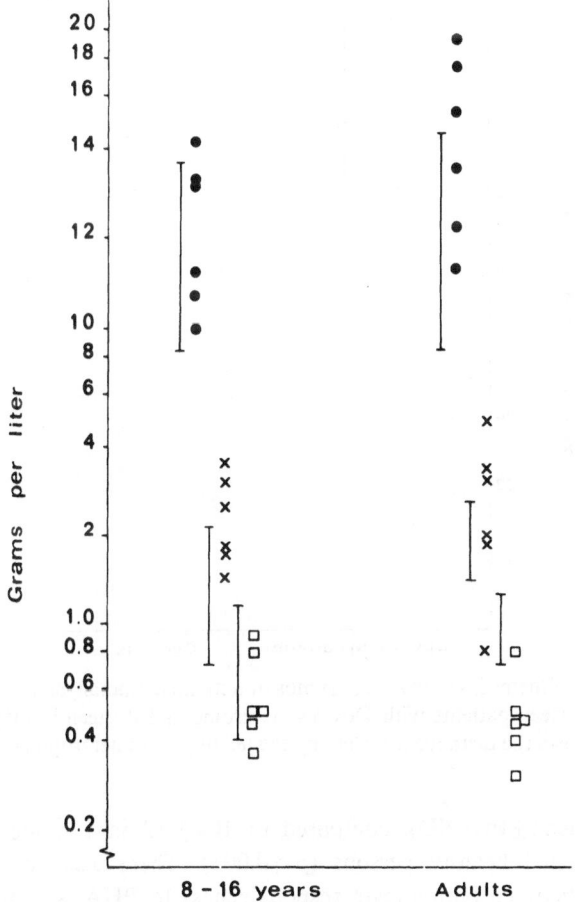

Figure 13.2   Immunoglobulin levels of IgG (●), IgA (×) and IgM (□) in DS compared to the range in normal persons (± two SD)

leukocytes and neutrophil chemiluminescence were normal in all patients investigated (Figure 13.1. Table 13.2).

Neutrophil chemotactic responsiveness was significantly depressed (Figure 13.3). The mean chemotaxis towards activated serum was 71 ± 15

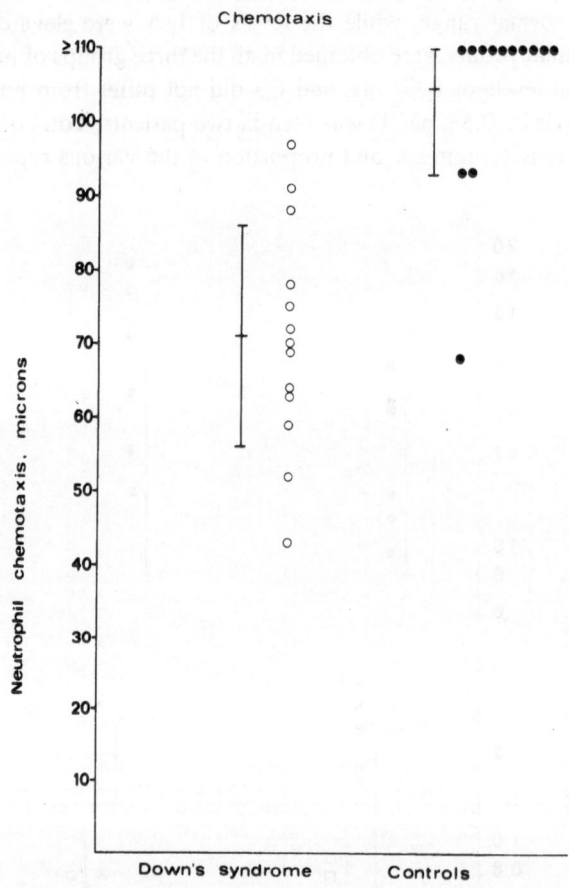

Figure 13.3 Chemotaxis towards zymosan-activated human serum of neutrophils from thirteen patients with Down's syndrome and thirteen healthy controls. The figure shows the distance travelled by the leading front neutrophils

microns, (mean ± two SD), compared to 104 ± 12 in a group of simultaneously tested healthy persons ($p < 0.001$). There was no significant correlation between lymphocyte responsiveness to PHA, serum IgM and neutrophil chemotaxis in the patients. The three groups of patients did not differ with regard to the test results.

DISCUSSION

Patients with DS have an increased morbidity in infectious diseases[1]. This was also shown in the present study; 24% of our patients had suffered from severe infectious diseases, 30% from chronic sinusitis or otitis media whereas 46% of the patients had no history of increased infection morbidity. Thus patients with DS apparently vary markedly with respect to frequency and severity of infections. We found no correlation between congenital heart defect and infection. We were not able to demonstrate any difference in the morbidity of infections between patients living in institutions and those living at home. Øster et al.[1], however, found a tendency to increased mortality in institutionalized patients. The reason for this discrepancy may be that our sample was too small to demonstrate any relationship between infections and care in institutions.

Lymphocytes from the patients with DS showed an impaired response to various doses of PHA when compared to those from healthy controls which confirms previous reports[3, 4, 17]. PHA mainly stimulates T lymphocytes. The impaired response was not due to a low percentage of T cells since we found the proportion of E rosette-forming lymphocytes to be normal. This is in accordance with a previous study[18]. Possible explanations for the impaired responsiveness include a shift in the relative proportions of helper and suppressor T lymphocytes or a subcellular defect of the responding T lymphocytes. Such a defect could involve any of numerous cellular events of the stimulation process, such as receptor function, phospholipid turnover of the membrane, levels of cyclic nucleotides and macromolecule synthesis, which all are known to be critical. The defect would however be only partial, since T lymphocytes from patients with DS do respond to PHA, although subnormally (Figure 12.1). The finding of abnormal skin reactivity to DNCB also suggests that T cell function in DS is abnormal.

Most patients in the present study had low levels of IgM. This is in agreement with previous reports[3, 19]. Abnormal T cell function, low IgM levels and recurrent infections are also present in the Wiskott–Aldrich syndrome, suggesting the possibility of a connection between the two immunological abnormalities.

The chemiluminescence assay provides a sensitive and reproducible technique for measuring neutrophil phagocytosis and postphagocytic metabolism[16, 20]. Using the yeast zymosan as stimulus of chemiluminescence we found DS neutrophils to have normal phagocytosis. This supports the findings of Seger et al.[5], who reported normal phagocytosis of C. albicans by DS neutrophils. However others have reported abnormal phagocytosis of *S. aureus*[6,7] and very recently of *C. albicans*[8]. Methodological differences may possibly explain the conflicting results. Gregory *et al.*[6] using bactericidal assay found defective killing of *S. aureus* in 16% of the patients. Kretschmer *et al.*[7] used NBT reduction as a measurement of phagocytosis. Since the normal increase in NBT reduction after phagocytosis is based on the ingestion of cophagocytized NBT solution[21], a diminished increase can also be caused by an impairment of phagocytosis in the presence of intact oxidative metabolism. Normal chemiluminescence proves the oxidative metabolism to be normal independent of host serum factors but does not exclude the possibility of delayed ingestion of microorganisms attached to the plasma membrane. Thus our data would indicate that the abnormal phagocytosis and killing of bacteria and fungi reported by others[6-8] are caused by depressed or delayed ingestion and not by defective oxidative metabolism.

Significantly depressed chemotaxis was found in DS. Chemotaxis in contrast to phagocytosis depends on normal function of microtubules[22,23]. Abnormal neutrophil chemotaxis and T cell function could possibly be explained by impaired function of contractile elements in the leukocytes. An intact function of microtubules seems to be crucial for a normal PHA response[24] as well as for neutrophil chemotaxis[22].

We were not able to relate the severity of immune deficiency to history of infections in the individual patients. Also there was no correlation between the degree of depressed PHA-stimulation, skin test results, neutrophil chemotaxis and IgM levels in the individual patients. Possibly the abnormalities of immunity reported here are only moderate and can usually be compensated for *in vivo*. Components of the defence system against infection other than those investigated in the present study may be responsible for the severity and frequency of infections in certain patients with DS.

Although several studies indicate an impaired cellular and humoral immune capacity in DS the underlying cause of the increased rate of infections in those patients remains unknown. The search for an underlying cause is complicated by the fact that the various deficiencies are only partial and vary between patients. Further studies of this problem may not only explain the increased incidence of infections in DS but also increase our knowledge of immune regulatory mechanisms in normal persons.

References

1. Øster, J., Mikkelsen, M. and Nielsen, A. (1975). Mortality and life-table in Down's syndrome. *Acta Paediatr. Scand.*, **64**, 322

2. Miller, M. E. (1970). Neoplasia and Down's syndrome. *Ann. N.Y. Acad. Sci.*, **171**, 637

3. Burgio, G. R., Ugazio, A. G., Nespoli, L., Marcioni, A. F., Botteli, A. M. and Pasquali, F. (1975). Derangements of immunoglobulin levels, phytohemagglutinin responsiveness and T and B cell markers in Down's syndrome at different ages. *Europ. J. Immunol.*, **5**, 600

4. Whittingham, S., Pitt, D. B., Sharma, D. L. B. and Mackay, I. R. (1977). Stress deficiency of the T-lymphocyte system exemplified by Down's syndrome. *Lancet*, **i**, 163

5. Seger, R., Buchinger, G. and Stroder, J. (1977). On the influence of age on immunity in Down's syndrome. *Europ. J. Pediat.*, **124**, 77

6. Gregory, L., Williams, R. and Thompson, E. (1972). Leukocyte function in Down's syndrome and acute leukaemia. *Lancet*, **i**, 1359

7. Kretschmer, R., López-Osuna, M., Dela Rosa, L. and Armendares, S. (1974). Leukocyte function in Down's syndrome. Quantitative NBT reduction and bactericidal capacity. *Clin. Immunol. Immunopathol.*, **2**, 449

8. Costello, C. and Webber, A. (1976). White cell function in Down's syndrome. *Clin. Genet.*, **9**, 603

9. Gustavson, K. H., Holmgren, G., Jonsell, R. and Blomquist, K. H. (1977). Severe mental retardation in children in a Northern Swedish county. *J. Mental Defic. Res.* (in press)

10. Jondal, M., Holm, G. and Wigzell, H. (1972). Surface markers on human T and B lymphocytes. I. A large population of lymphocytes forming non-immune rosettes with sheep red blood cells. *J. Exp. Med.*, **136**, 207

11. Böyum, A. (1968). Isolation of mononuclear cells and granulocytes from human blood. Isolation of mononuclear cells by one centrifugation. *Scand. J. Clin. Lab. Invest.*, **21 (suppl.)**, 27

12. Tärnvik, A. and Löfgren, S. (1975). Stimulation of human lymphocytes by a vaccine strain of *Francisella tularensis*. *Infect. Immunol.*, **12**, 951

13. Mancini, G., Carbonara, A. O. and Heremans, J. F. (1965). Immunochemical quantitation of antigens by single radial immune diffusion. *Int. J. Immunochem.*, **2**, 225

14. Bennet, C. W. (1968). *Clinical serology*. (Springfield, Ill.: Charles C. Thomas)

15. Wilkinson, P. C. (1974). *Chemotaxis and inflammation*, p. 163. (London: Churchill, Livingstone)

16. Allen, R. C., Stjernholm, R. L. and Steele, R. H. (1972). Evidence for the generation of an electronic excitation state(s) in human polymorphonuclear leukocytes and its participation in bactericidal activity. *Biochem. Biophys. Res. Commun.*, **47**, 679

17. Rigas, D. A., Elsasser, P. and Hecht, F. (1970). Impaired *in vitro* response of circulating lymphocytes to phytohemagglutinin in Down's syndrome: Dose- and time-response curves and relation to cellular immunity. *Int. Arch. Allergy Appl. Immunol.*, **39**, 587

18. Reiser, K., Whitcomb, C., Robinson, K. and MacKenzie, M. R. (1976). T and B lymphocytes in patients with Down's syndrome. *Am. J. Mental Def.*, **80**, 613

19. Stiehm, E. R. and Fudenberg, H. H. (1966). Serum levels of immune globulin in health and disease: a survey. *Pediatrics*, **37**, 715

20. Quie, P. G., Mills, E. L. and Holmes, B. (1977). Molecular events during phagocytosis by human neutrophils (in press)
21. Segal, A. W. and Levi, A. J. (1975). Factors influencing the entry of dye into neutrophil leukocytes in the nitroblue tetrazolium test. *Clin. Sci. Molec. Med.*, **48**, 201
22. Wilkinson, P. C. (1974). *Chemotaxis and inflammation*, p. 66 (London: Churchill, Livingstone)
23. Berlin, R. D. C. (1972). Effect of concanavalin A on phagocytosis. *Nature New Biol.*, **235**, 44
24. Wang, J. L., Gunther, G. R., Yahara, I., Cunningham, B. A. and Edelman, G. M. (1975). Receptor-cytoplasmic interactions and lymphocyte activation. In A. S. Rosenthal (ed.). *Immune Recognition*, p. 473

SECTION THREE

Disorders of Non-specific Immunity

14

Morphological and biochemical alterations of polymorphonuclear neutrophil (PMN) leukocytes from patients with inborn errors of phagocytic function: a comprehensive review
R. L. Baehner and L. A. Boxer

The purpose of this review is:

(1) to describe the cellular alterations in blood PMN during infection leading to phagocytic killing of bacteria at the site of infection;

(2) to separate these *in vivo* cellular alterations into specific sequential phases and to link selective *in vitro* tests of PMN function to each phase;

(3) to relate alterations of these tests to disorders of PMN phagocytic function; and

(4) to present examples of inborn errors of phagocytic function including

chronic granulomatous disease, Chediak–Higashi syndrome, actin dysfunction, and humoral deficiencies of complement components and specific immunoglobulins.

The blood phagocytes include PMN, monocytes, and eosinophils; each cell type is capable of carrying out all phases of the phagocytic act. However, the chief phagocytic cell is the PMN and it predominates in the bloodstream and bone marrow and participates extensively in eradication of pyogenic bacteria and certain fungi from extravascular sites. As pointed out by Rebuck[1] the PMN arrives at inflammatory sites rapidly after the inciting stimulus has been applied and continues to accumulate for 6–12 h before an influx of mononuclear cells occurs. This remarkable response of blood phagocytes to inciting stimuli such as tissue injury or infection has held the attention of investigators since the days of Eli Metchnikoff[2], the astute Russian biologist who injured a starfish larva with a thorn and observed the phagocytic process in its entirety.

Three related humoral systems are activated during bacterial infection; complement, kinin and plasmin play an integrative role in the inflammatory response[3]. Before the tissue becomes hyperaemic by the action of bradykinin, the circulating PMN marginates to the endothelial surface and adheres to it until finally it emigrates through the vascular endothelium

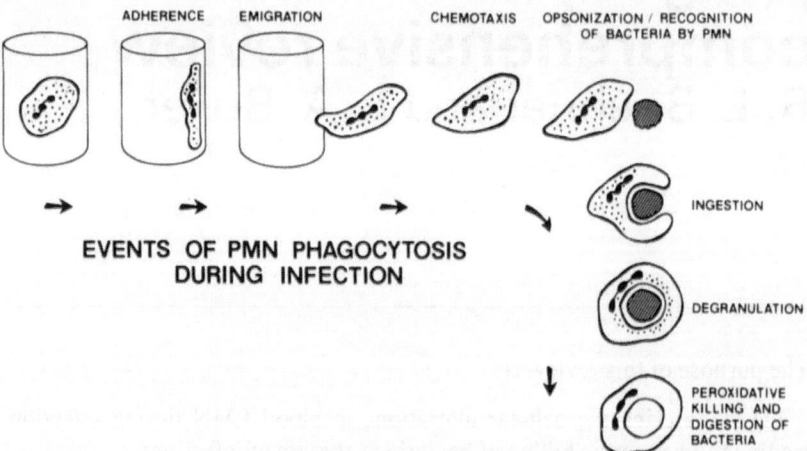

Figure 14.1   The phagocytic events include the following sequence of responses in the blood PMN: adherence to the endothelial surface, emigration out of the vascular tree, chemotaxis or directed movement to the site of the infection, opsonization of the bacteria and recognition of the opsonized bacteria by the PMN, ingestion, degranulation, and subsequent peroxidative killing of the bacteria by the PMN

and into the tissue (Figure 14.1). PMN movement through tissue is directed by a variety of chemotactic factors. As the PMN moves to the inflammatory site, it assumes a wide blunted front devoid of scintillating cytoplasmic granules so prevalent in the body of the cell and trails a tail reminiscent of a rodent on its way to kill its prey[4]. Meanwhile, the bacteria are involved in a preliminary but necessary reaction with antibody and complement, called opsonization, which prepares the bacteria so that they may be recognized by the oncoming phagocyte[5]. As contact is established between the PMN and the opsonized bacteria, the broad front of the PMN is cleaved when the deformed plasma membrane holding the bacteria invaginates forming a vacuole that becomes completely internalized as the newly created 'arms' fuse together[6]. Even before fusion takes place, the cytoplasmic granules begin discharging or degranulating their hydrolytic and peroxidative contents on the bacteria within the phagocytic vacuoles.

Although not required for phagocytic uptake, a series of redox reactions occurs during phagocytosis leading to the formation of several reduced products of oxygen that participate in the peroxidative killing of the bacteria[7]. As noted in Figure 14.2, in phagocytic PMN, oxygen is reduced univalently by rapid single electron transfer to form superoxide anion, hydrogen peroxide, and hydroxyl radicals; singlet oxygen forms from the shift of an electron to an orbital with a higher energy state. Only H_2O_2 is stable but all may be important for bacterial destruction. Activation of the PMN membrane by opsonized bacteria, latex particles, antigen–antibody complexes, chemotactic C_{5a} fragment, and non-ionic detergent results in a 3-fold increase in consumption and reduction of oxygen by the PMN[8]

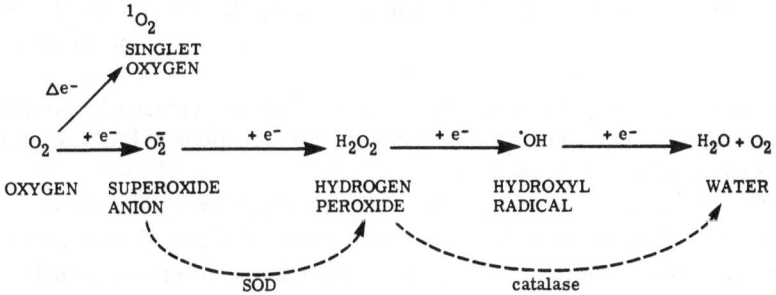

THE PRODUCTS OF OXYGEN REDUCTION BY PHAGOCYTIZING LEUKOCYTES

Figure 14.2   Redox reactions in PMN. Oxygen is reduced in univalent steps to superoxide anion, hydrogen peroxide, and hydroxyl radical. Singlet oxygen forms from a shift of an electron to an orbital of higher energy state. Superoxide dismutase and catalase catalyse the conversion of superoxide anion to H_2O_2 and of H_2O_2 to H_2O and O_2

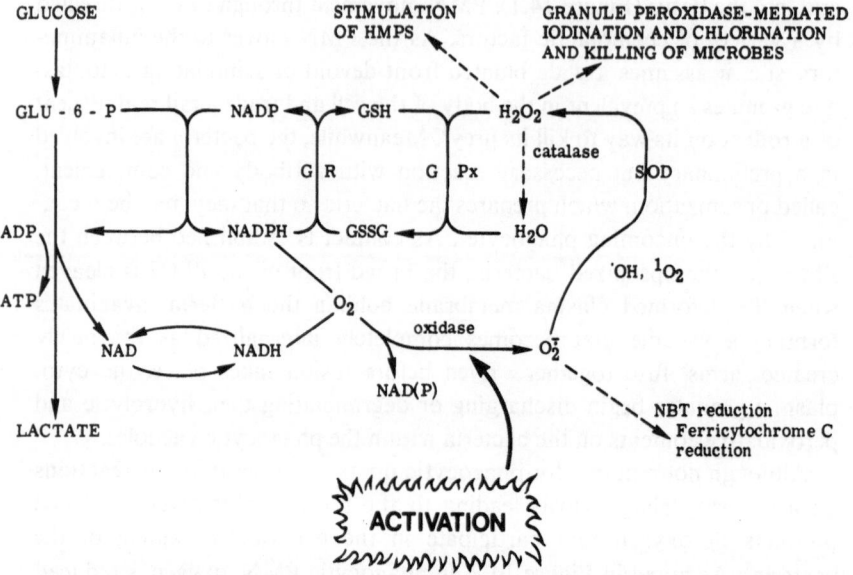

Figure 14.3   Metabolic reactions in PMN. Oxygen is reduced to superoxide anion by the enzymatic action of NADH and NADPH oxidase. Hydrogen peroxide generated from the dismutation of O_2^- stimulates the hexose monophosphate shunt by oxidation of NADPH either directly or indirectly through the glutathione system and participates in the iodination and chlorination reactions that lead to killing of bacteria

catalysed by one or more cyanide-insensitive oxidases requiring NADH[9] formed in glycolysis and NADPH formed in the hexose monophosphate shunt as substrates[10]. Superoxide anion is dismutated by superoxide dismutase to H_2O_2, which, in turn, stimulates the hexose monophosphate shunt by oxidation of NADPH either directly or indirectly through the glutathione pathway. Killing of microbes by H_2O_2 is enhanced by granule peroxidase-mediated iodination and chlorination reactions in PMN. Figure 14.3 summarizes these reactions.

An enlarging group of diseases categorically known as disorders of phagocytic function have been described during the past decade and in each case, one or more alterations in the capacity of the patient's PMN to carry out the expected function has been observed *in vitro*[11]. The development of a profile of *in vitro* phagocytic tests has enabled the clinician to begin to link *in vitro* defects to specific disease states (Table 14.1). There are at least fifteen tests of neutrophil function and they represent attempts to study in an isolated fashion one or more phases of phagocytic function[12]. We shall discuss briefly *in vitro* tests for PMN adherence, chemotaxis,

TABLE 14.1 *In vitro* **tests of phagocytic function**

Microtubule related:
  Adherence
  Chemotaxis
  Degranulation
    Phagocytic vacuole
    Secretion from cell
  Capping by fluoresceinated Concanavalin-A
Microfilament related:
  Phagocytic uptake oil red O paraffin oil coated with *E. coli* lipopolysaccharide
Oxidase activation:
  Oxygen consumption
  Superoxide anion
    Ferricytochrome *c* reduction
    Nitroblue tetrazolium reduction
  Hydrogen peroxide
    Scopoletin fluorescence
    $[^{14}C]$formate $\rightarrow ^{14}CO_2$
    Glucose-l-$^{14}C \rightarrow ^{14}CO_2$
    ^{125}Iodination of ingested particles
    Peroxidative bactericidal activity
    Chemiluminescence
Opsonization of bacteria and recognition by phagocyte
  C_{3b} coated RBC or bacterial rosettes
  IgG coated RBC or bacterial rosettes

Adapted from Baehner, R. L. (1977). In P. L. Altman and D Katz (eds.). *Human Health and Disease. Fed. Am. Soc. for Exp. Biol.*[12]

phagocytic ingestion, oxidase activation and bacterial killing as well as opsonization and recognition of bacteria by PMN. Usually PMNs are isolated from the peripheral blood by collection of venous blood in heparin, gravity sedimentation of the red cells, and transfer of the leukocyte-rich supernatant plasma to a plastic conical tube where the preparations can be freed from gross contamination of (a) red cells by hypotonic lysis, (b) platelets by differential centrifugation, and (c) lymphocytes and mono-nuclear cells by centrifugation through a Ficoll–Hypaque density gradient.

ADHERENCE

Probably less is known about the factors regulating PMN adherence than any other phase of phagocytosis (Table 14.2). Glycoproteins on the surface form hydrogen bonds that contribute to the adhesive property of the PMN. Treatment of PMN with (a) calcium chelating agents, (b) polycationic local anaesthetics, (c) pharmacological agents which raise intracellular

TABLE 14.2   Factors regulating PMN adherence

Glycoproteins on membrane surface
Calcium
Anionic regions
Cellular cyclic nucleotides
Cellular microtubules

cyclic AMP levels, and (d) drugs that inhibit the assembly of cytoplasmic microtubules all decrease the adherence of PMNs to nylon wool columns. Quantification of cellular adherence by PMNs can be performed simply by passing either whole blood or leukocyte suspensions through a micro-column of pre-weighed nylon fibres as described by MacGregor[13]. In this test, the percentage of PMNs that adhere to the nylon fibre is determined by assessing the PMN count before and after exposure of the suspensions to the column.

CHEMOTAXIS

Chemotaxis is the movement of cells in one direction toward the inciting stimulus rather than movement of cells in random directions. The principal chemotactic stimulants to PMNs include the complement fragments C_{3a}, C_{5a}, and C_{567}, bacterial factors that may give rise to formyl-methionyl tripeptides, and a lymphocyte-derived chemotactic factor[14]. The responding PMN must contain surface receptors to the stimulants, an energy source in the form of ATP utilized as fuel to propel the cell, and a function-

TABLE 14.3   Factors regulating chemotaxis

Humoral:
   C_{3a}, C_{5a}, C_{567}
   Formyl-methionine tripeptides
   Bacterial products
   Lymphocyte-derived chemotaxin
   Fibrinopeptides and fibrin split products
Cellular:
   Surface receptors
   Energy–ATP
   Contractile proteins
      Actin, myosin, actin-binding protein
   Microtubule assembly proteins
      Tubulin
      Microtubule associated proteins

ing cytoskeletal machinery including the contractile proteins actin, myosin and actin-binding proteins and the microtubule assembly protein, tubulin, and the high molecular weight microtubule-associated proteins (Table 14.3). *In vitro* assays of chemotaxis are used to estimate the capacity of blood PMNs or monocytes to move toward a source of chemotactic attractants. A 5 micron filter (Millipore, Nucleopore) is placed on a glass slide and PMNs from a suspension are gently layered on the filter. The cytocentrifuge method described by Hill[15] provides a homogeneous layer of cells on the filter. The Boyden chamber[16] consists of a lower chamber filled with chemotactic attractant, a filter placed above the lower chamber, and an upper chamber filled with buffer to establish a chemotactic gradient between the lower and upper chambers. Following a 3 h incubation, the filter is removed, the PMNs stained, and the number that crawled through the pores to the under surface of the filter determined. In our laboratory, a chemotactic score is determined by counting the number of PMNs in ten random oil immersion fields. Disorders of chemotaxis in Table 14.4 may be due to decreased chemotactic factors or to impaired cellular response to normal chemotactic stimuli[17].

TABLE 14.4 Disorders of chemotaxis

Serum
C_3 deficiency
C_5 deficiency
Inhibitors
Absent antagonist to inhibitors
PMN—Selective defect
Lazy leukocyte syndrome
Congenital ichthyosis and infection
Dermatitis with hyper IgE
Job's syndrome
Dermatitis with hyper IgA and respiratory infection
Allergic rhinitis and furunculosis
Chronic renal disease
Diabetes mellitus
Rheumatoid arthritis
Malnutrition
PMN—Associated with other defects of function
Chediak–Higashi syndrome
Chronic mucocutaneous candidiasis
Wiscott–Aldrich syndrome
Actin dysfunction

Opsonization

The mechanism for bacterial opsonization is determined by the immune status of the host as well as the biochemical nature of the bacterial surface[18]. *Staphylococcus aureus* requires activation of direct complement pathway since the deficiency of C_2 results in defective opsonization where as *Diplococcus pneumonia* requires activation of the alternative complement pathway. In both situations, prior sensitization to the specific micro-organisms must have occurred since small amounts of specific IgG antibody are required to activate the complement cascade. IgG alone is

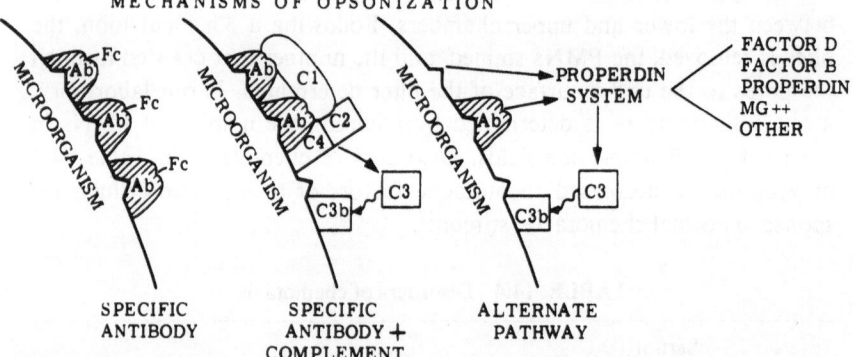

Figure 14.4   Mechanisms of opsonization. Three mechanisms for opsonization of bacteria are possible. In the hyperimmune state, specific antibody IgG may serve as the only source of opsonin and the F_c portion will attach the bacteria to the PMN surface (panel 1). Usually, the complement system participates either through activation of the direct pathway (panel 2), or through activation of the alternative pathway (panel 3)

opsonic in the immediate post-immune state following vaccination and infection. PMNs contain both F_c and C_{3b} receptors on their surfaces and this enables them to recognize and bind opsonized bacteria. The basis for severe life-threatening infection in patients with agammaglobulinaemia and complement (C_3 and C_5) deficiencies is due to faulty opsonization of infecting bacteria by the patient's serum. The sera of some children with sickle cell disease fail to support normal opsonization of type-specific pneumococci due to a poorly defined defect in the alternative complement pathway[19]. Type 25 pneumococci opsonized by sickle cell sera are not ingested by normal PMNs[20]. We have determined physico-chemical differences between F_c and C_3 receptor recognition by PMN to opsonized bacteria[21]. *Salmonella typhimurium* and *Streptococcus pneumonia* were directly stained with fluorescein and then the salmonella were opsonized with fresh serum which led to deposition of C_{3b} on the bacteria. After thorough washing, the bacteria were incubated with the PMNs and examined for bacterial rosettes under the fluorescence microscope. In a similar manner. Type 2-specific pneumococcal antiserum was used to opsonize type-specific pneumococcus with IgG. A brilliant fluorescence is evident when the bacteria bind to the PMNs. We observed the C_{3b}-bound bacteria became detached by exposure to 4 °C by H_2O_2 and by an oxidant-generating system whereas F_c-bound bacteria remained attached under these conditions.

PHAGOCYTIC INGESTION

The mechanism for ingestion of opsonized bacteria by PMNs has been clarified by the recent studies of Stossel and co-workers[22]. These investigators have pointed out that actin microfilaments form the structural framework in the 'arms' which developed from the cleavage in the leading front of the PMN by the deformed plasma membrane attached to the bacteria as it invaginates into the cell to form the phagocytic vacuole. Actin-binding protein associated with the cytoplasmic surface of the plasma membrane[23] cross-links the actin and transforms the cytosol to a gel. This reaction is blocked by cytochalasin B and this compound also blocks uptake of particles by PMNs[24]. Contraction of the gel requires activation of myosin magnesium-dependent ATPase. Similar to chemotaxis, ingestion requires expenditure of cellular energy by the contractile apparatus of the PMN but in contrast to chemotaxis, inhibition of microtubule assembly with colchicine does not affect the ingestion process. The rate of ingestion of oil red O by PMNs is one *in vitro* test that measures the kinetic uptake of particles opsonized by C_{3b}[25]. Phagocytic cells isolated from human blood ingest *E. coli* lipopolysaccharide-coated paraffin oil droplets stained with oil red O. Droplets are emulsified by a brief sonication, opsonized with fresh serum, and incubated for 5 min with the PMN. The reaction is stopped by addition of *N*-ethylmaleimide and the cells containing the ingested paraffin oil are pelleted by centrifugation and the oil red O is extracted with dioxane. Ingestion rate over the first 5 min is linear and is expressed as the amount of paraffin oil taken up by 10^7 PMNs/min. Primary disorders of PMN ingestion are rare. To date, a single patient had been described by Boxer and co-workers[26] and this infant had a fatal infection. The patient's PMN had a dysfunction of actin polymerization. The PMN from the infant failed to ingest oil red O particles and failed to move in a Boyden chamber. Sodium dodecyl sulphate polyacrylamide gel electrophoresis studies of PMN extracts showed that control PMN actin polymerized normally in response to KCl whereas the patient's PMN actin failed to polymerize. Similar studies of the parents of this child are in progress.

OXIDASE ACTIVATION

The prototype disease of the phagocytic dysfunction syndromes is chronic granulomatous disease. To date, 162 cases have been described in the world literature[27] since its initial description in 1957 by Dr Good and coworkers[28]. The defect appears to be due to a failure to activate PMN oxidase[9, 29, 30] during phagocytosis and this results in the defective peroxidative killing of catalase-positive bacteria. Activation of oxidase activity in normal phagocytizing PMN results in a 3-fold increase in oxygen consumption, stimulation of the hexose monophosphate shunt, iodination of ingested particles, hydrogen peroxide, superoxide anion, hydroxyl radical and singlet oxygen production, and reduction of nitroblue tetrazolium to formazan[31]. The NBT reduction to formazan is due to O_2^- in phagocytizing PMNs since the addition of SOD markedly decreases this response[32]. The NBT test[33] is one of a large variety of tests that reflects oxidase activation in PMN during phagocytosis. A 2% solution of yellow NBT is added to a suspension of resting and phagocytizing PMNs. During a 15 min incubation period, purple formazan forms at the site of attachment of opsonized paricles to the PMNs and subsequently the entire phagocytic vesicle becomes stained by purple formazan[34]. The PMN of patients with CGD failed to reduce NBT after a 15 min incubation. The extent of NBT reduction by resting and phagocytic cells is quantified by extraction of the precipitated formazan with either pyridine or dioxane. The test serves as a sensitive assay to detect patients and carriers of the X-linked form of chronic granulomatous disease.

PEROXIDATIVE KILLING

There are two major antimicrobial systems in PMNs; one requires oxygen and the other remains operative even in the absence of oxygen[7] (Table 14.5). Klebanoff was the first to show that myeloperoxidase, an enzyme contained in the primary azurophilic granules of PMN and also found at one-third of the PMN activity in monocytes, will enhance the killing of bacteria by H_2O_2 in the presence of a suitable halide ion such as iodide or chloride. There is evidence that the other unstable products of oxygen reduction may also contribute to the killing of ingested bacteria in the absence of myeloperoxidase. Phagocytic vacuole pH falls to 5.0 which is the pH optimum for most of the hydrolytic enzymes of the PMN[35]. Lyso-

TABLE 14.5   Antimicrobial system in PMN

Oxygen-dependent
    H_2O_2-halide-myeloperoxidase system
    H_2O_2
    Superoxide (O_2^-)
    Hydroxyl radical ($\cdot OH$)
    Singlet oxygen ($^1O_2$)
Phagocytic vacuole acidosis pH 5.0
Granule
    Lysozyme
    Lactoferrin
    Cationic proteins

---

zyme is bactericidal for unencapsulated bacteria and for Gram-negative bacteria exposed to complement or to a hydrogen peroxide generating system[36]. It is equally distributed in specific and secondary granules of the PMN and is transferred into the phagocytic vacuole. Lactoferrin is totally confined to specific granules and is transferred into the phagocytic vacuole and has recently been shown to have bactericidal properties partially related to its chelating capacity for iron which may be required for bacterial growth[37]. Antibacterial activity of cationic proteins from human PMN has also been described recently[38].

H_2O_2 plays a central role in oxidative metabolism and bacterial killing in the PMN. About 15% of the peroxide formed during O_2 reduction diffuses out of the cell, unknown quantities are available to stimulate the hexose monophosphate shunt and to diffuse into the phagocytic vacuole. The phagocytic vacuole is the only area of the cell lacking catalase. Ingested bacteria become iodinated and killed by the action of H_2O_2, peroxidase and halide ion[39] but the precise molecular mechanism for bacterial death remains unknown at present. Hydrogen peroxide producing bacteria such as *Streptococcus fecalis* and *Streptococcus viridans* are killed normally by chronic granulomatous disease PMNs[40] compared to their impaired killing against *Staphylococcus aureus*. Results of these *in vitro* tests correlate with the clinical observation that catalase-positive non-peroxide-producing bacteria are the major source of infection in chronic granulomatous disease patients. The children are plagued by suppurative infections of the skin and lymphoreticular organs. The lymph nodes about the head and neck are a frequent source of recurrent infection. The *in vitro* bactericidal assay is an essential test in any patient suspected to have a defect in PMN microbicidal activity[41]. Generally, equal concentrations of PMNs and bacteria are placed in an incubation tube containing 10% fresh serum as a source of opsonin. Incubation is carried out on a rotating wheel at

37 °C for 120 min. Aliquots from the patient and control tubes are removed at 30 min intervals, diluted in sterile tubes and mixed in a Petri dish with soft agar. After an overnight incubation, the number of viable bacterial colonies are counted with a grid or electronic counter. The extent of killing by normal PMNs is easily identified by this technique. Normal PMNs kill greater than '1 log' of the bacteria during the first 60 min of incubation. Patients with myeloperoxidase deficiency of the primary granules, and patients with Chediak–Higashi syndrome have a delayed killing during the initial 30 min of incubation, but thereafter, the rate of

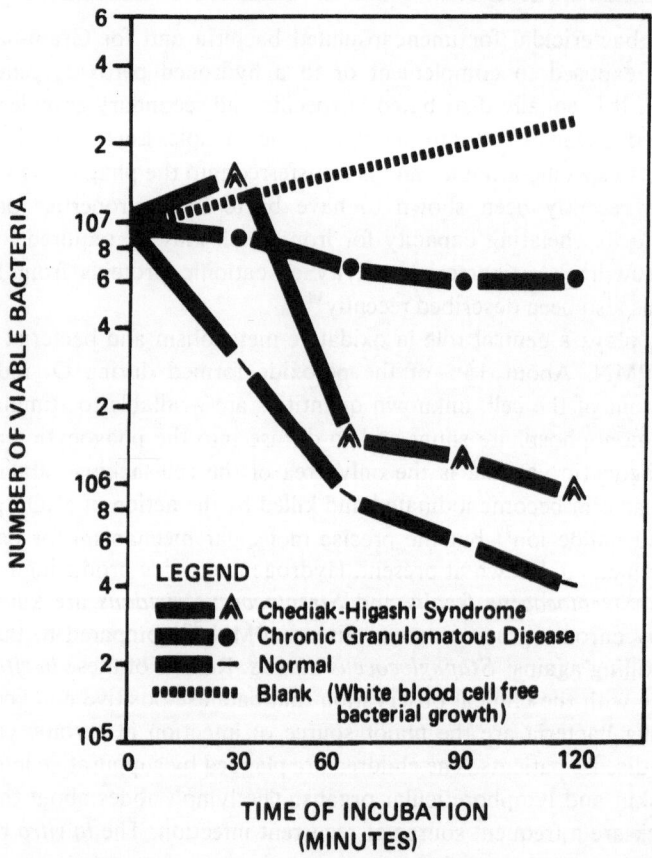

BACTERIAL KILLING STUDY |Organism: Staph Aureus (502A)|

TIME OF INCUBATION (MINUTES)

Figure 14.5 Bactericidal curve of chronic granulomatous disease, Chediak–Higashi syndrome, and normal PMN. Note the delayed killing in CHS PMN and the absence of killing in CGD PMN compared to the 1½ log reduction of bacteria by normal PMN

killing returns toward normal. Chronic granulomatous disease PMN kill less than '$\frac{1}{2}$ log' of bacteria over the entire 120 min period of incubation. Bacteria without PMN continue to grow 'logarithmically' during the incubation period (Figure 14.5). In CGD, both the bactericidal test and the metabolic test reflecting oxidase activation are abnormal.

We have recently attempted to restore oxidase activity in chronic granulomatous disease PMNs by incorporating glucose oxidase into artificial liposomes using the technique of Weissman[42]. The liposomes were opsonized with heat-aggregated IgG and ingested by CGD PMNs. The PMN granules discharge digestive enzymes into the phagocytic vacuole and the entrapped glucose oxidase is then released from the liposome and will generate H_2O_2. Under these conditions, response of the hexose monophosphate shunt, iodination and bactericidal activity by CGD PMN should become normal. Hydrogen peroxide release from the cell increased to normal levels, glucose-1-[^{14}C] oxidation to $^{14}CO_2$, a measure of the activity of the hexose monophosphate shunt, also increased toward normal values, and iodination activity was improved. However, the *in vitro* bactericidal activity against *Staphylococcus aureus* improved but was not totally corrected. These studies suggest that correction of this life-threatening disease may be possible in the future when effective *in vivo* restoration of oxidase activity in the CGD cells becomes a reality.

Patients with Chediak–Higashi syndrome[43] have a myriad of PMN phagocytic defects; *in vitro* adherence, emigration, chemotaxis, degranulation, and peroxidative killing of bacteria are faulty. The phenotypic manifestations include oculocutaneous albinism brought about through aggregation of melanin granules, enlarged lysosomes of granulocytes and most other body cells, decreased resistance to bacterial infection and a mild platelet function defect. The hair has a silver sheen and is several shades lighter than the other family members. The disorder occurs in Aleutian mink, beige mice, white killer whales, cows and cats. The blood PMNs contain enlarged granules that stain for peroxidase by both light microscopy as well as by electron microscopy. The patients die at an early age due to infection and bleeding, most often associated with the accelerated phase of the disease. In contrast to patients with CGD both catalase-positive and catalase-negative bacteria including pneumococcus and beta-haemolytic streptococcus cause infections in patients with Chediak–Higashi syndrome.

The recognition by Oliver and her co-workers[44] that the defect of phagocytic function resembled the defect evident in normal PMNs after treatment with the microtubule disassembly agent colchicine led to a series of remarkable experiments that has clarified the basis for the PMN dysfunction and has provided an effective *in vivo* therapy for the disease. Microtubule-related functions in PMN include capping, movement and degranulation. Capping refers to the response of the PMN after incubation with fluorescein-ated Concanavalin-A (Con-A). Fluoresceinated Con-A binds homogeneously over the surface of the PMN and induces the assembly of many microtubules in the pericentriolar area of the cell. Exposure of the PMN to colchicine results in disassembly of cytoplasmic microtubules and the receptors for Con-A move laterally in the fluid membrane to a polar area of the cell to form a cap. PMN from patients with Chediak–Higashi syndrome cap spontaneously indicating a defect in microtubule assembly[45]. Indeed, elec-tron microscopy study of Chediak–Higashi syndrome PMNs reveals a lack of microtubules after they are exposed to Con-A. However, pre-incubation of Chediak–Higashi syndrome PMNs with high concentrations of cGMP restores microtubule assembly and corrects the capping defect in the cells. Since microtubules play a role in degranulation and secretion, we quantitated the rate of release of the lysosomal enzyme beta-glucuronidase from PMNs rendered secretory by cytochalasin B[46], and confirmed the diminished release of lysosomal enzymes in response to opsonized zymosan in Chediak–Higashi syndrome PMN compared to normal cells. The de-granulation defect was corrected by incubation of the patient's cells with high concentrations of cyclic GMP[47]. Attempts to treat patients with the cholinergic agonist carbamyl methylcholine resulted in toxicity. However, based on the observation by Gallin and co-workers that ascorbic acid en-hances normal PMN movement[48], three patients with Chediak–Higashi syndrome were treated with 100–200 mg of ascorbic acid daily or their cells were incubated in the presence of 10 mM ascorbic acid *in vitro*. Both *in vitro* and *in vivo* treatment corrected the chemotactic defects as deter-mined in the Boyden chamber. Quantitation of cyclic nucleotide levels in three patients revealed a 5–15-fold increase in cAMP which returned toward normal following a 1 month treatment with ascorbate. There was no alteration in cGMP levels in these cells. Release of beta-glucuronidase was also corrected by ascorbic acid therapy. We have also demonstrated a relationship between PMN capping and adherence[49]. A larger percentage of normal non-adherent PMN after passage over the nylon filter column were capped compared to PMNs eluded from the filter. Similarly, Chediak–Higashi PMNs from patients, beige mice and mink were also less adherent to the filter. Ascorbic acid, both *in vitro* and *in vivo*, restored adherence in all three species. Finally, the delay in *in vitro* bacterial killing was also corrected in Chediak–Higashi syndrome PMNs obtained from patients on ascorbic acid treatment (Table 14.6).

These studies point to a fundamental defect of microtubule function in

TABLE 14.6   Effects of ascorbic acid on Chediak–Higashi PMN

Fluoresceinated Concanavalin-A caps reduced to normal
Enhanced degranulation of lysosomal enzymes
Correction of chemotactic defect in Boyden chamber
Increased cellular adherence to nylon fibres
Correction in the early phase of delayed bacterial killing
Return of 5–15-fold increases in cyclic AMP to normal range
Microtubule assembly corrected as shown by electron microscope
Abnormal granule morphology persists

Chediak–Higashi syndrome PMNs resulting in PMNs that are less adherent, slower to move and respond to chemotactic stimuli and to degranulate normally, and faulty in their ability to kill catalase-positive and catalase-negative bacteria at a normal rate. Cyclic AMP levels are markedly elevated in these cells and microtubules fail to assemble in response to Con-A and this abnormal response allows migration of Con-A receptors to a polar area on the cell's surface to form caps. Both cyclic GMP *in vitro* and ascorbic acid *in vitro* and *in vivo* correct these functional defects.

In vitro tests evaluating selective phases of phagocytic function have provided information to allow a better understanding of normal cellular and biochemical events occurring in phagocytizing PMNs. The tests have also proven useful in establishing new disorders of phagocytic function and in evaluating newer therapies designed to correct phagocytic defects.

SUMMARY

The phagocytic process in the PMN can be separated into cellular events regulated (a) by assembly of microtubules, (b) by polymerization, gelation, and contraction of microfilaments, (c) by activation of oxidase, and (d) by opsonization of bacteria leading to their recognition by C_{3b} and F_c cellular surface receptors. Altered microtubule function occurs in PMN from patients with Chediak–Higashi syndrome (CHS) and explains the diminished adherence, chemotaxis, degranulation and delayed peroxidative killing observed in CHS PMN. Altered microfilament function occurred in the PMN of an infant with actin dysfunction (AD) and explains the diminished chemotaxis and phagocytic ingestion of oil red O observed in AD PMN. The PMN from patients with chronic granulomatous disease (CGD) fail to activate oxidase during phagocytosis leading to an absence of all redox reactions involving molecular oxygen. The serum of patients with agammaglobulinaemia, complement (especially C_3 and C_5) deficiencies, and some patients with sickle cell disease fail to opsonize bacteria for their subsequent recognition and ingestion by the phagocytic PMN. The *in vitro* tests for phagocyte function have provided a rationale for the design and evaluation of effective therapies for patients with disorders of phagocytic function. Gammaglobulin and plasma infusions have improved the opsonic defects in agammaglobulinaemia and some complement deficiencies, respectively. Restoration in metabolic and bactericidal function in chronic granulomatous disease PMN has been accomplished by oxidase replacement *in vitro* employing glucose oxidase impregnated liposomes. Daily administration of 200 mg ascorbic acid to patients and animals with Chediak–Higashi syndrome has resulted in complete correction of all phases of microtubule-regulated function.

Acknowledgements

This investigation was supported by grant numbers PHS RO1 10892-05, PHS RO1 A1 13586-01, and PHS T32 AM 719301 awarded by the National Institute of Health, and by grants from the James Whitcomb Riley Memorial Association. Dr Boxer is an established investigator of the American Heart Association.

References

1. Rebuck, J. W. and Crowley, J. H. (1955). A method of studying leukocytes function *in vivo*. *Ann. N.Y. Acad. Sci.*, 59, 757
2. Metchnikoff, E. (1968). Lecture on the comparative pathology of inflammation. Translation by Dover Publication, New York
3. Ryan, G. B. and Majno, G. (1977). *Inflammation*. B. A. Thomas (ed.). (Kalamazoo: Upjohn)
4. Hirsch, J. G. and Cohn, Z. A. (1960). Degranulation of polymorphonuclear leukocytes following phagocytosis of microorganisms. *J. Exp. Med.*, 112, 1005
5. Winkelstein, J. A. (1973). Opsonins: Their function, identity, and clinical significance. *J. Ped.*, 82, 747
6. Stossel, T. P. (1974). Phagocytosis. *N. Engl. J. Med.*, 290, 717
7. Klebanoff, S. J. (1975). Antimicrobial mechanisms in neutrophilic PMN. *Semin. Hematol.*, 12, 117
8. Karnovsky, M. L. (1968). The metabolism of leukocytes. *Semin. Hematol.*, 5, 156
9. Briggs, R. T., Karnovsky, M. L. and Karnovsky, M. J. (1977). Hydrogen peroxide production in CGD: A cytochemical study of reduced pyridine nucleotide oxidases. *J. Clin. Invest.*, 59, 1088
10. Patriarca, P., Cramer, R., Moncalvo, Ross F. and Romer, D. (1971). Enzymatic basis of metabolic stimulation in leukocytes during phagocytosis: The role of activated NADPH oxidase. *Arch. Biochem. Biophys.*, 145, 255
11. Baehner, R. L. (1972). Disorders of leukocytes leading to recurrent infection. *Ped. Clin. N. Am.*, 19, 935

12. Baehner, R. L. (1977). In P. L. Altman and D. D. Katz (eds.). *Human Health and Disease.* p. 61. *Fed. Amer. Soc. for Exp. Biol.*
13. MacGregor, R. P., Spagnuolo, R. J. and Lentnek, A. L. (1974). Inhibition of granulocyte adherence by ethanol, prednisone, and aspirin measured with an assay system. *N. Engl. J. Med.,* 291, 642
14. Ward, P. A. (1971). Leukotactic factors in health and disease. *Am. J. Path.,* 64, 521
15. Hill, H. R., Hogan, N. A. and Thomas, G. M. (1974). Evaluation of a cytocentrifuge method for measuring neutrophil granulocyte chemotaxis. *J. Lab. Clin. Med.,* 86, 703
16. Boyden, S. (1962). Chemotactic effect of mixtures of antibody and antigen on PMN. *J. Exp. Med.,* 115, 453
17. Quie, P. G. (1978). Disorders of chemotaxis. *Am. J. Path.* (In press)
18. Scribner, D. J. and Fahrney, D. (1976). Neutrophil receptors for IgG and complement: Their roles in the attachment and ingestion phases of phagocytosis. *J. Immunol.,* 116, 892
19. Johnston, R. B. Jr., Newman, S. L. and Struth, B. S. (1973). An abnormality of the alternate pathway of complement activation in sickle cell disease. *N. Engl. J. Med.,* 288, 803
20. Winkelstein, J. A. and Drachman, R. H. (1968). Deficiency of pneumococcal serum opsonizing activity in sickle-cell disease. *N. Engl. J. Med.,* 279, 459
21. Boxer, L. A., Richardson, S. B. and Baehner, R. L. (1978). Effects of surface active agents on neutrophil receptors. *Infect. Immunol.,* 21, 28
22. Stossel, T. P. and Hartwig, J. H. (1976). Interaction of actin, myosin, and a new actin-binding protein of rabbit pulmonary macrophage. II. Role of cytoplasmic movement in phagocytosis. *J. Cell. Biol.,* 68, 602
23. Boxer, L. A., Richardson, S. and Floyd, A. (1976). Identification of actin-binding protein in membrane of polymorphonuclear leukocytes. *Nature (London),* 263, 249
24. Keller, H. V., Hess, M. W. and Cottier, H. (1975). Physiology of chemotaxis and random motility. *Semin. Hematol.,* 12, 47
25. Stossel, T. P. (1973). Evaluation of opsonic and leukocyte function with a spectrophotometric test in patients with infection and phagocytic disorders. *Blood.* 42, 121
26. Boxer, L. A., Hedley-White, E. T. and Stossel, T. P. (1974). Neutrophil actin dysfunction and abnormal neutrophil behaviour. *N. Engl. J. Med.,* 291, 1093
27. Johnston, R. B. Jr. and Newman, S. L. (1977). Chronic granulomatous disease. *Ped. Clin. N. Am.,* 24, 365
28. Berendes, H., Bridges, R. A. and Good, R. A. (1957). Fatal granulomatous disease of childhood. Clinical study of a new syndrome. *Minn. Med.,* 40, 309
29. Curnutte, J. T., Kipnes, R. S. and Babior, B. M. (1975). Defect in pyridine nucleotide dependent superoxide production by a particulate fraction from the patients with chronic granulomatous disease. *N. Engl. J. Med.,* 293, 628
30. Hohn, D. C. and Lehrer, R. I. (1975). NADPH oxidase deficiency in X-linked chronic granulomatous disease. *J. Clin. Invest.,* 55, 707
31. Baehner, R. L. (1975). The growth and development of our understanding of chronic granulomatous disease. In J. A. Bellanti and D. H. Dayton (eds.). *The Phagocytic Cell and Host Resistance.* p. 173. (New York: Raven Press)

32. Baehner, R. L., Murrmann, S. K., Davis, J. and Johnston, R. B., Jr. (1975). The role of superoxide anion and hydrogen peroxide in phagocytosis-associated oxidative metabolic reactions. *J. Clin. Invest.*, 56, 571

33. Baehner, R. L. and Nathan, D. G. (1968). Quantitative nitroblue tetrazolium test in chronic granulomatous disease. *N. Engl. J. Med.*, 278, 971

34. Nathan, D. G., Baehner, R. L. and Weaver, D. K. (1969). Failure of nitro-blue tetrazolium reduction in the phagocytic vacuoles in chronic granulomatous disease. *J. Clin. Invest.*, 48, 1895

35. Mandell, G. L. (1970). Intraphagosomal pH of human polymorphonuclear neutrophils. *Proc. Soc. Exp. Biol. Med.*, 134, 447

36. Miller, T. E. (1969). Killing and lysis of Gram-negative bacteria through the synergistic effect of hydrogen peroxide ascorbic acid, and lysozyme. *J. Bacteriol.*, 98, 949

37. Arnold, R. R., Cole, M. F. and McGhee, J. R. (1977). A bactericidal effect for human lactoferrin. *Science*, 197, 263

38. Odeberg, H. and Olsson, I. (1975). Antibacterial activity of cationic proteins from human granulocytes. *J. Clin. Invest.*, 56, 1178

39. Klebanoff, S. J. (1968). Myeloperoxidase-halide-hydrogen peroxide anti-bacterial system. *J. Bacteriol.*, 95, 2131

40. Kaplan, E. L., Laxdal, T. and Quie, P. G. (1968). Studies of PMN in patients with CGD of childhood bactericidal capacity for streptococci. *Pediatrics*, 41, 591

41. Quie, P. G., White, J. G., Holmes, B. and Good, R. A. (1967). *In vitro* bactericidal capacity of human PMN: Diminished activity in chronic granulomatous disease of childhood. *J. Clin. Invest.*, 46, 668

42. Ismail, G., Boxer, L. A. and Baehner, R. L. (1977). Utilization of liposomes for correcting the metabolic deficiencies in chronic granulomatous disease (CGD). *Ped. Res.*, 11, 779A

43. Blume, R. S. and Wolff, S. M. (1972). The Chediak–Higashi syndrome: Studies in four patients and a review of the literature. *Medicine*, 51, 247

44. Oliver, J. M., Zurier, R. B. and Berlin, R. D. (1975). Concanavalin-A cap formation on PMN of normal and beige (C–H) mice. *Nature (London)*, 253, 471

45. Zurier, R. B., Weissmann, G., Hoffstein, S., Kammerman, S. and Tai, H. H. (1974). Mechanisms of lysosomal release for human leukocytes. II. Effects of cAMP and cGMP autonomic agonists and agents which affect micro-tubular function. *J. Clin. Invest.*, 53, 297

46. Boxer, L. A., Rister, M., Allen, J. M. and Baehner, R. L. (1977). Improvement of Chediak–Higashi leukocyte function by cyclic guanosine mono-phosphate. *Blood*, 49, 9

47. Sandler, J. A., Gallin, J. I. and Vaughan, M. (1975). Effects of serotonin, carbomylcholine, and ascorbic acid on leukocyte cyclic GMP and chemo-taxis. *J. Cell. Biol.*, 67, 480

48. Boxer, L. A., Watanabe, A. M., Rister, M., Besch, H. R. Jr., Allen, J. and Baehner, R. L. (1976). Correction of leukocyte function in Chekiak–Higashi syndrome by ascorbate. *N. Engl. J. Med.*, 295, 1041

49. Provisor, D., Boxer, L. A., Strawbridge, R., Allen, J. M., Watanabe, A. M., Besch, H. R. and Baehner, R. L. (1977). Granulocyte adherence in the Chediak–Higashi syndrome. *Clin. Res.*, 25, 382A

15

Experimental approaches to the role of mononuclear phagocytes in non-specific immunity
G. G. MacPherson

INTRODUCTION

The majority of chapters concerning non-specific immunity contained in this book have been devoted to polymorphonuclear leukocytes (PMNs). This is not difficult to understand. PMNs are a homogeneous population of fully mature cells which can be easily collected in large numbers for biochemical and functional investigations. Disorders of these cells produce well-defined clinical syndromes and much work is being carried out in an endeavour to understand the underlying mechanisms.

In contrast, mononuclear phagocytes, MNP, are an extremely hetero-geneous cell population (Figures 15.1 to 15.4). They emerge from the bone marrow as immature monocytes, migrate into the tissues and differentiate into macrophages. Many of their properties are dependent upon the site from which they are extracted. In addition we have little idea how MNP kill pathogens.

The types of infections in which MNP are important differ from those

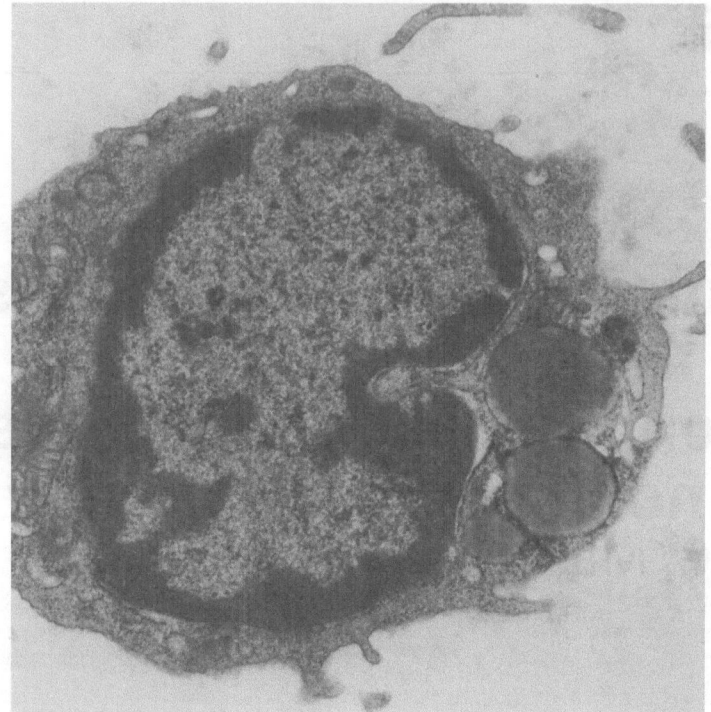

Figure 15.1   Electron micrograph of a rat monocyte ($\times$ 20 400)

where PMN act. They are caused by pathogens such as mycobacteria, many viruses and some parasites which live a preferentially intracellular existence. It is now clear that in considering immunity to these organisms, one cannot separate non-specific from specific immunity. The expression of immunity is non-specific but is dependent on the recognition of antigen by specific lymphocytes[1].

MECHANISMS OF CELL-MEDIATED IMMUNITY (CMI)

Figure 15.5 shows, in a simplified form, a model that may be used to understand CMI. Antigen is presented to specific T cells, probably on the surface of MNP in association with Ia histocompatibility antigens[2]. The T cell transforms into a lymphoblast, divides clonally and releases humoral factors[3], the number of which appears to depend mainly on the ingenuity of the investigator in devising tests to recognize them. However, some of these factors are at least partially defined as molecular entities. The most

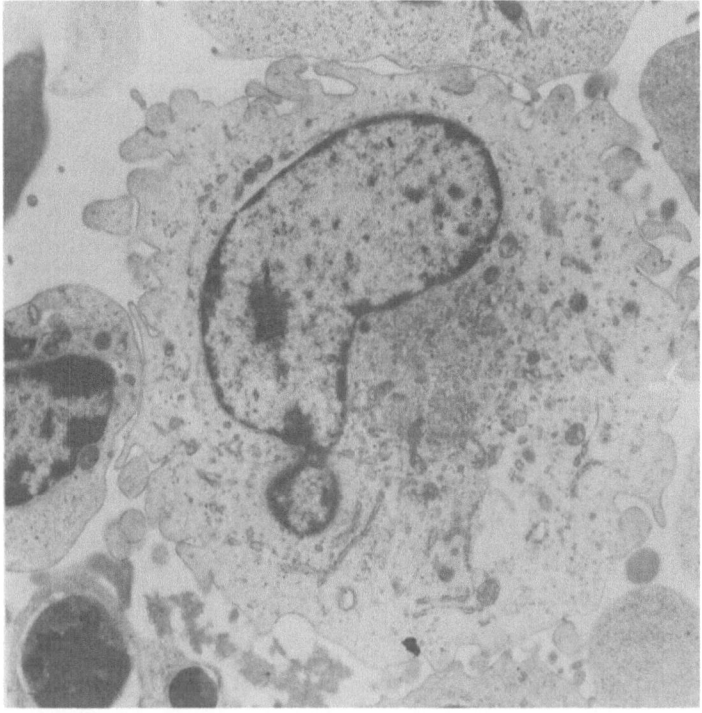

Figure 15.2   Electron micrograph of a mature sheep macrophage in renal afferent lymph. Golgi apparatus is conspicuous in the perinuclear area (× 6000)

important so far as this model of CMI is concerned are those acting on MNP (macrophage chemotactic factor – MCF, migration inhibition factor – MIF, and macrophage activating factor – MAF), and those which act as mitogens for non-specific lymphocytes, stimulation of which probably acts to increase the local concentration of lymphokines.

Thus it is considered that specifically sensitized T lymphocytes act to recruit MNP to the sites of pathogen localization, and to cause the differentiation and activation of the MNP. Only in this state of activation are MNP able to kill ingested pathogens.

Useful as this model is, there are still many gaps to be filled before we have a thorough understanding of CMI. Amongst these are the nature of the antigen-specific T cell factor, the structure and mechanisms of action of lymphokines and the microbicidal mechanisms of MNP. Some of these will be discussed later.

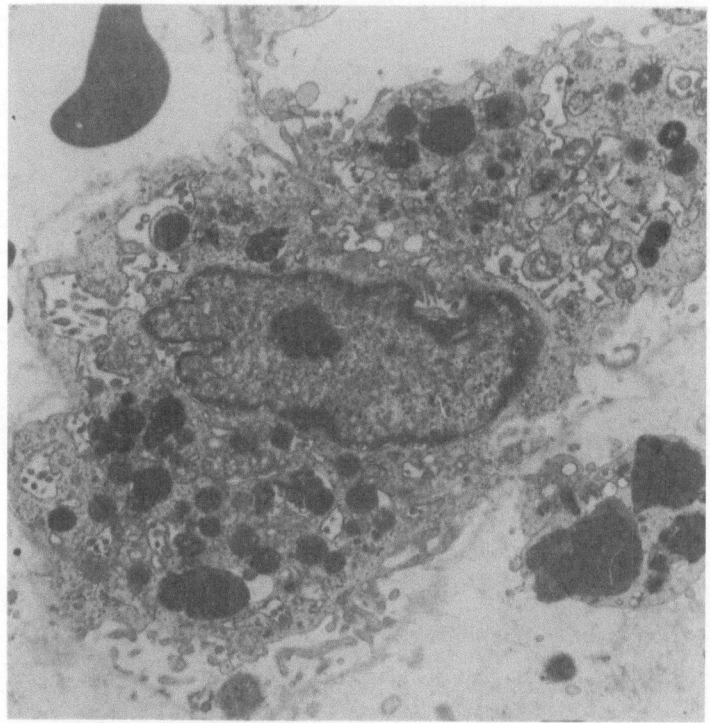

Figure 15.3 Electron micrograph of a 'stimulated' macrophage in a rejecting rat cardiac allograft. Numerous intracytoplasmic organelles are present, and there is a conspicuous nucleolus (× 7200)

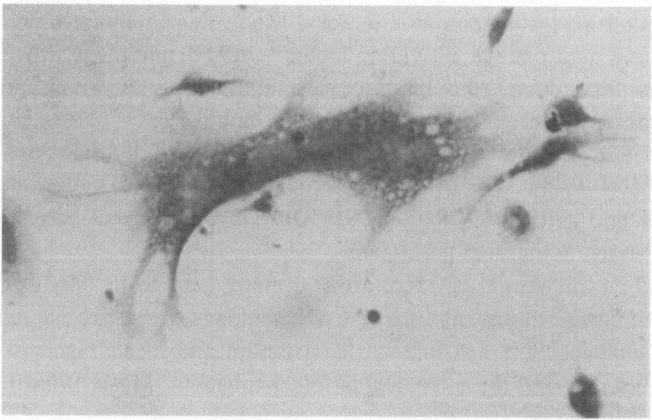

Figure 15.4 Light micrograph of a giant cell formed by fusion of sheep macrophages. Approximately 20 nuclei are present (× 360)

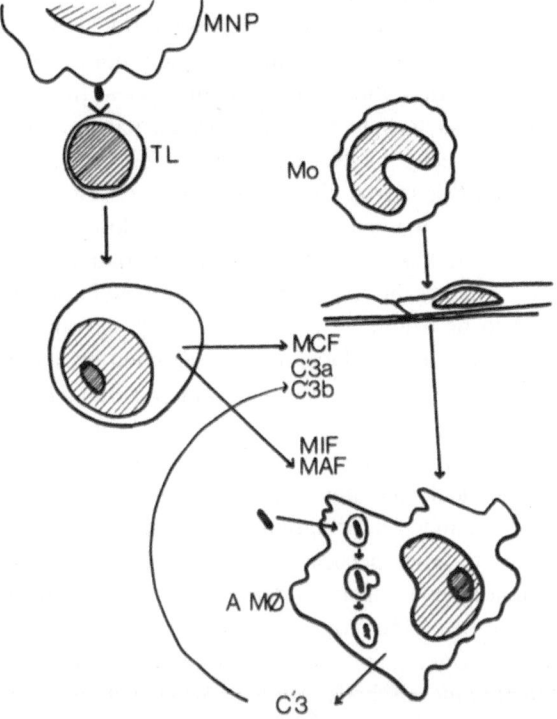

Figure 15.5   Diagram illustrating a current model for cell-mediated immunity.
TL: thymus-derived lymphocyte; MNP: mononuclear phagocyte; Mo: monocyte;
MCF: macrophage chemotactic factor; MIF: migration inhibition factor; MAF:
macrophage activating factor; AM: activated macrophage

POSSIBLE SITES FOR DEFECTS IN CMI

The investigation and characterization of defects in CMI is dependent
upon a clear understanding of the mechanisms operating in the normal
state. However, the description and analysis of defects in immunity is
itself a powerful means of gaining insight into these mechanisms. It is
quite possible that only major defects will be easily recognizable and thus
in order to recognize minor defects, one should try to predict sites where
they could or should occur if the current model for CMI is correct.

Some possible sites for defects in non-specific CMI can be indicated
and ways in which such defects might be investigated can be suggested. As
we are only just beginning to understand T cell–MNP interactions in the
generation of CMI, many of these suggestions are necessarily speculative.

The first non-specific site for a defect in CMI might be in the MNP responsible for the presentation of antigen to the T cell. However, the rigorous non-specificity of MNP in Ag presentation has recently been called into question by the suggestion that Ir gene products may be present on the MNP surface[4]. In addition, it is becoming clear that T cells do not recognize antigen as such, but recognize it in association with histocompatibility antigens, usually Ia. Recent work by Zinkernagel and his co-workers[5] shows that this is true also of immunity to Listeria. This field is still in its infancy, but it would be interesting to look for resistance to infection in terms of linkage to particular histocompatibility antigens and then to determine whether the resistance was expressed in MNP.

The next area to be examined is that of the lymphokines. It would be quite possible for there to be defects in their secretion by activated T cells or in their molecular structure. However, this area is difficult to investigate for two reasons. Firstly we do not know details of the structure of these substances and secondly because we cannot accurately quantitate them. To say that a chemical mediator is a glycoprotein of molecular weight 50 000 does not give much information, and neither are the bioassays for lymphokines able to give accurate quantitative data. Further understanding of lymphokines is likely to derive from two approaches. Firstly the chemical definition of the molecules, and secondly the development of quantitative assays. Both these approaches would be greatly helped if a specific anti-lymphokine antibody could be produced, and recent reports suggest that this might be possible[6]. If the Kohler and Milstein[7] technique for producing monoclonal antibody were utilized, then rapid advances might be made.

A further site for a defect might be in the lymphokine–MNP interaction. Again we know so little about the molecular nature of these interactions, or about the relative importance of different lymphokines in the initiation of these reactions that it is not at present technically possible to design experiments to analyse them. Much of the difficulty stems from a deep lack of understanding of the biological role of the mediators in *in vivo* CMI. Take the example of MIF. This, the first lymphokine to be described[8] causes MNP to round up and stop migration *in vitro*. It was thus thought that its action *in vivo* would be to prevent MNP from leaving the site of the response. However, it is quite clear that in cell-mediated immune responses *in vivo*, MNP in all stages of differentiation do leave these sites in large numbers in the lymph[9,10]. It now seems possible that the MAF may be the same molecule as MIF, and that the role of MIF *in vivo* is the activation of MNP.

This leads to the question of MNP activation. Unlike neutrophils, normal MNP are not strongly microbicidal towards pathogenic organisms;

although they phagocytose them avidly, they are not able to destroy them. However, MNP from an animal recovering from a sublethal infection with one of these organisms show a greatly increased microbicidal activity. MNP such as these also show metabolic and functional changes, for example increased respiratory activity[11], increased content of lysosomal enzymes, increased secretion of lysosomal[12] and neutral[13] enzymes and increased phagocytic capability. A major problem facing us is how all these well-described parameters relate to each other and to the increased microbicidal capacity.

There is some evidence that they may not all necessarily be present at the same time or all be needed for the increase in microbicidal capability. Thus thioglycollate is a potent stimulator of phagocytosis, of metabolic changes and of enzyme secretion, but makes little if any difference to microbicidal capabilities. On the other hand, the peritoneal MNP from a mouse recovering from a Listeria infection appear to be less stimulated than thioglycollate MNP, yet show a markedly increased microbicidal capability. This dichotomy could be the answer to a longstanding problem, the relationship between delayed hypersensitivity and cellular immunity. Are these two phenomena always found together? Clinical and experimental evidence suggests that in some cases there may be relatively more tissue-destructive delayed hypersensitivity. For instance, why are most infective episodes with *Mycobacterium leprae* and tuberculosis subclinical, with but a few cases reaching clinical significance because of the development of marked delayed hypersensitivity? Is it possible that particular antigens or antigens presented in a particular manner tend to lead to the stimulation of the secretory activity of MNP rather than the microbicidal? This then might be another example of a defect in MNP function, but perhaps one that is open to investigation at the present time.

EXPERIMENTAL INVESTIGATION OF CMI

Two separate types of experimental approach are available for investigating defects in CMI in experimental animals. The first is to look for differences in resistance to infection between families or inbred lines of animals.

The other method is to introduce artificial defects into a CMI model that works efficiently under normal circumstances. At the moment we are rather limited in the ways that this method can be applied. T cell manipulation is possible to some extent, but only in a few cases are we able to deplete or select a specific T cell population. The use of lymphokine inhibitors[6] is just commencing but may prove to be a most rewarding approach.

The field which holds most promise at the moment lies in the manipulation of MNPs. The action of the MNP as the final effector cell depends on the heightening of its microbicidal powers via antigen-specific T cells. One may then predict that agents which interfere with MNP activation will depress resistance to infection while those which stimulate MNP will increase resistance.

That this is true in general terms is well recognized, but some aspects of the techniques involved need to be examined. Agents that depress MNP function are of several kinds. Some, mainly inert chemicals, are thought to be specifically cytotoxic to MNP. These are exemplified by silica, carrageenan and dextran sulphate. Another presumably cytotoxic agent is antimacrophage serum. Other methods are much less specific, for example corticosteroids, which certainly depress MNP function[14] but also have profound effects on the specific immune system.

The mechanism by which these agents act *in vitro* are reasonably well understood. For example silica damages the lysosomal membrane after phagocytosis causing the release of hydrolases into the cytoplasm of the cell[15]. However, their action *in vivo* is less well defined. There are many reports which show that these agents can depress the expression of CMI in terms of delayed hypersensitivity and resistance to infection, but in many cases there is no attempt made to show that the changes are caused by a cytotoxic action on MNP. These agents initiate widespread chronic inflammatory lesions and it is possible that MNP are recruited into these lesions preferentially, resulting in a decrease in MNP migration to the other areas.

The situation is even less clear with antimacrophage serum which unabsorbed has activity against lymphocytes and PMN as well as MNP[16]. The antilymphocyte activity can be absorbed relatively easily, but it is very difficult to absorb anti-PMN activity without also removing anti-MNP activity. Figure 15.6 shows the *in vivo* effects of rabbit antirat macrophage serum on absolute numbers of circulating blood leukocytes. This serum had been absorbed ×2 with lymphocytes and peritoneal exudate PMN. However, the intravenous injection of the serum still caused striking changes in the numbers of PMN and lymphocytes as well as a marked diminution in the numbers of monocytes. Despite the lowering of monocyte numbers by 80–90%, the accumulation of MNP on a coverslip skin window was not significantly decreased. Thus it is clear that claims that alterations in CMI following the administration of antimacrophage serum are due to effects on MNP must be viewed with caution.

Finally I should like to turn to the other experimental approach to the study of defects in CMI, the use of inbred strains which demonstrate differ-

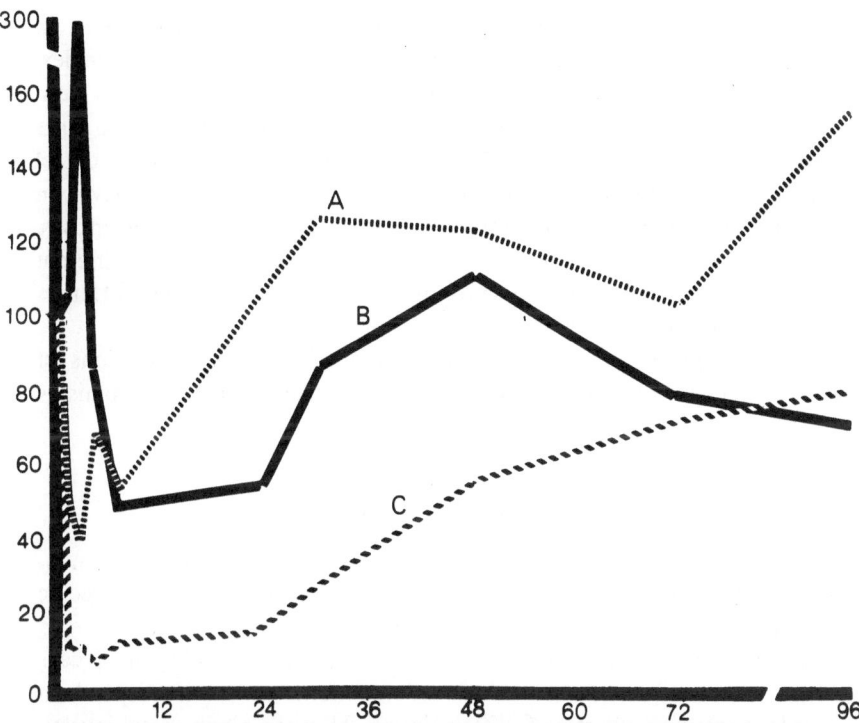

Figure 15.6   Effects of a single 0.5 ml intravenous dose of antimacrophage serum on numbers of circulating leukocytes. A. Neutrophil polymorphs; B. Lymphocytes; C. Monocytes

ences in immunity to infection. A genetic basis for susceptibility to infection has long been recognized in animals. as exemplified by the work of Lurie with families of rabbits[17]. However, it is only recently that analytical techniques have become available to permit the investigation of the mechanisms underlying these defects. Some of these defects are probably under the control of genes linked to the major histocompatibility complex and are probably concerned with specific antigen responsiveness, but others probably are not, and several models under current investigation are of interest[18-20]. In two of these studies the natural resistance of different mouse strains to *Salmonella typhimurium*[18] and *Leishmania donovani*[19] was compared. In both cases, strains were found to be resistant or nonresistant in terms of the ability of the pathogens to grow within the mice; no strains were of intermediate resistance. The same strains were resistant both to *S. typhimurium* and to *L. donovani*. Breeding experiments with *L. donovani* showed that resistance behaved as a Mendelian dominant characteristic. Most interestingly, the gene controlling resistance to *L. donovani* clearly does not map with the major histocompatibility complex. In other studies, natural resistance to virus infection in mice has been investigated[20]. These studies illustrate quite clearly that resistance to virus infection is mediated via macrophages and that it is under genetic control with a single Mendelian dominant gene conferring resistance. However, in the case of viruses, different strains may be resistant to different viruses, and it has been shown that the genes controlling resistance to different viruses may segregate independently. In one case, the resistance to Herpes simplex virus has been shown to be X-linked[21].

Thus it appears that there exist different phenotypic expressions of genetic resistance to infection. and that the elucidation of the mechanisms underlying this resistance is of the utmost importance.

CONCLUSIONS

(1) The expression of cell-mediated immunity to many pathogens is non-specific, but depends on a complex series of interactions between specific T lymphocytes, humoral mediators and mononuclear phagocytes.

(2) Mononuclear phagocytes are a heterogeneous population of cells whose morphological, biochemical and functional properties depend on their localization and state of differentiation. Thus the biochemical investigation of defects in cell-mediated immunity is greatly hampered.

(3) The analysis of defects in cell-mediated immunity depends on the development of techniques allowing investigation of individual components of the immune response.

(4) Studies of genetic differences which are not linked to the major histocompatibility complex in resistance to infection may provide valuable information concerning defects in non-specific CMI and may be relevant to susceptibility in humans.

References

1. Mackaness, G. B. (1970). Cellular immunity. In R. van Furth (ed.). *Mononuclear Phagocytes in Immunity, Infection and Pathology*. (Oxford: Blackwell Scientific Publications)
2. Thomas, D. W. and Shevach, E. M. (1977). Nature of the antigenic complex recognized by T lymphocytes: specific sensitization by antigens associated with allogenic macrophages. *Proc. Natl. Acad. Sci., USA,* **74**, 2104
3. Dumonde, D. C., Kelly. R. H., Preston, P. M. and Wolstencroft, R. A. (1975). Lymphokines and macrophage function in the immunological res-

ponse. In R. van Furth (ed.). *Mononuclear Phagocytes in Immunity, Infection and Pathology*. (Oxford: Blackwell Scientific Publications)

4. Rosenthal, A. S., Barcinski, M. A. and Blake, J. T. (1977). Determinant selection is a macrophage-dependent immune response gene function. *Nature (London)*, **267**, 156

5. Zinkernagel, R. M., Althage, A., Adler, B., Blanden, R. V., Davidson, W. F., Kees, U., Dunlop, M. B. C. and Shreffler, D. O. (1977). H-2 Restriction of cell-mediated immunity to an intracellular bacterium. *J. Exp. Med.*, **145**, 1353

6. Geczy, C. L., Friedrich, W. and De Weck, A. L. (1975). Production and *in vivo* effect of antibodies against guinea-pig lymphokines. *Cell. Immunol.*, **19**, 65

7. Kohler, G. and Milstein, C. (1976). Derivation of specific antibody-producing tissue culture and tumour lines by cell fusion. *Europ. J. Immunol.*, **6**, 511

8. Bloom, B. R. and Bennett, B. (1966). Mechanism of a reaction *in vitro* associated with delayed-type hypersensitivity. *Science NY*, **153**, 80

9. Smith, J. B., McIntosh, G. H. and Morris, B. (1970). The migration of cells through chronically inflamed tissues. *J. Pathol.*, **100**, 21

10. MacPherson, G. G., Murphy, M. J., Jr. and Morris, B. *Transplantation*, **24**, 16

11. Nathan, C. F., Karnousky, N. L. and David, J. R. (1971). Alterations of macrophage functions by mediators from lymphocytes. *J. Exp. Med.*, **133**, 1356

12. Davies, P. and Allison, A. C. (1976). Secretion of macrophage enzymes in relation to the pathogenesis of chronic inflammation. In D. S. Nelson (ed.). *Immunobiology of the Macrophage*. (New York: Academic Press)

13. Werb, Z. and Gordon, S. (1975). Secretion of a specific collagenase by stimulated macrophages. *J. Exp. Med.*, **142**, 346

14. Thompson, J. and van Furth, R. (1970). The effect of glucocorticosteroids on the kinetics of mononuclear phagocytes. *J. Exp. Med.*, **131**, 429

15. Allison, A. C., Harington, J. S. and Birbeck, M. (1966). An examination of cytotoxic effects of silica on macrophages. *J. Exp. Med.*, **124**, 141

16. MacPherson, G. G. Unpublished results

17. Lurie, M. B. (1964). *Resistance to Tuberculosis: Experimental Studies in Nature and Acquired Defence Mechanisms*. (Cambridge, Mass.: Harvard University Press)

18. Plant, J. and Glynn, A. A. (1974). Natural resistance to *Salmonella* infection, delayed hypersensitivity and *Ir* genes in different strains of mice. *Nature (London)*, **248**, 345

19. Bradley, D. J. (1974). Genetic control of natural resistance to *Leishmania donovani*. *Nature (London)*, **250**, 353

20. Allison, A. C. (1974). Interactions of antibodies, complement components and various cell types in immunity against viruses and pyogenic bacteria. *Transplant Rev.*, **19**, 3

21. Mogensen, S. Personal communication

16

Molecular bases of the metabolic excitability of phagocytes
D. Romeo, P. Dri, P. Bellavite and F. Rossi

A number of oxidative reactions, lethal to many bacteria, fungi, certain viruses and mycoplasmas, are activated by phagocytosis in polymorphonuclear leukocytes (PMNL) and macrophages[1-4].

The efficiency of these microbicidal systems depends on the continuous supply of hydrogen peroxide (H_2O_2) and superoxide anion (O_2^-), the main products of the increased O_2 reduction in phagocytosing leukocytes[3, 5-14]. The mechanism of generation and utilization of these compounds has been the subject of extensive investigation in several laboratories. Suitable techniques have been set up to measure the rate and extent of O_2 consumption and of concomitant generation of O_2^-, H_2O_2 and $NADP^+$, especially in the early stage following cell exposure to phagocytosable particles.

METHODOLOGY

The most appropriate way of measuring the consumption of O_2 by phagocytes is that of following the rate of respiration of a cell suspension, before and after addition of particulate objects, by means of an oxygen elec-

231

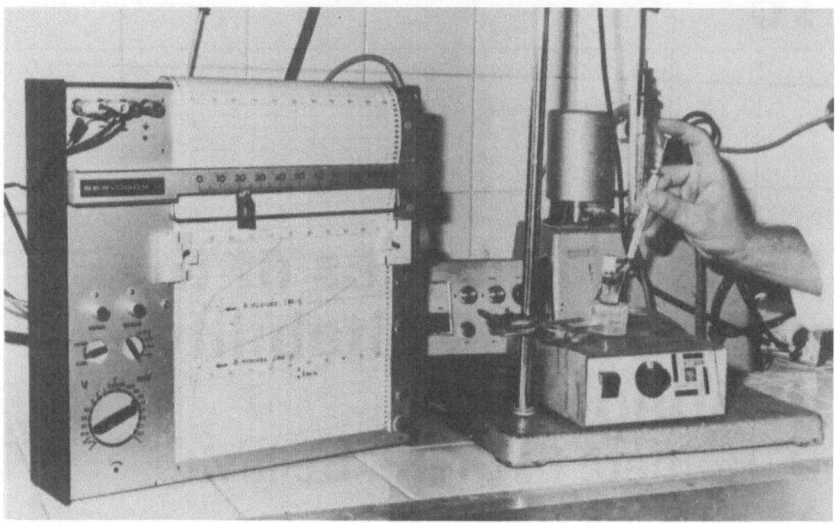

Figure 16.1   Polarographic assembly and recorded traces of oxygen consumption by PMNL

trode[15]. We currently use a Clark-type oxygen electrode attached to a thermostatically controlled (37 °C) plastic vessel. Each sample contains 2 ml of cell suspension ($1-2 \times 10^7$ cells) stirred magnetically and additions of activators of cell metabolism are made through a narrow puncture in the lid covering the vessel. Our polarographic set-up and a typical polarographic trace are shown in Figure 16.1.

The rate of hydrogen peroxide release from the cells can be measured fluorometrically by the decrease of scopoletin fluorescence in the presence of horseradish peroxidase (HRP)[12]. Scopoletin (7-hydroxy-6-methoxy-coumarin) emits a blue fluorescence when excited with light of 350 nm wavelength (emission 460 nm). In the presence of H_2O_2 it is oxidized by HRP yielding a loss of fluorescence which is directly proportional to the peroxide concentration in the medium. Hydrogen peroxide can also be determined colorimetrically with the ferrithiocyanate method[16]. Briefly, portions of a cell suspension are treated with trichloroacetic acid and, after removal of precipitated protein by centrifugation, reacted with ferrous ammonium sulphate and potassium thiocyanate. The absorption of the red thiocyanate complex formed in the presence of H_2O_2 is read at 480 nm. With the two methods, determinations of H_2O_2 on standard H_2O_2 solutions as well as on samples of phagocytes provide results which match very closely each other[14].

The assay of O_2^- is in general confined to the amount of this radical which is recovered outside the cell, where it reacts with exogenous ferricytochrome c in a stoichiometric relationship of $1:1$[10]. The amount of O_2^--dependent reduction of cytochrome c is calculated from the difference of absorbance between the cytochrome c reduced in the absence of superoxide dismutase (SOD) and the cytochrome c reduced in the presence of SOD, by using an extinction coefficient[14] of $21.1\ mM^{-1}\ cm^{-1}$; O_2^- production can also be determined by measuring SOD-sensitive reduction of nitroblue tetrazolium (NBT) to formazan at 530 nm, by using an E_m M for formazan of 18.3 and a stoichiometric relationship between O_2^- formation and NBT reduction of two to one[4,17].

Dri et al.[14] have combined these techniques to obtain a simultaneous determination of O_2 consumption and recovery of O_2^- and H_2O_2 in the same cell suspension. Briefly, they measured the consumption of O_2 in the absence or in the presence of cytochrome c (to trap O_2^-) and of NaN_3 (to inhibit the peroxidatic and catalatic degradation of H_2O_2). At 2 min from the addition of phagocytosable particles to the leukocytes, portions of the cell suspension are quickly transferred from the vessel, where O_2 consumption is recorded, into an Eppendorf microtube and centrifuged (when measuring O_2^-, the microtubes contain SOD to prevent further cytochrome c reduction). The cell free supernatants are then used for the determination of H_2O_2 and of the extent of O_2^--dependent ferricytochrome c reduction.

Coupled to the enhanced O_2 reduction in phagocytosing leukocytes there is also an increased utilization of glucose in the oxidative route of the hexose monophosphate pathway (HMP)[18-23]. The yield of $^{14}CO_2$ from 1-[^{14}C]glucose can be evaluated either after a suitable incubation time or by continuous sampling from the O_2 electrode vessel[9]. In the former case, the leukocyte suspension is added to Erlenmeyer flasks, which are shaken at 37 °C in a Dubnoff incubator. After addition of labelled glucose and of suitable metabolic stimulants, the flasks are rapidly covered with a rubber cap. The reaction is terminated by injecting H_2SO_4 through the cap and $^{14}CO_2$, trapped in a centre well containing KOH, is quantitated by liquid scintillation spectrometry. Alternatively, labelled glucose can be added to the oxygen electrode vessel; in the course of the measurement of oxygen consumption, small portions of the cell suspension are withdrawn at suitable time intervals with a microsyringe, and rapidly injected into rubber-capped flasks containing H_2SO_4.

KINETICS OF STIMULATION OF THE OXIDATIVE METABOLISM OF PHAGOCYTES

The methods described above allow a continuous recording of the process of activation of oxidative metabolism in phagocytosing leukocytes. This has permitted us to observe that the onset of phagocytosis-associated stimulation of O_2 reduction to O_2^- and H_2O_2 and of HMP activity falls a few seconds after exposure of leukocytes to the phagocytosable objects. This is shown by the representative experiments of Figures 16.2 and 16.3.

The overall rate of the oxidative route of HMP is dependent on the cellular NADP$^+$ concentration[24]. Thus one would expect that the increased rate of glucose oxidation by phagocytosing PMNL is sustained by a sudden increase in the steady-state concentration of NADP$^+$. Rossi et al.[23] have indeed shown that 3 min after the exposure of leukocytes to bacteria there is a 3-fold increase in the NADP$^+$:NADPH ratio, whereas the steady-state concentrations of NAD$^+$ and NADH vary very slightly (Table 16.1).

Continuous monitoring of O_2 disappearance from the cell-suspending medium in the electrode vessel (Figures 16.1 and 16.2) indicates that the

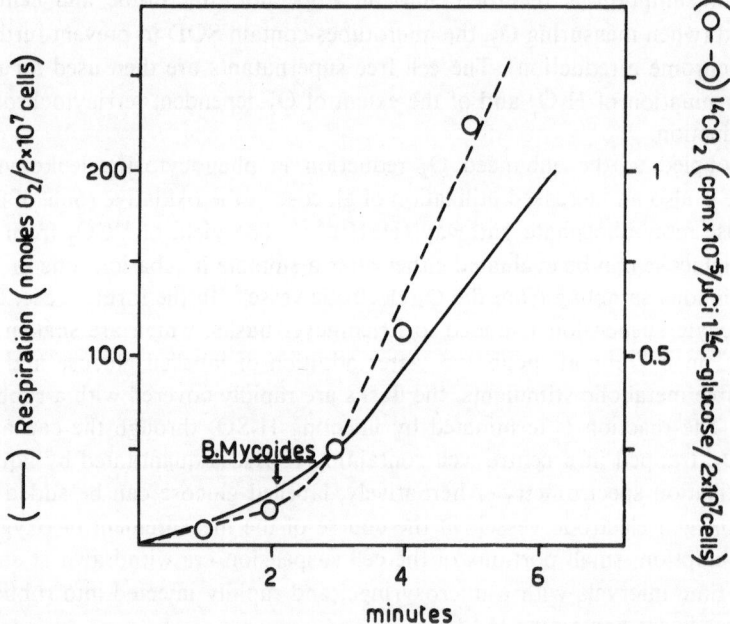

Figure 16.2   Simultaneous evaluation of the kinetics of stimulation of O_2 consumption and hexose monophosphate pathway activity in PMNL exposed to heat-killed opsonized bacteria

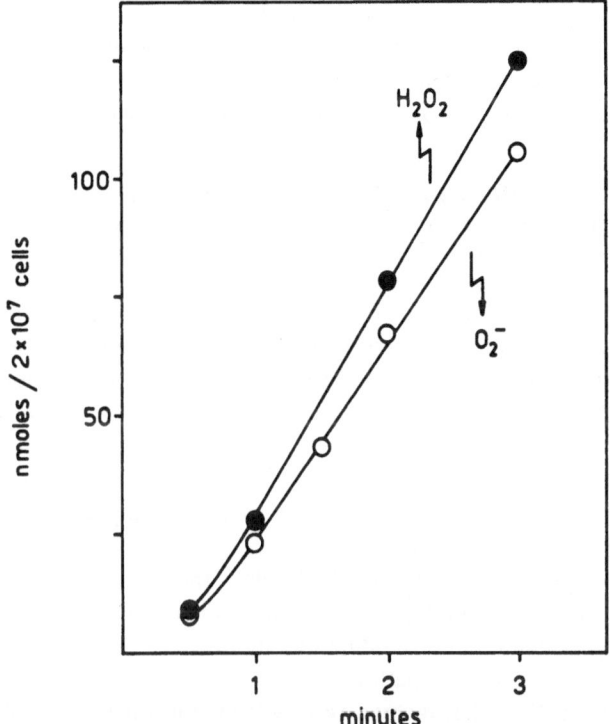

Figure 16.3 Recovery of O_2^- and H_2O_2 ($+ NaN_3$) generated by phagocytosing PMNs (heat-killed opsonized *B. mycoides* added at time zero)

TABLE 16.1 Nicotinamide adenine nucleotide concentrations in resting and phagocytosing (3 min) PMNL*.

| | Resting cells | | Phagocytosing cells | |
	mM†	*Ratio*	*mM†*	*Ratio*
NADP⁺	0.031	0.11	0.065	0.31
NADPH	0.273		0.211	
NAD⁺	0.434	7.11	0.448	7.72
NADH	0.061		0.058	

* Data taken from Patriarca *et al.*[25]
† Based on a value of 0.35 μl cell water/million PMNL (Hawkins and Berlin[57])

rate of activated oxygen consumption is linear for at least a few minutes. Concomitantly, the sampling technique for determination of HMP activity, O_2^- and H_2O_2 (Figures 16.2 and 16.3) also confirms that the rate of activated metabolism is linear for a few minutes after exposure of leukocytes to phagocytosable particles. This linearity of the rate of the metabolic events very likely reflects a linearity of the rate of the phagocytic process, which with increasing time involves an increasing number of cells and leads to increased number of surface membrane invaginations[26].

STOICHIOMETRIC RELATIONSHIP BETWEEN CONSUMPTION OF O_2 AND GENERATION OF O_2^- AND H_2O_2

The steady-state rate of consumption of O_2 and generation of O_2^- and H_2O_2 by a leukocyte population challenged with phagocytosable objects depends on a number of factors. First of all, as mentioned above, it depends on the rate at which an increasing number of cells become engaged in phagocytosis and on the rate at which the metabolism-activating endocytic events take place. For example, cytochalasin B causes a depression in O_2 consumption by reducing the number of phagocytic events and the rate of surface internalization[26].

Secondly, it depends on the activity levels of the primary O_2 reductase(s) and on the rates at which O_2^- and H_2O_2 are utilized in the cells and in the surrounding medium. In the assumption that the reduction of O_2 essentially proceeds via a one-electron pathway[13], the steady-state rate of oxygen consumption by activated leukocyte results from the rates of the following reactions:

$$1. \quad O_2 + RH \rightarrow O_2^- + H^+ + R^{\cdot}$$
$$1'. \quad O_2 + R^{\cdot} \rightarrow O_2^- + R$$
$$2. \quad 2O_2^- + 2H^+ \rightarrow O_2 + H_2O_2$$
$$3. \quad H_2O_2 \rightarrow \tfrac{1}{2}O_2 + H_2O$$

Reactions 1 and 1' have not yet been defined precisely and, as we will discuss below, the identity of RH, the cell localization and the nature of the oxidase (or O_2^--generating enzyme) have not yet been fully clarified. Reaction 2 may either proceed spontaneously or be catalysed by SOD, whose presence in the cytosol and in the granule fraction of PMNL has been detected by several investigators[4, 27-31]. Finally, the rate of reaction 3 is controlled by catalase, an enzyme which in phagocytes is either soluble or particulate[8, 23, 32, 33].

In the presence of ferricytochrome c, the extracellularly released O_2^-, instead of undergoing dismutation (reaction 2), is oxidized to molecular oxygen:

$$4. \quad O_2^- + cyt\ c\ (Fe^{3+}) \rightarrow O_2 + cyt\ c\ (Fe^{2+})$$

This duplicates the amount of O_2^- converted back to O_2 (see reaction 2). Thus, addition of ferricytochrome c to O_2^--releasing phagocytes is expected to diminish the overall rate of O_2 consumption, this effect being neutralized by exogenous SOD.

Treatment of phagocytosing leukocytes with poisons of haem-enzymes, such as sodium azide (NaN_3), causes the inhibition of catalatic breakdown of H_2O_2 (reaction 3), thereby somewhat increasing the overall rate of O_2 consumption. Hydrogen peroxide may be utilized in other reactions, such as that catalysed by NaN_3-sensitive peroxidase(s):

$$5. \quad H_2O_2 + AH_2 \rightarrow 2H_2O + A$$

and that catalysed by NaN_3-insensitive glutathione peroxidase[21]:

$$6. \quad H_2O_2 + 2GSH \rightarrow GSSG + 2H_2O$$

Thus, the higher the rate of reaction 3 (catalase) with respect to reactions 5 (peroxidase) and 6 (glutathione peroxidase) the larger will be the effect of NaN_3 on the rate of overall oxygen consumption.

With their sampling technique, carried out under appropriate conditions of assay linearity with respect to time and cell concentration, Dri et al.[14] have recently carried out a number of measurements of O_2 consumption and recovery of generated O_2^- and H_2O_2, which allow an experimental control of the stoichiometric relationships shown in the above reactions. Data referring to phagocytosing guinea-pig PMNs are summarized in Table 16.2. The table shows that, consistently with the expectations, the addition of NaN_3 increases the overall O_2 consumption, which is on the contrary decreased by cytochrome c. By virtue of the NaN_3-insensitivity of the O_2^--generating enzyme(s)[17, 31], the recovery of O_2^- is virtually unaffected by this inhibitor. Conversely, the inhibition of catalase and peroxidase by NaN_3 causes a great increase in the accumulation of H_2O_2.

TABLE 16.2 O_2 consumption, extracellular O_2^- recovery and H_2O_2 accumulation in phagocytosing PMNL*

	$-NaN_3$		$+NaN_3$	
	$-$	$+ cyt\ c\ddagger$	$-$	$+ cyt\ c\ddagger$
O_2 Consumption†	72.7 ± 10.6	56.3 ± 8.8	94.5 ± 15.8	64.0 ± 14.0
O_2^- Recovery†	$-$	65.5 ± 15.5	$-$	63.7 ± 14.2
H_2O_2 Accumulation†	<2	<2	84.8 ± 7.4	59.9 ± 11.1

* Data taken from Dri et al.[14]
† nmol/2 min/2 × 10^7 cells (increments with respect to resting cells)
‡ The effects of cytochrome c were neutralized by exogenous SOD

In the presence of NaN_3, the only back-production of O_2 should derive from decay of O_2^- (1 mol of O_2 generated per 2 mol of O_2 reduced in reactions $1 + 1'$). Thus, the total amount of O_2 reduced should be twice that actually measured, i.e. by using the data of Table 16.2, an average of $94.5 \times 2 = 189$ nmol/2 min/2 $\times 10^7$ cells. The reduction of this amount of O_2 should ultimately lead to the generation of 94.5 nmol of H_2O_2 (reactions $1 + 1' + 2$), of which about 90% are recovered. This suggests that not more than 10% of the produced H_2O_2, at least in the early phase of metabolic stimulation of PMNs, is disposed through NaN_3-insensitive pathways, including the glutathione-metabolizing pathway.

Table 16.2 also shows that the presence of NaN_3 causes an increment in O_2 consumption of 21.8 nmol/2 min/2 $\times 10^7$ cells. On account of reaction 3, this means that 43.6 nmol of H_2O_2/2 $\times 10^7$ cells are degraded by catalase in the first 2 min following the metabolic stimulation. This value represents about 46% of the H_2O_2 actually produced during this time, thereby suggesting that the residual 44% of H_2O_2 is utilized in NaN_3-sensitive peroxidative reactions.

From Table 16.2 it also emerges that the addition of cytochrome c to phagocytosing cells does not fully suppress O_2 consumption, as would be expected if, under this condition, reactions $1 + 1'$ and 4 prevailed over the other reactions. The possibility that this might be due to competition between O_2^- dismutation and oxidation by cytochrome c seems very unlikely. In fact, although at pH 7.4 the two reactions have comparable rate constants[34, 35], the steady-state extracellular concentration of O_2^- should be several-fold lower than that of cytochrome c. A more likely explanation is that only a portion of O_2^- is accessible to cytochrome c extracellularly, the remaining part of it being subjected to dismutation either in the cytoplasm or in the phagocytic vacuoles. From the data of Table 16.2, which refer to measurements carried out in the early stage of the phagocytic stimulus, it appears that the amount of O_2^- oxidized by cytochrome c is about 34% of that produced according to the one-electron mechanism of reduction of O_2 (reactions $1 + 1'$). An additional explanation is that, in contrast to our assumption, part of O_2 is reduced by a two-electron mechanism with direct generation of H_2O_2.

Some interesting considerations might finally be made on the stoichiometric relationship between the decrease of O_2 consumption caused by cytochrome c and O_2^- recovered extracellularly. By adding reactions 2 and 3, one ends up with the following overall reaction:

$$7. \quad 2O_2^- + 2H^+ \rightarrow \tfrac{3}{2}O_2 + H_2O$$

which shows that for $2O_2$ reduced to $2O_2^-$ only $\frac{1}{2}O_2$ is actually consumed. Thus, the ratio between the decrease of O_2 consumption caused by cytochrome c and the extracellularly recovered O_2^- should be $1:4$. This calculated ratio is fully verified by the experimental data of Table 16.2. When catalase is prevented from acting on H_2O_2 because of the presence of NaN_3, this ratio should become $1:2$ (see reaction 2). This is also fully consistent with the data of Table 16.2.

To summarize, our conclusions are that, at least in the early stage following the PMN exposure to phagocytosable particles, not more than one-third of the O_2 reduced in reactions $1 + 1'$ is recovered extracellularly as O_2^-, and that most of the H_2O_2 produced, either by dismutation of O_2^- or as primary product of O_2 reduction, is utilized in NaN_3-sensitive peroxidatic and catalatic reactions.

SUBSTRATE AND LOCALIZATION OF THE OXIDASE (O_2^--GENERATING ENZYME)

The coupling of enhanced O_2 reduction to stimulation of HMP, sustained by an increased $NADP^+$: NADPH ratio, requires that an NADPH oxidative pathway is activated in phagocytosing leukocytes. Following the original discovery of an NADPH oxidase in PMNs by Iyer and Quastel[36], Rossi and his co-workers have described a particulate NADPH oxidase, whose activity is several-fold increased in phagocytosing cells[9, 23, 25, 37, 38]. This enzyme, which is recovered in the 20 000 g granule fraction of leukocytes, has been originally assayed both polarographically and spectrophotometrically at pH 7.2 and shown to lead to the generation of H_2O_2[37]. Subsequently, Patriarca *et al.*[25, 38] demonstrated that NADPH oxidation by the granule fraction is maximal at pH 5.5 and is activated by Mn^{2+}. The low pH optimum has been thought to support a role for the NADPH oxidase in the metabolic activation of PMNs, since the phagocytic vacuole, where the enzyme should exert its activity, is rapidly acidified after interiorization[39].

At pH 5.5 the oxidation of NADPH is inhibited by SOD[38], thereby suggesting that the oxidation of the nucleotide is O_2^--dependent. This finding is consistent with the observation later reported by Babior *et al.*[17, 40] that the granule fraction of PMNL exhibits an NADPH-dependent O_2^--generating enzyme activity (pH 5.5), which is increased more than 30 times by phagocytosis.

Both NADPH oxidase (pH 5.5, Mn^{2+})[41, 42] and NADPH-dependent O_2^- generating enzyme (pH 5.5)[40] have been reported to be insensitive to the phagocytic stimulus in PMNs of CGD patients, thereby suggesting that the inability of these cells to carry out the respiratory burst may be due to lack of activation of O_2^--generating NADPH oxidation.

The localization of the NADPH-dependent O_2^--generating enzyme is still unclear. The granule fraction, to which it is associated, presumably contains, beside the two main populations of granules of PMNs[43], vesicles derived from the plasma membrane and other subcellular organelles. Takanaka and O'Brien[44] and Roos[45] have suggested that the enzyme is a component of the plasma membrane. A generation of O_2^- and H_2O_2 at the PMNs surface, which is favoured also by Baehner, Johnston, Root, Goldstein and their associates[4, 49, 50], would directly result in synthesis of these reactive compounds within the phagosome upon membrane internalization during particle ingestion. Furthermore, since the oxidative metabolism of phagocytes is excited not only by particulate objects but by a variety of surface-reactive stimuli, a plasma membrane localization of the oxidase would simplify the problem of understanding the mechanism of its activation[26].

This postulated localization of the NADPH oxidase appears, however, to be in contrast with some experimental observations. In fact, Rossi et al.[46] have shown that the specific activity of NADPH oxidase (pH 5.5, Mn^{2+}) in purified plasma membrane preparations of guinea-pig PMNs is lower than that of the nuclei + granules fraction. Furthermore, Patriarca et al.[47] and Segal and Peters[31] have demonstrated, by sucrose density zonal centrifugation, that in rabbit exudate and human blood PMNs, respectively, the enzyme is associated to the azurophilic granules.

The conclusions reached by Rossi, Babior, Lehrer, De Chatelet and their associates on the key role of NADPH oxidase in the metabolic stimulation of PMNL are not shared by other investigators. In particular, Karnovsky, Segal and their associates believe not only that the site of O_2 reductase activity is the plasma membrane, but also that the reduction of O_2 is accomplished by NADH[31, 48]. They base their conclusions on the observations that NADH stimulates the production of H_2O_2 within the phagosomes and on the plasma membrane of phagocytosing PMNL, as shown by cytochemical identification of H_2O_2 oxidation products, and that purified plasma membrane preparations of resting PMNL exhibit a SOD-inhibitable NBT reductase with high affinity for NADH. So far, however, no isolation of a plasma membrane fraction with stimulated NADH-dependent O_2^--generating activity has been described.

An NADH-dependent reduction of O_2 as a key event in the respiratory burst of phagocytes makes it necessary to postulate secondary pathways to account for the increased generation of $NADP^+$ from NADPH. One such secondary pathway involves the existence in PMNL of a nicotinamide nucleotide transhydrogenase-catalysed reaction[51] that transfers hydrogen from NADPH to newly formed NAD^+. The activity of this enzyme, however, is too low[23, 51, 52] to account for an adequate supply of $NADP^+$ to the HMP[19]. Alternatively, a glutathione-metabolizing pathway has been proposed[21], whose net effect is to reduce a portion of H_2O_2 generated in the metabolic burst. The contribution of this pathway to the generation of $NADP^+$, however, does not appear to be very large, at least in the early stage of the metabolic activation. In fact, Weening et al.[53] have shown that in phagocytosing PMNs of a patient severely deficient in glutathione reductase activity the initial stimulation of HMP activity is only somewhat less than normal.

A third possibility would be that O_2^- generated by the reduction of O_2 by NADH at the plasma membrane oxidizes NADPH via a non-enzymatic chain reaction in the cytosol. This possibility, however, seems rather unlikely, because O_2^- is presumably very rapidly converted to O_2 and H_2O_2 by cytoplasmic SOD[4, 27-30]. Furthermore, the O_2^--dependent oxidation of NADPH is markedly inhibited by NADH at concentrations close to the physiological ones[54].

In conclusion, there are arguments for both a granular NADPH-dependent and a plasma membrane NAD(P)H dependent O_2^- generation, but the problem of the localization and substrate specificity of the O_2 reductase in the intact cell has not yet been conclusively solved, nor has the possibility been ruled out that phagocytosis activates more than one oxidase.

CONCLUSIONS

The main reactions which are thought to lead to generation and utilization of O_2^- and H_2O_2 by phagocytosing leukocytes are illustrated in the scheme of Figure 16.4. The scheme represents a cycle that can be interrupted by a deficient activity of enzymes catalysing either the generation or the detoxification of O_2^- and H_2O_2. Both a failure in the activation of an NADPH-dependent O_2 reductase[41, 42] and the absence of an NADH-dependent O_2 reductase[31] have been suggested to be the defect which interrupts the cycle in PMNL of CGD patients. On the other hand, a defective detoxification of excess H_2O_2 has been proposed to cause O_2 consumption to stop, which was observed after a normal initial stimulation in PMNL of patients with severe glutathione reductase activity[53]. Furthermore, the decreased or absent respiratory burst in glucose-6-phosphate dehydrogenase-deficient PMNs[55] is likely to be ascribed to a decreased rate of NADPH regeneration from $NADP^+$, which would cause a drop in the rate of NADPH-dependent O_2

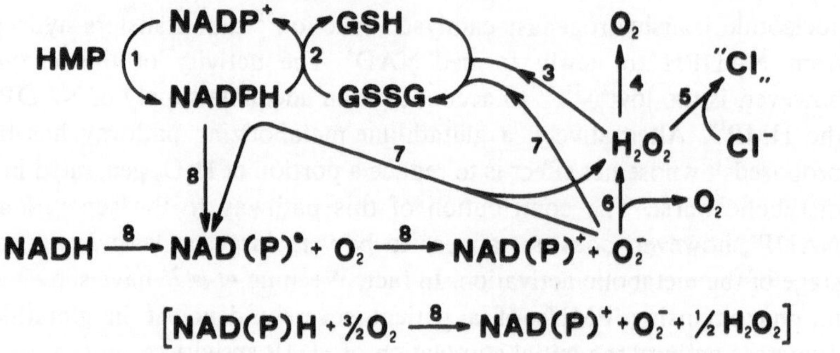

1. Gluc-6-P DH & 6-P-Glucon DH   2. Glutathione Reductase
3. Glutathione Peroxidase   4. Catalase
5. Myeloperoxidase   6. Superoxide Dismutase
7. O_2^- - Dependent Non-Enzymatic Oxidations
8. NAD(P)H-Dependent O_2 Reductase

Figure 16.4 Scheme of metabolism of O_2^- and H_2O_2 in phagocytes (the reaction in square brackets refers to a hypothetical simultaneous monovalent and divalent reduction of O_2)

reduction (O_2^--generation) and of glutathione reduction (H_2O_2 detoxification).

Reagents and products of the reactions shown in the scheme of Figure 16.4 may interact in a rather complex way. The effects of inhibition or activation of any enzyme of the cycle can, therefore, be amplified by these interactions. For example, a drug added to phagocytosing PMNL can decrease O_2 consumption by simply causing an oxidative back-conversion of O_2^- to O_2 or by inhibiting the dehydrogenases of the HMP[56], without any interaction with the primary oxidase. On the contrary, an increase in O_2 consumption may be caused by inhibition of catalatic breakdown of H_2O_2 or by an increased reduction of O_2^-, thereby preventing the conversion of H_2O_2 and O_2^- to O_2, respectively. A stimulation of PMNL respiration caused by cell exposure to reduced nicotinamide nucleotides might be due to O_2^--dependent chain reactions[38] and not to supply of exogenous substrate to an oxidase[44]. In view of these considerations, conclusions concerning the role of enzymes of the cycle of Figure 16.4, based on measurements of a single biochemical parameter (O_2 consumption, for example) carried out with intact cells, are to be drawn with great caution.

Acknowledgements

The research carried out at the Departments of General Pathology and Biochemistry of the University of Trieste was supported by grants of the National Research Council of Italy (CNR). P. Bellavite is a recipient of a fellowship of the A. Villa Rusconi Foundation.

References

1. Klebanoff, S. J. (1975). Antimicrobial mechanisms in neutrophilic polymorphonuclear leukocytes. *Semin. Hematol.*, **12**, 117
2. Sbarra, A. J., Paul, B. B., Jacobs, A. A., Strauss, R. R. and Mitchell, G. W. Jr. (1972). Role of the phagocyte in host–parasite interactions. XXXVIII. Metabolic activities of the phagocyte as related to antimicrobial action. *J. Reticuloendothel. Soc.*, **12**, 109
3. Paul, B. B., Strauss, R. R., Selvaraj, R. J. and Sbarra, A. J. (1973). Peroxidase mediated antimicrobial activities of alveolar macrophage granules. *Science*, **181**, 849
4. Johnston, R. B. Jr., Keele, B. B. Jr., Misra, H. P., Lehmeyer, J. E., Webb, L. S., Baehner, R. L. and Rajagopalan, K. V. (1975). The role of superoxide anion generation in phagocytic bactericidal activity. Studies with normal and chronic granulomatous disease leucocytes. *J. Clin. Invest.*, **55**, 1357
5. Iyer, G. Y. N., Islam, D. M. F. and Quastel, J. H. (1961). Biochemical aspects of phagocytosis, *Nature (London)*. **192**, 535
6. Paul, B. and Sbarra, A. J. (1968). The role of the phagocyte in host–parasite interactions. XIII. The direct quantitative estimation of H_2O_2 in phagocytizing cells. *Biochim. Biophys. Acta*, **156**, 168
7. Zatti, M., Rossi, F. and Patriarca, P. (1968). The H_2O_2 production by polymorphonuclear leucocytes during phagocytosis. *Experientia*, **24**, 669
8. Gee, J. B. L., Vassallo, C. L., Bell, P., Kaskin, J., Basford, R. E. and Field, J. (1970). Catalase-dependent peroxidative metabolism in the alveolar macrophage during phagocytosis. *J. Clin. Invest.*, **49**, 1280
9. Romeo, D., Zabucchi, G., Marzi, T. and Rossi, F. (1973). Kinetic and enzymatic features of metabolism stimulation of alveolar and peritoneal macrophages challenged with bacteria. *Exp. Cell. Res.*, **78**, 423
10. Babior, B. M., Kipnes, R. S. and Curnutte, J. T. (1973). Biological defense mechanisms. The production by leukocytes of superoxide, a potent bactericidal agent. *J. Clin. Invest.*, **52**, 741
11. Drath, D. B. and Karnovsky, M. L. (1975). Superoxide production by phagocytic leukocytes. *J. Exp. Med.*, **141**, 257
12. Root, R. K., Metcalf, J., Oshino, N. and Chance, B. (1975). H_2O_2 release from human granulocytes during phagocytosis. I. Documentation, quantitation, and some regulating factors. *J. Clin. Invest.*, **55**, 945
13. Weening, R. S., Wever, R. and Roos, D. (1975). Quantitative aspects of the production of superoxide radicals by phagocytizing human granulocytes. *J. Lab. Clin. Med.*, **85**, 245
14. Dri, P., Bellavite, P., Bocton, G. and Rossi, F. (1977). Interrelationships between oxygen consumption, superoxide anion and hydrogen peroxide

in phagocytosing guinea pig polymorphonuclear leucocytes. *Mol. Cell. Biochem.* (In press)

15. Rossi, F. and Zatti, M. (1966). The mechanism of the respiratory stimulation during phagocytosis in polymorphonuclear leucocytes. *Biochim. Biophys. Acta,* 113, 395

16. Thurman, R. G., Ley, H. G. and Scholz, R. (1972). Hepatic microsomal ethanol oxidation. Hydrogen peroxide formation and the role of catalase. *Eur. J. Biochem.,* 25, 420

17. Babior, B. M., Curnutte, J. T. and Kipnes, R. S. (1975). Pyridine nucleotide-dependent superoxide production by a cell-free system from human granulocytes. *J. Clin. Invest.,* 56, 1035

18. Sbarra, A. J. and Karnovsky, M. L. (1959). The biochemical basis of phagocytosis. I. Metabolic changes during the ingestion of particles by polymorphonuclear leukocytes. *J. Biol. Chem.,* 234, 1355

19. Rossi, F. and Zatti, M. (1966). Effect of phagocytosis on the carbohydrate metabolism of polymorphonuclear leukocytes. *Biochim. Biophys. Acta,* 121, 110

20. Morton, D. J., Moran, J. F. and Stjernholm, R. L. (1969). Carbohydrate metabolism in leucocytes. XI. Stimulation of eosinophils and neutrophils. *J. Reticuloendothel. Soc.,* 6, 525

21. Reed, P. (1969). Glutathione and the hexose monophosphate shunt in phagocytizing and hydrogen peroxide-treated rat leukocytes. *J. Biol. Chem.,* 244, 2459

22. Baehner, R. L., Gilman, N. and Karnovsky, M. L. (1970). Respiration and glucose oxidation in human and guinea-pig leukocytes: comparative studies. *J. Clin. Invest.,* 49, 692

23. Rossi, F., Romeo, D. and Patriarca, P. (1972). Mechanism of phagocytosis-associated oxidative metabolism of polymorphonuclear leucocytes and macrophages. *J. Reticuloendothel. Soc.,* 12, 127

24. Beck, W. S. (1958). Occurrence and control of the phosphogluconate oxidation in normal and leukemic leucocytes. *J. Biol. Chem.,* 232, 271

25. Patriarca, P., Cramer, R., Moncalvo, S., Rossi, F. and Romeo, D. (1971). Enzymatic basis of metabolic stimulation in leucocytes during phagocytosis: The role of activated NADPH oxidase. *Arch. Biochem. Biophys.,* 145, 255

26. Romeo, D., Zabucchi, G. and Rossi, F. (1977). Surface modulation of oxidative metabolism of polymorphonuclear leucocytes. In F. Rossi, P. Patriarca and D. Romeo (eds.). *Movement, Metabolism and Bactericidal Mechanisms of Phagocytes,* p. 153. (Padua: Piccin Medical Books)

27. De Châtelet, L. R., McCall, C. E., McPhail, L. C. and Johnston, R. B. Jr. (1974). Superoxide dismutase activity in leukocytes. *J. Clin. Invest.,* 53, 1197

28. Patriarca, P., Dri, P. and Rossi, F. (1974). Superoxide dismutase in leukocytes. *FEBS Lett.,* 43, 247

29. Salin, M. L. and McCord, J. M. (1974). Superoxide dismutases in polymorphonuclear leukocytes. *J. Clin. Invest.,* 54, 1005

30. Patriarca, P., Dri, P. and Snidero, M. (1977). Interference of myeloperoxidase with the estimation of superoxide dismutase activity. *J. Lab. Clin. Med.,* 90, 289

31. Segal, A. W. and Peters, T. J. (1977). Analytical subcellular fractionation

of human granulocytes with special reference to the localisation of enzymes involved in microbicidal mechanisms. *Clin. Sci. Mol. Med.*, **52**, 429

32. Evans, W. H. and Rechcigl, M. Jr. (1967). Factors influencing myeloperoxidase and catalase activities in polymorphonuclear leukocytes. *Biochim. Biophys. Acta.* **148**, 243

33. Michell, R. H., Karnovsky, M. J. and Karnovsky, M. L. (1970). The distributions of some granule-associated enzymes in guinea-pig polymorphonuclear leucocytes. *Biochem. J.*, **116**, 207

34. Fridovich, I. (1975). Superoxide dismutases. *Ann. Rev. Biochem.*, **44**, 877

35. Simic, M. G., Taub, I. A., Tocci, J. and Hurwitz, P. A. (1975). Free-radical reduction of ferricytochrome-*c. Biochem. Biophys. Res. Commun.*, **62**, 161

36. Iyer, G. J. N. and Quastel, H. J. (1963). NADPH and NADH oxidation by guinea-pig polymorphonuclear leukocytes. *Can. J. Biochem. Physiol.*, **41**, 427

37. Rossi, F., Zatti, M. and Patriarca, P. (1969). H_2O_2 production during NADPH oxidation by the granule fraction of phagocytosing polymorphonuclear leucocytes. *Biochim. Biophys. Acta.* **184**, 201

38. Patriarca, P., Dri, P., Kakinuma, K., Tedesco, F. and Rossi, F. (1975). Studies on the mechanism of metabolic stimulation in polymorphonuclear leucocytes during phagocytosis. I. Evidence for superoxide anion involvement in the oxidation of $NADPH_2$. *Biochim. Biophys. Acta*, **385**, 380

39. Jensen, M. S. and Bainton, D. F. (1973). Temporal changes in pH within the phagocytic vacuole of the polymorphonuclear neutrophilic leukocyte. *J. Cell. Biol.*, **56**, 379

40. Curnutte, J. T., Kipnes, R. S. and Babior, B. M. (1975). Defect in pyridine nucleotide dependent superoxide production by a particulate fraction from the granulocytes of patients with chronic granulomatous disease. *N. Engl. J. Med.*, **293**, 628

41. Hohn, D. C. and Lehrer, R. I. (1975). NADPH oxidase deficiency in X-linked chronic granulomatous disease. *J. Clin. Invest.*, **55**, 707

42. De Chatelet, L. R., McPhail, L. C., Mullikin, D. and McCall, C. E. (1975). An isotopic assay for NADPH oxidase activity and some characteristics of the enzyme from human polymorphonuclear leukocytes. *J. Clin. Invest.*, **55**, 714

43. Bainton, D. F. and Farquhar, M. G. (1966). Origin of granules in polymorphonuclear leukocytes. Two types derived from opposite faces of the Golgi complex in developing granulocytes. *J. Cell. Biol.*, **28**, 277

44. Takanaka, K. and O'Brien, P. J. (1975). Mechanism of H_2O_2 formation by leukocytes. Evidence for a plasma membrane location. *Arch. Biochem. Biophys.*, **169**, 428

45. Roos, D. (1977). Oxidative killing of microorganisms by phagocytic cells. *Trends Biochem. Sci.*, **2**, 61

46. Rossi, F., Patriarca, P., Romeo, D. and Zabucchi, G. (1976). The mechanism of control of phagocytic metabolism. In S. M. Reichard, M. R. Escobar and H. Friedman (eds.). *The Reticuloendothelial System in Health and Disease: Functions and Characteristics*, p. 205. (New York: Plenum Publ. Corp.)

47. Patriarca, P., Cramer, R., Dri, P., Fant, L., Basford, R. E. and Rossi, F. (1973). NADPH oxidizing activity in rabbit polymorphonuclear leukocytes:

localization in azurophilic granules. *Biochem. Biophys. Res. Commun.*, **53**, 830

48. Briggs, R. T., Drath, B. D., Karnovsky, M. L. and Karnovsky, M. J. (1975). Localization of NADH oxidase on the surface of human polymorphonuclear leukocytes by a new cytochemical method. *J. Cell. Biol.*, **67**, 566

49. Root, R. K. and Stossel, T. P. (1974). Myeloperoxidase mediated by granulocytes. Intracellular site of operation and some regulating factors. *J. Clin. Invest.*, **53**, 1207

50. Goldstein, I. M., Cerqueira, M., Lind, S. and Kaplan, H. B. (1977). Evidence that the superoxide-generating system of human leukocytes is associated with the cell surface. *J. Clin. Invest.*, **59**, 249

51. Evans, H. W. and Karnovsky, M. L. (1962). The biochemical basis of phagocytosis. IV. Some aspects of carbohydrate metabolism during phagocytosis. *Biochemistry*, **1**, 159

52. Evans, A. E. and Kaplan, N. O. (1966). Pyridine nucleotide transhydrogenase in normal human and leukemic leucocytes. *J. Clin. Invest.*, **45**, 1268

53. Weening, R. S., Roos, D., van Schaik, M. L. J., Voetman, A. A., de Boer, M. and Loos, H. A. (1977). The role of glutathione in the oxidative metabolism of phagocytic leukocytes. Studies in a family with glutathione reductase deficiency. In F. Rossi, P. Patriarca and D. Romeo (eds.). *Movement, Metabolism and Bactericidal Mechanisms of Phagocytes*, p. 277 (Padua: Piccin Medical Books)

54. McPhail, L. C., De Châtelet, L. R. and Shirley, P. S. (1976). Further characterization of NADPH oxidase activity of human polymorphonuclear leukocytes. *J. Clin. Invest.*, **58**, 774

55. Cooper, M. R., De Chatelet, L. R., McCall, C. E., La Via, M. F., Spurr, C. L. and Baehner, R. L. (1972). Complete deficiency of leukocyte glucose-6-phosphate dehydrogenase with defective bactericidal activity. *J. Clin. Invest.*, **51**, 769

56. De Chatelet, L. R., Cooper, M. R. and McCall, C. E. (1971). Dissociation by colchicine of the hexose monophosphate shunt activation from the bactericidal activity of the leukocyte. *Infect. Immun.*, **3**, 66

57. Hawkins, R. A. and Berlin, R. D. (1969). Purine transport in polymorphonuclear leukocytes. *Biochim. Biophys. Acta*, **173**, 324

17

Chronic granulomatous disease – biochemistry with special reference to oxygen metabolism
A. W. Segal

Introduction

The metabolism of oxygen by polymorphonuclear leukocytes is enormously increased in association with phagocytosis[1]. This oxygen consumption is not inhibited by cyanide and is largely unconnected with the respiration of these cells which contain very few mitochondria[2] and derive most of their energy from glycolysis[3]. The oxygen is reduced and activated to form superoxide (O_2^-)[4], hydrogen peroxide (H_2O_2)[5,6] hydroxyl radicals (OH^-)[7] and other reactive species which are generated in the specialized microbicidal system of neutrophils[8,9].

The oxygen-dependent microbial system has received considerable attention from clinicians and scientists because of its fundamental biological importance. It is a clearly defined system which is relatively amenable to investigation as the cells and organisms are readily obtained and can be highly purified, and many of the biochemical steps can be independently measured and controlled. Although the importance of this oxygen-free radical generating system has only been proven in relation to the killing of bacteria[10] it has much wider implications as similar free radical reactions may be involved in the killing of other cells, including foreign and malignant cells, by lymphocytes[11] and monocytes[12], the pathogenic effects of microbes, and the therapeutic effects of ionizing radiation[13]. Elucidation of the exact mechanisms by which the microbes are damaged might indicate the strengths and weaknesses of the system and allow therapeutic manipulation of these processes.

Chronic granulomatous disease[14] (CGD) is characterized by a specific failure of this oxygen-dependent microbicidal system[15]. The study of the pattern of disease in these patients indicates the protection normally afforded against infection by this system, and their cells form an ideal experimental control with which to compare studies on the biochemistry of oxygen metabolism by normal neutrophils.

THE CLINICAL SYNDROME OF CLASSICAL CGD

Recurrent, chronic or unduly virulent infection by unusual organisms in a male infant or child, often from a family in whom a male sib has died of infection, is usually the pattern that alerts the clinician to the possibility of this inherited defect of immunity[14, 16]. The infections usually present as a suppurative lymphadenitis, pneumonia, osteitis, or liver abscess and these patients often have eczematous skin rashes. They are usually slightly anaemic and may have a leukocytosis and markedly elevated serum gammaglobulin levels. Histology of the site of infection shows a chronic suppurative inflammation with granuloma formation and an infiltration by large numbers of plasma cells; non-suppurative granulomata are often seen in distant organs such as the liver[14, 16].

In the initial description it was postulated that CGD was caused by a collagen type of disease of the reticuloendothelial system[14]. It was later shown that the defect lay in the inability of the neutrophils of these patients to kill certain bacteria[17, 18] and that these cells did not exhibit the normal burst of metabolic activity in association with phagocytosis[15]. Furthermore the pattern of infection in these patients correlates well with the efficiency with which their cells kill the organisms *in vitro*[10], which can be related to the metabolism of H_2O_2 by the bacteria[19]. They are particularly susceptible to organisms like staphylococci which produce catalase and can degrade H_2O_2, and resistant to organisms such as streptococci, lactobacilli and pneumococci which themselves generate H_2O_2[19].

The syndrome of CGD gives insight into the general role of phagocytes in fighting infection. Although their cells are often totally unable to kill common saprophytes such as staphylococci, overwhelming septicaemia, which is almost the rule in the presence of severe neutropenia[20], is relatively uncommon in these patients. Thus it seems likely that the prime role of the phagocyte is to clear organisms from the blood and that the cells of these patients perform this task admirably. The bacteria must then be digested, which sometimes requires prior killing of the organism, and it is here that the defect in CGD manifests itself as persistence of the organism resulting in granuloma formation around the accumulated foreign material and, if it multiplies, in local sepsis. The common sites of infection in these patients – the lymph nodes, liver, lungs and bone marrow[14, 16] – are probably the organs in which neutrophils terminate when they leave the circulation.

The classical syndrome of CGD is generally inherited in an X-linked fashion[14, 21]. It occurs in young boys whose mothers may be carriers and in whom the Lyon effect, where random suppression of one of the X chromosomes results in the expression of the defect in half of the carrier's cells, has been demonstrated[22]. A small proportion of the patients are female[16, 23], and in these cases the mode of inheritance is thought to be autosomal recessive. It is possible that an abnormality is present in both the mothers and fathers of patients suggesting an autosomal recessive pattern with sex modification[24, 25].

BIOCHEMICAL CHANGES ASSOCIATED WITH PHAGOCYTOSIS AND THE DIAGNOSIS OF CGD

Phagocytosis is followed after approximately 30 sec by a dramatic burst of oxygen consumption. The exact sequence of reactions is uncertain, but superoxide (O_2^-)[4], hydrogen peroxide (H_2O_2)[5, 6] and hydroxyl radicals $(OH^{\cdot})$[7] are generated. The hydrogen peroxide probably acts as a substrate for myeloperoxidase-mediated oxidation of ingested microbes[9], which results in the emission of light[26]. In association with these processes, there is a dramatic increase in the activity of the hexose monophosphate shunt[27] (HMP shunt) which generates reducing equivalents either for the production[28], or for the scavenging and detoxification[29], of free radicals, or for both these processes.

The definitive diagnosis of CGD rests upon a clear demonstration of a defective burst of oxygen metabolism by neutrophils which have been adequately stimulated – opsonized bacteria and latex particles must be shown to have been phagocytosed, and soluble stimuli such as cytochalasin E[30] and phorbol myristate acetate[31] may be more reliable. Oxygen consumption can be measured directly, but this requires a relatively large number of cells and has been largely replaced by indirect methods; O_2^- production can be measured by the inhibition of the reduction of cytochrome c[4] or nitroblue tetrazolium (NBT)[32] by superoxide dismutase. The reduction of NBT can be used as a screening test[32,33] for this condition, but care must be taken because the dye is toxic to cells[34], and because it is the failure of the enhancement of dye reduction which normally follows phagocytosis by neutrophils that must be assessed[34]; H_2O_2 production can be measured directly or indirectly by myeloperoxidase-dependent bacterial iodination[35]. HMP shunt activity can be measured by $^{14}CO_2$ production from $1-[C^{14}]$ glucose[36] and in CGD cells in which shunt activity remains low after stimulation, the integrity of the shunt itself, which is generally normal in these patients[37], can be established by stimulating it artificially with an oxidizing agent such as methylene blue[37].

THE CAUSAL LESION IN CGD

There is no direct evidence that O_2^- is generated by an enzymic reaction. There are a number of compounds including ascorbate[38] and glutathione which could react chemically to form O_2^- particularly in the presence of iron[39] which is bound to lactoferrin[40] and released from the specific granules into the phagocytic vacuole. Whatever the process, it is defective in CGD which thus becomes an important tool in the verification of any putative oxidase system. However, this is not without its problems because CGD is almost certainly a syndrome in which the final common metabolic derangement could result from defects in a number of independent, but interrelated, processes. Also, the clinical severity of the disease is variable[24,41], and the less severely affected patients, with less complete metabolic abnormalities, are those that are more likely to survive and hence to be available for study. It does seem likely that at least part of the process is enzymic and that, as in the case of many other oxidase enzymes, a flavin-containing enzyme is involved[42]. Much of the work on this oxidase enzyme has been done with the reduced pyridine nucleotides as substrate, and this can lead to difficulties in interpretation because neutrophils contain many dehydrogenase[43] and transhydrogenase[37] enzyme systems, and because these nucleotides can interact directly with, and can themselves form, free radicals[44], and because NADH and NADPH can sometimes substitute for each other as substrate for the same enzyme[43].

Another difficulty encountered when working on these enzymes is to reproduce accurately the natural conditions under which they normally function. The plasma membrane seems to be important in the generation of activated oxygen[43], and it forms a partition between the cytosol, which contains the substrate and has a relatively high pH, and the vacuole cavity which rapidly becomes acidic[45]. Similarly, there is surprisingly little space between the wall of the phagocytic vacuole and the engulfed object, and the local concentration of products discharged into the vacuole will be relatively high, and these high concentrations may be important for product interactions such as free radical chain reactions. It is thus very difficult to reproduce accurately these compartmentalized conditions and to obtain reliable quantitative data on these membrane enzymes.

HMP shunt and NADPH oxidases

There is no doubt that in normal neutrophils the HMP shunt is markedly stimulated by phagocytosis[1], and it seems likely that part of this activity is involved in the catabolism of H_2O_2 by glutathione peroxidase and the subsequent reduction of oxidized glutathione reductase[29]. What is uncertain is whether the shunt generates NADPH to be utilized by the primary oxidase in the afferent limb of the process.

If the O_2^- generating system is entirely dependent on NADPH from the HMP shunt for its reducing equivalents, then it should be inactivated by malfunction of the shunt. Similarly, if the shunt is only stimulated as a secondary event by O_2^- produced by some other source, then a scavenging system which removes the O_2^- directly it is generated should prevent the enhancement of HMP shunt activity. Unfortunately the data on both these points are conflicting. Glucose-6-phosphate dehydrogenase (G6PD) is a key enzyme in the HMP shunt and deficiency of this enzyme, which is a fairly common genetic defect, limits shunt activity. In general, reduction of the enzyme activity to 20% of normal does not seem to affect neutrophil function[37, 46]. A few patients have been reported in whom neutrophil G6PD activity was unrecordable[47, 48]. These patients had many of the metabolic characteristics of CGD but seemed less susceptible to infection and generally killed bacteria more efficiently than patients with classical CGD[48]. It is difficult to assess how much the neutrophil function is indirectly modified by G6PD deficiency – in the face of severe enzyme deficiency reducing equivalents may be transferred from NADH to NADPH by a transhydrogenase, thereby reducing the concentration of NADH, low levels of which have been demonstrated in a patient with only 5% of the normal G6PD activity[37], and possibly interfering with NADH oxidase function. Colchicine, which markedly inhibits G6PD and HMP shunt activity[49], does not interfere with bacterial killing. In general it would seem that although the malfunction of G6PD and the consequently reduced HMP shunt activity can seriously disturb neutrophil behaviour, the resulting defect is not consistent and does not accurately mimic that observed in CGD.

Nitroblue tetrazolium is reduced[50] by O_2^- to a diformazan, and acts as an irreversible scavenger of its free electron. Thus, if the HMP shunt is stimulated by O_2^- or one of its reaction products as a secondary event, NBT should scavenge the O_2^- and inhibit the phagocytosis induced HMP shunt activity. The two studies performed with this object in mind have come to completely different conclusions; in the one case HMP shunt activity was inhibited[51] and in the other it was unaffected[52].

It has generally been accepted that the natural spontaneous consequence of O_2^- generation is the formation of H_2O_2. Two pieces of evidence argue against this. The first is a series of elegant studies by Tsan and colleagues[53], using the non-penetrating sulphydryl inhibitor p-chloromercuriphenyl sulphonate. After incubation with this compound, the generation of super-oxide by stimulated cells remained normal and could be dissociated from H_2O_2 production and HMP shunt activity, which were almost completely inhibited. These results are not in agreement with studies by Goldstein et al.[54] in which O_2^- generation was also inhibited by p-CMPSA; however, the cells in the latter experiments had also been treated with cytochalasin B, and the conditions were thus less physiological. The second piece of evidence comes from the description by Roos and his colleagues[55] of studies on a patient with a deficiency of neutrophil glutathione reductase. The O_2^- generation and bacterial killing were found to be normal, H_2O_2 generation was initially normal but rapidly fell off, and HMP shunt activity was reduced. Although the authors relate this discrepancy to the experimental conditions and in particular to the protective effect of cytochrome c acting as a superoxide scavenger, it is possible that the production of O_2^- is distinct from H_2O_2 formation.

So much for the supporting evidence – what of the direct evidence of an NADPH oxidase in neutrophils? In 1961 Iyer, Islam and Quastel described an NADPH oxidase in dialysed neutrophil homogenates[5]. This enzyme was markedly stimulated by Mn^{2+} ions and had a pH optimum of 5.5. Further work was done on this enzyme by Rossi and co-workers who localized it to the azurophil granules and noted that a marked drop in its K_m was induced by phagocytosis[56,57]. Hohn and Lehrer[58] and De Châtelet and colleagues[59] measured the activity of this enzyme in human neutrophil homogenates and in subcellular fractions of unstimulated cells or cells which had been stimulated by the phagocytosis of zymosan particles. An enzyme was detected which had oxidase activity with both NADH and NADPH but with much greater activity with the latter, which was markedly stimulated by phagocytosis and which was optimally active in the presence of Mn^{2+} at a pH of 5.5. The activity of this enzyme was found to be grossly defective in patients with CGD.

It has recently been shown that in the presence of Mn^{2+}[44] and/or Cn^- [60], and O_2^-, NAD(P)H can react in a non-enzymic free radical chain reaction. Thus the difference between the normal and CGD cells in these studies could lie in the lack of the initiating O_2^- which we know to be deficient in phagocytosing neutrophils from these patients. The O_2^- could come from a few residual intact cells, or could be produced by an NAD(P)H oxidase whose properties would be obscured by the more obvious properties of the amplified non-enzymic chain reaction. This might explain the non-linear relationship between the reaction rate and the amount of leukocyte protein that has been described[59]. Another weakness of these studies, also present in those of Curnutte, Kipnes and Babior[61], is that the phagocytosed zymosan that is used to stimulate the cells is not removed from the fractionated neutrophil preparations in which the enzyme activity is measured. Phagocytosed zymosan is oxidized by the microbicidal free radicals[26, 62], and it is well known that peroxidized lipid undergoes auto-oxidation and free radical chain reactions[39]. The zymosan phagocytosed by CGD neutrophils is not oxidized to the same extent as that phagocytosed by normal neutrophils[62] – the difference in the zymosan present in the incubation mixture could be responsible for the observed differences in NAD(P)H oxidase activity.

NADH oxidases

The concept of an NADH oxidase was first proposed by Cagan and Karnovsky[42] in 1964 when they found a cyanide-insensitive NADH oxidase in the supernatant fraction of homogenates of guinea-pig neutrophils. It was subsequently found that in five patients with CGD the activity of this enzyme was approximately 25% of normal[63], although other investigators have been unable to reproduce these results[16].

Segal and Peters determined the subcellular distribution of NAD(P)H oxidoreductase enzymes in human neutrophils[43]. It was found that at high substrate concentrations (1–2.5 mmol/l) there was a multifocal distribution with most of the activity in the regions of the cytosol, plasma membrane and mitochondria, and that this pattern was observed in both CGD and normal neutrophils[64]. The properties of the plasma membrane enzyme were investigated further and it was shown that the K_m of this enzyme was much lower for NADH (± 2 μmol/l) than for NADPH (± 2 mmol/l). The subcellular distribution of this enzyme was again measured, but this time a more physiological concentration of NADH (25 μmol/l) was used – almost all the activity in normal cells was observed as a single peak with the same distribution as the plasma membrane, and in all four patients with CGD the plasma membrane peak of activity was markedly reduced[64,65]. The location of this enzyme in the plasma membrane, which invaginates to form the wall of the phagocytic vacuole, appears optimal as it lies between its substrate and inhibitors in the cytosol, and the target in the vacuole cavity[43]. A problem with the early localization of the NADH oxidase of Cagan and Karnovsky to the cytosol[42] was that any superoxide or H_2O_2 produced here would be immediately catabolized – it now seems likely that this enzyme was eluted from the plasma membrane by the high salt concentration of the medium in which the cells were homogenized (M. L. Karnovsky – personal communication).

Unfortunately it appears that the picture may be confused by the presence in the neutrophil plasma membrane of yet another enzyme that metabolizes NADH. This is an ectoenzyme, first identified by Briggs, *et al.* by measuring the NADH-dependent precipitation of cerium ions by H_2O_2 on the outer surface of intact cells[66]. Using electron microscopic morphological criteria they have found a patchy inconsistent defect in CGD[67]. Quantitative studies by Segal, Leoni and Allison on NAD(P)H dependent reduction of NBT by intact neutrophils[68] confirm that there is a diaphorase enzyme on the outside of human neutrophils, but indicate that it is also present on the surface of lymphocytes and other cell lines, and that the activity, which accounts for approximately 25% of the total plasma membrane activity and the K_m of this enzyme with regard to NADH, were found to be entirely normal in three patients with CGD. Thus this extrinsic enzyme does not appear to be specific for neutrophils, has normal activity in CGD, and seems to be a different enzyme from the intrinsic NADH oxidase. Both the ectoenzyme and intrinsic enzyme are present in cell homogenates and this ectoenzyme could be responsible for the small amount of NADH oxidase activity that is found in patients with CGD and which should be possible to eradicate with non-penetrating inhibitors.

Glutathione peroxidase deficiency and other defects

There are a number of abnormalities that have been reported in CGD that do not fit neatly into current biochemical concepts of its pathogenesis. The first of these is the finding of grossly reduced levels of glutathione peroxidase in two girls with CGD, but normal levels in male patients[69]. Glutathione peroxidase should be involved in the catabolism of H_2O_2, and as the defect in CGD appears to be in its generation, it is difficult to see how defective removal of H_2O_2 could result in the CGD syndrome. Glutathione peroxidase deficiency is not confined to girls and has been described in a boy[70], and as one of a number of interrelated enzyme defects affecting several members of a family[71]. It is possible that glutathione peroxidase deficiency is an associated rather than the primary causal defect, but as this enzyme is assayed in the presence of both H_2O_2 and NADPH, a more direct relationship to the oxidase may exist.

In some experiments it appears that in CGD there is some delay of early degranulation of the cytoplasmic granules into the phagocytic vacuoles[72], although in other studies degranulation was normal[73]. The phagocytic vacuoles may be smaller than normal[17], and Kell Kx antigen seems to be missing from the surface of CGD neutrophils[74]. These findings indicate that there may be a basic abnormality of the plasma membrane in these patients, and as it seems likely that the primary oxidase enzyme is closely related to the plasma membrane, its malfunction could result from excessive constraint or failure of activation of an inherently normal enzyme situated within an abnormal plasma membrane.

A proposed scheme of the neutrophil oxidase system

The primary oxidase, probably an NADH oxidase, is located in the plasma membrane and activated by a conformational change[75] as it invaginates to form the wall of the phagocytic vacuole. It *initiates* the process by generating O_2^- radicals which are released on the external face of the membrane where they are reduced to H_2O_2 by sulphydryl (SH) groups located on the surface of the membrane to protect it from oxidative damage. The H_2O_2 reacts, either spontaneously or enzymatically, with further O_2^- in a *propagating reaction* which greatly enhances the throughput of the reaction and the overall consumption and generation of oxygen. The hydroxyl radicals, or other oxygen-free radical species which are formed, either react with the phagocytosed microbe, or with each other, or are detoxified by reactions with protective SH groups which line the vacuole. The oxidized sulphydryl groups (S–S) are transferred to the cytoplasmic surface of the membrane where they are spontaneously reduced back to SH groups by glutathione with reducing equivalents which originate from the HMP shunt. Thus the primary oxidase, which produces O_2^- and is defective in CGD, is probably independent of the HMP shunt. However, its products interact with reducing equivalents which originate in the shunt to boost the activity of the primary oxidase and to produce a more efficient bactericidal system and, as a result, defective function of this second limb of the system can produce similar biochemical and microbicidal defects.

References

1. Sbarra, A. J. and Karnovsky, M. L. (1959). The biochemical basis of phago-cytosis. I. Metabolic changes during the ingestion of particles by polymor-phonuclear leukocytes. *J. Biol. Chem.*, **234**, 1355
2. Kirschner, R. H., Getz, G. S. and Evans, A. E. (1972). Leukocyte mito-chondria: Function and biogenesis. *Enzyme*, **13**, 56
3. Selvaraj, R. J. and Sbarra, A. J. (1966). Relationship of glycolytic and oxidative metabolism to particle entry and destruction in phagocytosing cells. *Nature (London)*, **211**, 1272
4. Babior, B. M., Kipnes, R. S. and Curnutte, J. T. (1973). Biological defence mechanisms. The production by leukocytes of superoxide, a potential bac-tericidal agent. *J. Clin. Invest.*, **52**, 741
5. Iyer, G. Y. N., Islam, M. F. and Quastel, J. H. (1961). Biochemical aspects of phagocytosis. *Nature (London)*, **192**, 535
6. Homan-Müller, J. W. T., Weening, R. S. and Roos, D. (1975). Production of hydrogen peroxide by phagocytizing human granulocytes. *J. Lab. Clin. Med.*, **85**, 198
7. Tauber, A. I. and Babior, B. M. (1977). Evidence for hydroxyl radical pro-duction by human neutrophils. *J. Clin. Invest.*, **60**, 374
8. De Châtelet, L. R. (1975). Oxidative bactericidal mechanisms of polymor-phonuclear leukocytes. *J. Infect. Dis.*, **131**, 295
9. Klebanoff, S. J. (1975). Antimicrobial mechanisms in neutrophilic poly-morphonuclear leukocytes. *Semin. Hematol.*, **12**, 117
10. Mandell, G. L. (1974). Bactericidal activity of aerobic and anaerobic polymorphonuclear neutrophils. *Infect. Immunol.*, **9**, 337
11. Sbarra, A. J., Selvaraj, R. J., Paul, B. B., Poskitt, P. K. F., Mitchell, G. W., Louis, F. and Asbell, M. A. (1977). Granulocyte biochemistry and a hydro-gen peroxide-dependent microbicidal system. In T. J. Greenwalt and G. A. Jamieson (eds.). *The Granulocyte Function and Clinical Utilisation*, pp. 44–48. (New York: Liss)
12. Weiss, S. J., King, G. W. and Lobuglio, A. F. (1977). Evidence for hydroxyl radical generation by human monocytes. *J. Clin. Invest.*, **60**, 370
13. Wills, E. D. and Wilkinson, A. E. (1966). Release of enzymes from lyso-somes by irradiation and the relation of lipid peroxide formation to enzyme release. *Biochem. J.*, **99**, 657
14. Berendes, H., Bridges, R. A. and Good, R. A. (1957). A fatal granuloma-tosus of childhood. The clinical study of a new syndrome. *Minn. Med.*, **40**, 309
15. Holmes, B., Page, A. R. and Good, R. A. (1967). Studies of the metabolic activity of leukocytes from patients with a genetic abnormality of phago-cytic function. *J. Clin. Invest.*, **46**, 1422
16. Holmes, B. and Good, R. A. (1971). Chronic granulomatous disease of childhood. In R. A. Good and D. W. Fisher (eds.). *Immunobiology*, p. 55. (Stamford: Sinauer Associates)
17. Holmes, B., Quie, P. G., Windhorst, D. B. and Good, R. A. (1966). Fatal granulomatous disease of childhood. An inborn abnormality of phagocytic function. *Lancet*, **i**, 1225
18. Quie, P. G., White, J. G., Holmes, B. and Good, R. A. (1967). *In vitro*

bactericidal capacity of human polymorphonuclear leukocytes: Diminished activity in chronic granulomatous disease of childhood. *J. Clin. Invest.*, **46**, 668

19. Mandell, G. L. and Hook, E. W. (1969). Leukocyte bactericidal activity in chronic granulomatous disease: correlation of bacterial hydrogen peroxide production and susceptibility to intracellular killing. *J. Bacteriol.*, **100**, 531

20. Body, G. P., Buckley, M., Sathey, S. and Freireich, E. J. (1966). Quantitative relationships between circulating leukocytes and infection in patients with acute leukaemia. *Ann. Intern. Med.*, **64**, 328

21. Windhorst, D. B., Page, A. R., Holmes, B., Quie, P. G. and Good, R. A. (1968). The pattern of genetic transmission of the leukocyte defect in fatal granulomatous disease of childhood. *J. Clin. Invest.*, **47**, 1026

22. Windhorst, D. B., Holmes, B. and Good, R. A. (1967). A newly defined X-linked trait in man with demonstration of the Lyon effect in carrier females. *Lancet*, i, 737

23. Quie, P. G., Kaplan, E. L., Page, A. R., Gruskay, F. L. and Malawista, S. E. (1968). Defective polymorphonuclear-leukocyte function and chronic granulomatous disease in two female children. *N. Engl. J. Med.*, **278**, 976

24. Thompson, E. N. and Soothill, J. F. (1970). Chronic granulomatous disease: Quantitative clinicopathological relationships. *Arch. Dis. Child.*, **45**, 24

25. Chandra, R. K., Cope, W. A. and Soothill, J. F. (1969). Chronic granulomatous disease. Evidence for an autosomal mode of inheritance. *Lancet*, ii, 71

26. Cheson, B. D., Christensen, R. L., Sperling, R., Kohler, B. E. and Babior, B. M. (1976). The origin of the chemiluminescence of phagocytosing granulocytes. *J. Clin. Invest.*, **58**, 789

27. Stjernholm, R. L. and Manak, R. C. (1970). Carbohydrate metabolism in leukocytes. XIV. Regulation of pentose cycle activity and glycogen metabolism during phagocytosis. *J. Reticuloendothel. Soc.*, **8**, 550

28. Zatti, M. and Rossi, F. (1965). Early changes of hexose monophosphate pathway activity and of NADPH oxidation in phagocytizing leucocytes. *Biochim. Biophys. Acta*, **99**, 557

29. Reed, P. W. (1969). Glutathione and the hexose monophosphate shunt in phagocytizing and hydrogen peroxide-treated rat leukocytes. *J. Biol. Chem.*, **244**, 2459

30. Nakagawara, A., Kakinuma, K., Shin, H., Miyazaki, S. and Minakami, S. (1976). Lack of cytochalasin E-induced superoxide release by polymorphonuclear leucocytes of patients with chronic granulomatous disease: a new diagnostic test. *Clin. Chim. Acta*, **70**, 133

31. Repine, J. E., White, J. G., Clawson, C. C. and Holmes, B. M. (1974). Effects of phorbol myristate acetate on the metabolism and ultrastructure of neutrophils in chronic granulomatous disease. *J. Clin. Invest.*, **54**, 83

32. Baehner, R. L. and Nathan, D. G. (1968). Quantitative nitroblue tetrazolium test in chronic granulomatous disease. *N. Engl. J. Med.*, **278**, 971

33. Segal, A. W. and Peters, T. J. (1975). The nylon column dye test: a possible screening test of phagocyte function. *Clin. Sci. Mol. Med.*, **49**, 591

34. Segal, A. W. and Levi, A. J. (1975). Cell damage and dye reduction in the quantitative nitroblue tetrazolium (NBT) test. *Clin. Exp. Immunol.*, **19**, 309

35. Klebanoff, S. J. and White, L. R. (1969). Iodination defect in the leukocytes of a patient with chronic granulomatous disease of childhood. *N. Engl. J. Med.*, **280**, 460

36. Beck, W. S. (1958). The control of leukocyte glycolysis. *J. Biol. Chem.*, **232**, 251

37. Baehner, R. L., Johnston, R. B. and Nathan, D. G. (1972). Comparative study of the metabolic and bactericidal characteristics of severely glucose-6-phosphate dehydrogenase-deficient polymorphonuclear leukocytes and leukocytes from children with chronic granulomatous disease. *J. Reticuloendothel. Soc.*, **12**, 150

38. De Châtelet, L. R., Cooper, M. R. and McCall, C. E. (1972). Stimulation of the hexose monophosphate shunt in human neutrophils by ascorbic acid: mechanism of action. *Antimicrob. Agents Chemother.*, **1**, 12

39. Mead, J. F. (1976). Free radical mechanisms of lipid damage and consequences for cellular membranes. In W. A. Pryor (ed.). *Free Radicals in Biology*, Vol. 1, pp. 51–68. (New York, San Francisco, London: Academic Press)

40. Gladstone, G. P. and Walton, E. (1970). Effect of iron on the bactericidal proteins from rabbit polymorphonuclear leukocytes. *Nature (London)*, **227** 849

41. Nathan, D. G., Baehner, R. L. and Weaver, D. K. (1969). Failure of nitro-blue tetrazolium reduction in the phagocytic vacuoles of leukocytes in chronic granulomatous disease. *J. Clin. Invest.*, **48**, 1895

42. Cagan, R. H. and Karnovsky, M. L. (1964). Enzymic basis of the respiratory stimulation during phagocytosis. *Nature (London)*, **204**, 255

43. Segal, A. W. and Peters, T. J. (1977). Analytical subcellular fractionation of human granulocytes with special reference to the localisation of enzymes involved in microbicidal mechanisms. *Clin. Sci. Mol. Med.*, **52**, 429

44. Curnutte, J. T., Karnovsky, M. L. and Babior, B. M. (1976). Manganese-dependent NADPH oxidation by granulocyte particles. *J. Clin. Invest.*, **57**, 1059

45. Mandell, G. L. (1970). Intraphagosomal pH of human polymorphonuclear neutrophils. *Proc. Soc. Exp. Biol. Med.*, **134**, 447

46. Schiliro, G., Russo, A., Mauro, L., Pizzarelli, G. and Marino, S. (1976). Leukocyte function and characterization of leukocyte glucose-6-phosphate dehydrogenase in Sicilian mutants. *Pediatr. Res.*, **10**, 739

47. Cooper, M. R., De Châtelet, L. R., McCall, C. E., La Via, M. F., Spurr, C. L. and Baehner, R. L. (1972). Complete deficiency of leukocyte glucose-6-phosphate dehydrogenase with defective bactericidal activity. *J. Clin. Invest.*, **51**, 769

48. Gray, G. R., Klebanoff, S. J., Stamatoyannopoulos, G., Austin, T., Naiman, S. C., Yoshida, A., Kliman, M. R. and Robinson, G. C. F. (1973). Neutrophil dysfunction, chronic granulomatous disease, and non-spherocytic haemolytic anaemia caused by complete deficiency of glucose-6-phosphate dehydrogenase. *Lancet*, **ii**, 530

49. De Châtelet, L. R., Cooper, M. R. and McCall, C. E. (1971). Dissociation by colchicine of the hexose monophosphate shunt activation from the bactericidal activity of the leukocyte. *Infect. Immunol.*, **3**, 66

50. Younes, M. and Weser, U. (1976). Inhibition of nitroblue tetrazolium reduction by cuprein (superoxide dismutase), Cu(tyr)$_2$ and Cy(lys)$_2$. *FEBS Lett.*, **61**, 209

51. Wilkinson, R. W., Powars, D. R. and Hochstein, P. (1975). New evidence for the role of NADH oxidase in phagocytosis by human granulocytes. *Biochem. Med.*, **13**, 83

52. De Châtelet, L. R. and Shirley, P. S. (1975). Effect of nitroblue tetrazolium dye on the hexose monophosphate shunt activity of human polymorphonuclear leukocytes. *Biochem. Med.*, **14**, 391

53. Tsan, M., Newman, B. and McIntyre, P. A. (1976). Surface sulphydryl groups and phagocytosis-associated oxidative metabolic changes in human polymorphonuclear leucocytes. *Br. J. Haematol.*, **33**, 189

54. Goldstein, I. M., Cerqueira, M., Lind, S. and Kaplan, H. B. (1977). Evidence that the superoxide-generating system of human leukocytes is associated with the cell surface. *J. Clin. Invest.*, **59**, 249

55. Weening, R. S., Roos, D., van Schaik, M. L. J., Voetman, A. A., de Boer, M. and Loos, H. A. (1977). The role of glutathione in the oxidation metabolism of phagocytic leukocytes. Studies in a family with glutathione reductase deficiency. In F. Rossi, P. L. Patriarca and D. Romeo (eds.). *Movement, Metabolism and Bactericidal Mechanisms of Phagocytes*, p. 277. (Padua: Piccin)

56. Rossi, F. and Zatti, M. (1964). Changes in the metabolic pattern of polymorphonuclear leucocytes during phagocytosis. *Br. J. Exp. Pathol.*, **45**, 548

57. Rossi, F., Romeo, D. and Patriarca, P. (1972). Mechanism of phagocytosis-associated oxidative metabolism in polymorphonuclear leucocytes and macrophages. *J. Reticuloendothel. Soc.*, **12**, 127

58. Hohn, D. C. and Lehrer, R. I. (1975). NADPH oxidase deficiency in X-linked chronic granulomatous disease. *J. Clin. Invest.*, **55**, 707

59. De Châtelet, L. R., McPhail, L. C., Mullikin, D. and McCall, C. E. (1975). An isotopic assay for NADPH oxidase activity and some characteristics of the enzyme from human polymorphonuclear leukocytes. *J. Clin. Invest.*, **55**, 714

60. De Châtelet, L. R., McPhail, L. C. and Shirley, P. S. (1977). Effect of cyanide on NADPH oxidation by granules from human polymorphonuclear leukocytes. *Blood*, **49**, 445

61. Curnutte, J. T., Kipnes, R. S. and Babior, B. M. (1975). Defect in pyridine nucleotide dependent superoxide production by a particulate fraction from the granulocytes of patients with chronic granulomatous disease. *N. Engl. J. Med.*, **293**, 628

62. Stossel, T. P., Mason, R. J. and Smith, A. L. (1974). Lipid peroxidation by human blood phagocytes. *J. Clin. Invest.*, **54**, 638

63. Baehner, R. L. and Karnovsky, M. L. (1968). Deficiency of reduced nicotinamide-adenine dinucleotide oxidase in chronic granulomatous disease. *Science*, **162**, 1277

64. Segal, A. W. and Peters, T. J. (1976). Characterisation of the enzyme defect in chronic granulomatous disease. *Lancet*, **i**, 1363

65. Segal, A. W. and Peters, T. J. (1977). Analytical subcellular fractionation of human neutrophils – The enzyme defect in chronic granulomatous disease. In F. Rossi, P. Patriarca and D. Romeo (eds.). *Movement, Metabolism and Bactericidal Mechanisms of Phagocytes*, p. 175. (Padua: Piccin)

66. Briggs, R. T., Drath, D. B., Karnovsky, M. L. and Karnovsky, M. J. (1975). Localisation of NADH oxidase on the surface of human polymorphonuclear leukocytes by a new cytochemical method. *J. Cell. Biol.*, **67**, 566

67. Briggs, R. T., Karnovsky, M. L. and Karnovsky, M. J. (1977). Hydrogen peroxide production in chronic granulomatous disease. *J. Clin. Invest.*, **59**, 1088

68. Segal, A. W., Leoni, P. and Allison, A. C. (19—). Reduced pyridine nucleotide-dependent reduction of nitroblue tetrazolium by intact neutrophils and other cells. (In preparation)

69. Holmes, B., Park, B. H., Malawista, S. E., Quie, P. G., Nelson, D. L. and Good, R. A. (1970). Chronic granulomatous disease in females. A deficiency of leukocyte glutathione peroxidase. *N. Engl. J. Med.*, **283**, 217

70. Matsuda, I., Oka, Y., Taniguchi, N., Furuyama, M., Kodama, S., Arashima, S. and Mitsuyama, T. (1976). Leukocyte glutathione peroxidase deficiency in a male child with chronic granulomatous disease. *J. Pediatr.*, **88**, 581

71. Rutenberg, W. D., Yang, M. C., Doberstyn, E. B. and Bellanti, J. A. (1977). Multiple leukocyte abnormalities in chronic granulomatous disease: a familial study. *Pediatr. Res.*, **11**, 158

72. Gold, S. B., Hanes, D. M., Stites, D. P. and Fudenberg, H. H. (1974). Abnormal kinetics of degranulation in chronic granulomatous disease. *N. Engl. J. Med.*, **291**, 332

73. Stossel, T. P., Root, R. K. and Vaughan, M. (1972). Phagocytosis in chronic granulomatous disease and the Chediak–Higashi syndrome. *N. Engl. J. Med.*, **286**, 120

74. Marsh, W. L., Øyen, R., Nichols, M. E. and Allen, F. H. (1975). Chronic granulomatous disease and the Kell blood groups. *Br. J. Haematol.*, **29**, 247

75. Takanaka, K. and O'Brien, P. J. (1975). Mechanisms of H_2O_2 formation by leukocytes. Evidence for a plasma membrane location. *Arch. Biochem. Biophys.*, **169**, 428

18

The protective role of glutathione

THE EFFECT OF CONGENITAL DEFECTS OF GLUTATHIONE METABOLISM ON THE FUNCTION OF ERYTHROCYTES, EYE LENS CELLS, AND PHAGOCYTIC LEUKOCYTES. A REVIEW AND SOME PERSONAL OBSERVATIONS

D. Roos, R. S. Weening and J. A. Loos

INTRODUCTION

Function of glutathione

Many biological oxidations proceed via formation of radicals and/or peroxides. The tripeptide γ-glutamylcysteinylglycine or reduced glutathione (GSH) is known to protect cells against oxidative damage. This function can be executed in three different ways:

1. GSH, like other thiols, can act as a radical acceptor[1], thereby forming the disulphide GSSG (oxidized glutathione):

$$GSH + R\cdot \quad \rightarrow \quad GS\cdot + RH$$
$$2\,GS\cdot \quad \rightarrow \quad GSSG$$

261

2. Peroxides may be eliminated either by catalase (in case of hydrogen (peroxide) or by GSH in the glutathione peroxidase reaction[2]:

$$2GSH + \begin{cases} ROOH \\ HOOH \end{cases} \xrightarrow[\text{peroxidase}]{\text{glutathione}} GSSG + \begin{cases} ROH + H_2O \\ 2H_2O \end{cases}$$

3. Oxidative reactions may also give rise to formation of disulphide bridges in proteins, often leading to unfolding and denaturation of these proteins. Glutathione is able to restore the function of these proteins by reduction of such disulphides, with formation of mixed disulphides as intermediates[3,4]:

$$GSH + R\text{-}S\text{-}S\text{-}R' \rightleftharpoons G\text{-}S\text{-}S\text{-}R + R'\text{-}SH$$
$$GSH + G\text{-}S\text{-}S\text{-}R \rightleftharpoons GSSG + R\text{-}SH$$

Although glutathione is, in some cell types, present in high amounts[5]. GSSG must be reduced again for effective cell protection. This process takes place in the glutathione reductase reaction, with NADPH as the reducing agent. Probably this enzyme can also accept mixed disulphides as the oxidant[5-7]:

$$\begin{rcases} G\text{-}S\text{-}S\text{-}G \\ R\text{-}S\text{-}S\text{-}G \end{rcases} + NADPH + H^+ \xrightarrow[\text{reductase}]{\text{glutathione}} \begin{rcases} 2GSH \\ RSH + GSH \end{rcases} + NADP^+$$

Thus, the complete glutathione cycle runs as depicted in Figure 18.1. In normal viable cells, glutathione is predominantly in the reduced form[8,9]. Only during periods of oxidative stress, a temporary shift from the reduced to the oxidized form is observed[9].

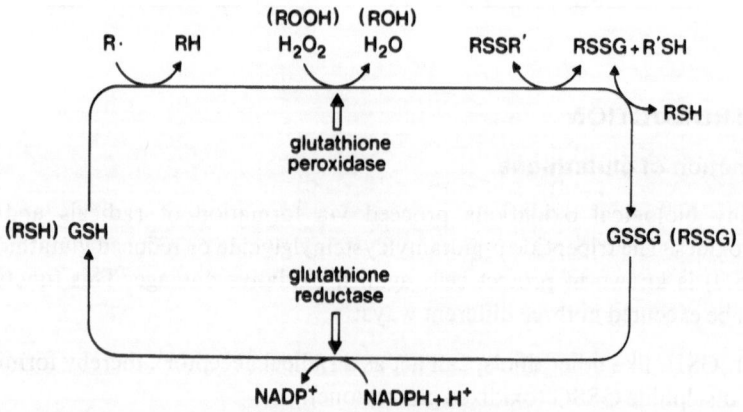

Figure 18.1   The glutathione cycle

Metabolism of glutathione

Glutathione is synthesized from its constituting amino acids in two steps[10,11]. First, γ-glutamylcysteine is formed from L-γ-glutamic acid and L-cysteine in a reaction catalysed by glutamylcysteine synthetase (Figure 18.2, reaction 1). This process is followed by reaction of γ-glutamylcysteine with glycine to glutathione, catalysed by glutathione synthetase (Figure 18.2, reaction 2).

For the reduction of GSSG to GSH in the glutathione reductase reaction, two enzymes are very important: glucose-6-phosphate dehydrogenase and 6-phosphogluconate dehydrogenase (Figure 18.2, reactions 5 and 6, respectively). In most cells, the hexose monophosphate shunt (HMP shunt) is one of the most important pathways to reduce NADP. Therefore, the capacity of these two enzymes is essential for the antioxidative action of glutathione.

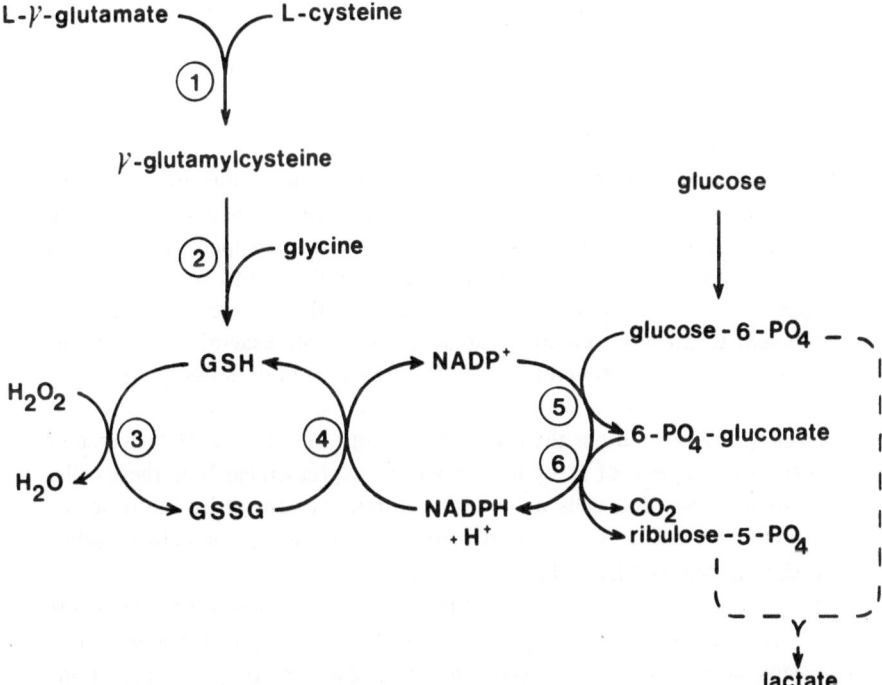

Figure 18.2 Glutathione synthesis and redox reactions. (1) glutamylcysteine synthetase; (2) glutathione synthetase; (3) glutathione peroxidase; (4) glutathione reductase; (5) glucose-6-phosphate dehydrogenase; (6) 6-phosphogluconate dehydrogenase

Breakdown of glutathione is effected mainly by two different pathways: the γ-glutamyl cycle[12, 13] and the formation of mercapturic acids[14, 15]. In the γ-glutamyl cycle glutathione combines with a wide variety of amino acids, thereby splitting off cysteinylglycine. The γ-glutamyl-amino acid product is reconverted to free amino acids and 5-oxoproline. In three steps, GSH is resynthesized from cysteinylglycine and 5-oxoproline. The whole cycle probably serves to transport amino acids across membranes, especially in the kidney.

In the liver, glutathione protects the organism against potentially harmful electrophilic compounds[14, 15]. Catalysed by several different S-transferases, glutathione conjugates with a large number of such compounds. These products are then converted in three steps to the N-acetylcysteine conjugates (mercapturic acids) and excreted in the bile or the urine.

Finally, when the capacity of the cell to keep glutathione in the reduced state is exceeded, GSSG may be released from the cell. This has been demonstrated in erythrocytes[16], eye lens cells[17], and perfused rat liver[18]. In erythrocytes and in the eye lens, transport of GSSG may be the major determinant in glutathione turnover[19].

Importance of glutathione

The red cell, for several reasons, is extremely vulnerable for oxidative damage. First, it cannot replace inactivated proteins by new ones. Second, oxyhaemoglobin can participate in the generation of superoxide radicals and hydrogen peroxide[20]. Although red cells contain both superoxide dismutase and catalase, it must be concluded that this defence is apparently insufficient to prevent oxidative damage, since acatalasaemic erythrocytes are not injured by hydrogen peroxide[21, 22], whereas glutathione peroxidase-deficient red cells are[23]. Third, erythrocytes have no alternative means of generating NADPH other than the HMP shunt; therefore, a disturbance in the first two enzymes of this pathway will be expressed easily in these cells. And finally, since red cells are under continuous control by the reticuloendothelial system, any deviation from the normal size or deformability will result in removal from the circulation.

Two other cell types also depend heavily on the glutathione system for protection against oxidation: eye lens cells and phagocytic leukocytes. Eye lens cells resemble red cells in many aspects: they are also non-nucleated, they also depend on anaerobic glycolysis as a source of NADPH, they can be damaged by oxidative stress, and they contain a high amount of glutathione which is kept reduced by a very active glutathione metabolism[5]. Moreover, eye lens cells do not contain catalase[24].

This article contains some data from the literature, therefore, on the effects of inborn errors of glutathione metabolism on the function of eye lens fibres.

Finally, during ingestion, phagocytic leukocytes generate enormous amounts of superoxide, hydrogen peroxide, and possibly other highly reactive oxidative reagents. Thus, these cells are stressed heavily during this process, and it may well be that reductive protection by glutathione is essential for adequate bactericidal capacity. Moreover, glutathione has also been proposed as a reactant in the *formation* of hydrogen peroxide by these cells[25]. Therefore, the interaction of the glutathione metabolism with the microbicidal process merits careful examination. Some of the recent results in this area are discussed in the last section of this article.

INBORN ERRORS OF GLUTATHIONE METABOLISM IN ERYTHROCYTES

Deficiencies in red cell glutathione metabolism have been recognized in all six enzymes shown in Figure 18.2. γ-glutamylcysteine synthetase deficiency has been identified with certainty in two patients only[26]. A defect in glutathione synthetase has been found in at least 14 patients[27-35]. Both defects result in a very low content of glutathione (less then 10% of normal) in the erythrocytes. The glutathione synthetase deficiency seems to occur in two different forms: a generalized deficiency accompanied by excessive production of 5-oxoproline[13, 32-35] and a deficiency predominantly limited to erythrocytes without 5-oxoprolinuria. In most cases decreased red cell viability during oxidative stress, both *in vivo* and *in vitro*, is found. Heterozygotes with 5-oxoprolinuria can be detected[33].

The second step in which a disturbance of glutathione metabolism has been recognized is in the glutathione cycle itself, i.e. a block in the glutathione peroxidase (Figure 18.2, reaction 3) or glutathione reductase reaction (Figure 18.2, reaction 4). Homozygous GSH peroxidase deficiency is extremely rare: only two cases have been identified[36, 37]. In these cases, *in vivo* and *in vitro* signs of increased haemolysis were seen during oxidative challenge. A number of heterozygous deficiencies of GSH peroxidase have also been described[37-41]. Except in case of newborns, no clinical or biochemical evidence is available to suggest that a moderate decrease in the activity of this enzyme will affect red cell survival.

Glutathione reductase is a flavoprotein with FAD as the prosthetic group. A deficiency of this enzyme has been found in a great number of patients[42] and has been associated with a wide variation of haematological disorders. However, in virtually all cases the enzyme activity could be restored to normal by FAD *in vitro* or riboflavin *in vivo*[43], whereas the clinical disorders remained unchanged[44]. Thus, the connection between glutathione reductase activity and red cell survival is not clear. Only a few cases of reduced glutathione reductase activity with insufficient response to FAD or riboflavin are known, sometimes associated with altered electrophoretic mobility of the enzyme[44] or a change in the affinity for FAD[45]. These patients too, suffered from various haematological disorders.

Recently, we have discovered a family with three homozygous-deficient children with no detectable glutathione reductase activity in their red cells[46]. The two (consanguineous) parents showed half-normal values for this enzyme in their erythrocytes (Table 18.1). No stimulation by FAD *in vitro* or riboflavin *in vivo* was detectable (Table 18.1). Clinically, this deficiency was manifested by haemolytic crises after eating fava beans[46]. Oxidative stress *in vitro* with acetylphenylhydrazine resulted in Heinz body formation[46] and decreased GSH stability (Table 18.2)*. Thus, these studies prove that the activity of glutathione reductase in red cells is directly related to the viability of these cells during oxidative stress.

TABLE 18.1   Glutathione reductase activity† in the erythrocytes of family M

| Subjects | | Addition in vitro | | Riboflavin in vivo (5 mg/d, 3 days) |
	FAD (1 μM)	FAD (5 μM)	FAD (1000 μM)	
Father	1.7	1.4	nt	nt	nt
Mother	1.7	1.5	nt	nt	nt
Brother	< 0.2	< 0.2	nt	nt	nt
Patient	< 0.2	< 0.2	< 0.2	< 0.2	< 0.2
Sister	< 0.2	< 0.2	nt	nt	nt
Control	3.5	3.9	5.2	3.3	nt
25 normals	2.4–4.8	—	—	—	—

† GSSG reductase activity in μmol/min/g haemoglobin at 25 °C
nt = not tested

Finally, decreased activity of two more enzymes in the glutathione metabolism has been found. One of these, glucose-6-phosphate dehydrogenase (Figure 18.2, reaction 5) has been studied very intensively and deficiencies in this enzyme comprise the most common metabolic defect

* It is noteworthy that the initial amount of GSH in these cells is normal, indicating that glutathione is either kept reduced by the extremely low GSSG reductase or by another, unknown mechanism. Alternatively, GSH oxidation may be compensated by an increased GSH synthesis and GSSG excretion.

TABLE 18.2   Glutathione stability* in the erythrocytes of family M

Subjects		Addition Acetylphenyl-hydrazine†
Father	57	23
Mother	63	32
Brother	59	6
Patient	59	7
Sister	56	7
25 normals	56–90	> 40

*GSH levels in mg/100 ml packed erythrocytes
† Incubation with acetylphenylhydrazine (5 mg/ml blood) for 2 h at 37 °C

in the red cell[42]. The other, 6-phosphogluconate dehydrogenase (Figure 18.2, reaction 6) has been found deficient only very rarely[42, 47] and the clinical effects of this disorder are poorly defined. The effect of these two enzymes on the glutathione metabolism is mediated through NADPH, which acts as a substrate for glutathione reductase (in the erythrocyte no other ways to generate NADPH are available).

An enormous variation in glucose-6-phosphate dehydrogenase deficiencies exists[42]. Some genetic variants do not lead to clinical effects, others only when the erythrocytes are exposed to an abnormal oxidative stress (drugs, infection, fava beans). The most severe deficiencies result in haemolysis without stress, leading to non-spherocytic congenital haemolytic anaemia. Due to the Lyonization phenomenon, heterozygotes may also show clinical symptoms.

Both partial and complete absence of 6-phosphogluconate dehydrogenase has been reported to affect red cell viability[42, 48, 49]. In another case, however, no evidence of haemolysis was present[50]. Possibly, NADPH production in the glucose-6-phosphate dehydrogenase reaction sometimes suffices for adequate glutathione reduction.

From the description of the haematological consequences of these abnormalities it may be concluded that glutathione fulfils an extremely important role in red cells. It protects haemoglobin against oxidation, which often results in unfolding, denaturation, and Heinz body formation[42]. Therefore, an intact glutathione system is essential for proper red cell functioning.

THE ROLE OF GLUTATHIONE IN THE EYE LENS

Ocular lens fibres are filled with a highly concentrated solution of the clear lens protein crystallin. Since no catalase is found in these cells[24], the protection of crystallin against oxidative damage must be executed largely by the glutathione system. It is to be expected, therefore, that deficiencies in this system will lead to clinical manifestations of lens fibre damage.

Thiol groups of crystallin are easily oxidized[51], either by photo-oxidation or by oxygen and hydrogen peroxide[52]. Such oxidation may cause unfolding and denaturation of crystallin; moreover, intermolecular cross-linking may cause insolubility of this protein. Clinically, this is manifested as cataracts.

For some time it has been recognized that glutathione may serve in the lens as a protectant against denaturation of lens proteins. The amount of glutathione in the lens is even higher than in erythrocytes and, as in other tissues, it is predominantly in the reduced form[5]. The enzymes to synthesize GSH are present in the lens. Moreover, GSH peroxidase and especially GSSG reductase are very active in the eye lens[51]. Oxidation of lens proteins is preceded or accompanied by reduction in the amount of GSH[51]. Finally, the concentration of GSH in the lens drops in concert with the progression of senile cataract[52]. Thus, it seems clear that the eye lens has a very active glutathione metabolism *because* it needs GSH to protect its proteins against oxidation.

The importance of glutathione in this respect may also be deduced from some published observations on patients with deficiencies in their glutathione metabolism. Several patients with severe deficiencies of glucose-6-phosphate dehydrogenase have been reported to present with cataracts[53-56]. In some of them, the levels of glucose-6-phosphate dehydrogenase activity in the lens were shown to be strongly depressed.

Boivin[30] reported one case of glutathione synthetase deficiency with cataracts. And finally, we found in the family with GSSG reductase deficiency, that two of the three homozygous deficient children developed cataracts, while the third suffers from an undiagnosed eye problem[46]. Thus, not only defects in the reducing system, but also defects in the glutathione cycle itself may lead to crystallin oxidation in the lens. This is a clear indication that GSH fulfils a vital protective role in these tissues too.

A DUAL ROLE OF GLUTATHIONE IN PHAGOCYTIC LEUKOCYTES?

The oxidative microbicidal system

Granulocytes, as well as monocytes, exhibit a characteristic increase in oxidative metabolism during phagocytosis. Contact with ingestible particles starts an accelerated oxygen uptake by these cells, up to 20 times the resting value of respiration. In a cyanide-insensitive, i.e. non-mitochondrial, reaction, the oxygen is reduced to superoxide (O_2^-), which then reacts with protons to form hydrogen peroxide (Figure 18.3). Both superoxide and hydrogen peroxide are released into the phagosomes, in close proximity to the ingested micro-organisms. The generation of these products is essential for the microbicidal function of the phagocytic leukocytes: if these reactions are absent, such as in chronic granulomatous disease, severe infec-

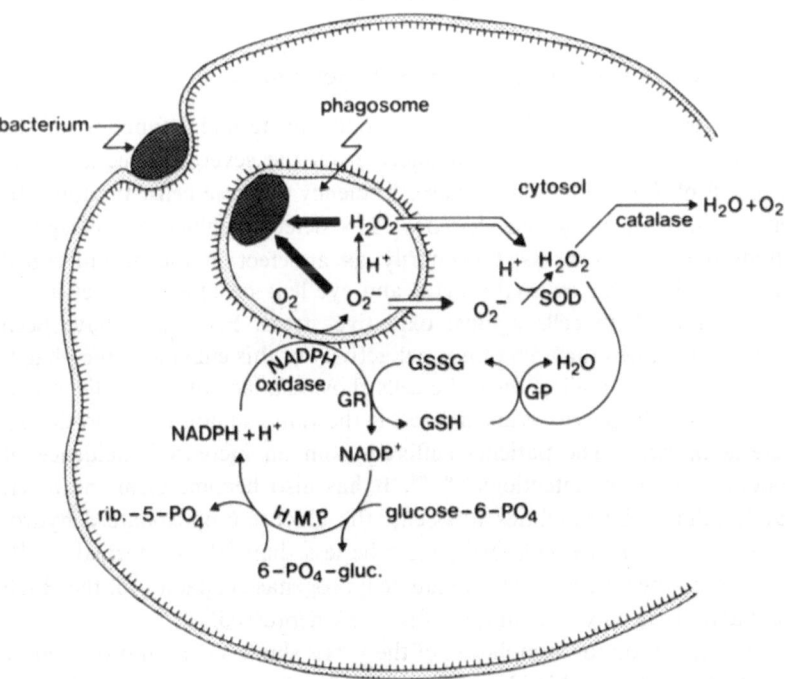

Figure 18.3   Formation of bactericidal oxygen products in the phagosomes of phagocytic leukocytes and protection of the cytosol against oxidative stress; →= reaction; ⇒ =attack; ⇒ =diffusion; GR, glutathione reductase; GP, glutathione peroxidase; SOD, superoxide dismutase; HMP, hexose monophosphate shunt

tions occur, often with fatal outcome. Moreover, the defect in bactericidal capacity of the phagocytic leukocytes of such patients is manifested only towards non-H_2O_2-producing bacteria, and this defect can be corrected by the introduction of a H_2O_2-generating system into the phagosomes of these cells[57].

The key enzyme in the conversion of oxygen to superoxide is probably an NADPH oxidase[58-60], as depicted in Figure 18.3, although NADH has also been cited as the reducing agent[61, 62]. The reader who is interested in this controversy, hotly debated for over a decade already, is referred to the reviews by Segal and by Romeo and colleagues (Chapters 16 and 17 in this volume). Most people agree, however, on glucose being the source of reducing equivalents for the ultimate reduction of oxygen to superoxide. The increase in hexose monophosphate (HMP) shunt activity, simultaneous with the increased respiration, is regarded, therefore, as necessary for the supply of NADPH which, either by itself or by reduction of NAD^+, serves in the superoxide-producing reaction.

Glucose-6-phosphate dehydrogenase deficiency

The importance of the HMP shunt in the bactericidal function of the phagocytic leukocytes can be deduced from the severe consequences of glucose-6-phosphate dehydrogenase deficiency in these cells. It should be realized that, in phagocytic leukocytes, a defect in glucose-6-phosphate dehydrogenase is expressed primarily as a defect in the antimicrobial activity and not (as in erythrocytes and eye lens cells) as a defect in the protection of these cells against oxidative stress. Five cases have been described with less than 5% of normal activity of this enzyme in the phagocytic leukocytes; in all of them the cells showed a lack of metabolic stimulation during phagocytosis and a defect in the killing of non-H_2O_2-producing bacteria *in vitro*. The patients suffered from an increased incidence of moderate to severe infections[56, 63, 64]. It has also become clear, however, that for these abnormalities to occur, the glucose-6-phosphate dehydrogenase activity in the leukocytes must be less than 20% of normal[63, 65, 66]. Apparently, the glucose-6-phosphate dehydrogenase capacity for the HMP shunt activity is only rate-limiting if severely depressed.

Another reason for stimulation of the HMP shunt has been proposed by Reed[67]. According to his idea, the excess of hydrogen peroxide, which can diffuse into the cytosol of the phagocytic cells and may cause oxidative injury to cell constituents, is detoxified in the glutathione cycle (Figure 18.3). For the regeneration of GSH, NADPH is required; therefore, the HMP shunt must be activated to cope with this increased demand. Although this concept is now generally accepted, the actual proof that the glutathione cycle is indeed operating in phagocytic leukocytes between H_2O_2 and the HMP shunt, is scarce.

Reed[67] and others[68,69] showed that addition of H_2O_2 to these cells activates the HMP shunt, a process which can be inhibited by the glutathione-

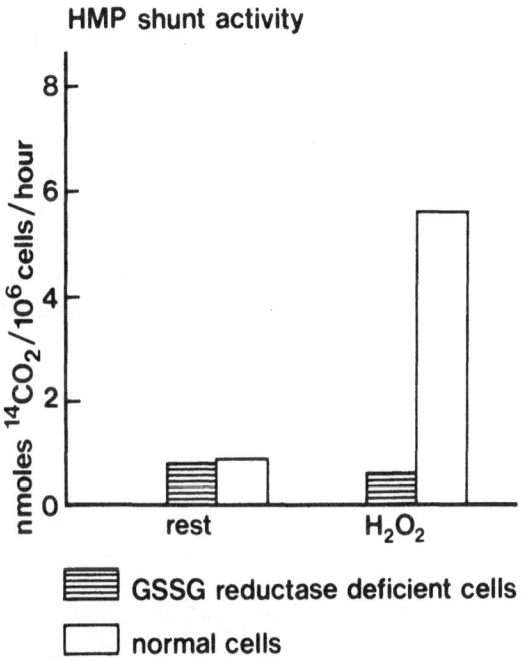

HMP shunt activity

Figure 18.4   Effect of H_2O_2 addition on $^{14}CO_2$ production from glucose-l-^{14}C by normal and GSSG reductase-deficient granulocytes

binding agent N-ethylmaleimide (NEM). This substance binds to other thiol groups as well, however, and is known to inhibit many metabolic and functional reactions in phagocytes[67-70]. Reed[67] also showed that the phagocytosis-induced HMP activation was inhibited by NEM, but stimulated by cyanide, azide, and aminotriazole, agents known to inhibit intracellular H_2O_2 breakdown. Finally, Noseworthy and Karnovsky[68] and Vogt *et al.*[69] found that addition of GSSG, or GSH plus H_2O_2, in combination with NADP(H), stimulated the HMP shunt activity in broken cell preparations.

Still, this does not prove that the system is operating in intact, phagocytizing cells. However, together with the presence of glutathione in large amounts[25, 69-71], and the existence of GSH peroxidase[25, 67, 69, 72, 73] and GSSG reductase[25, 67-69, 72-74] in these cells, it became highly likely that such is indeed the case. Direct proof has now been obtained from our observations on glutathione reductase deficient granulocytes: as Figure 18.4 shows, these cells are, in contrast to normal cells, unable to react with increased HMP shunt activity to H_2O_2 addition. Thus, this is clear evidence that an intact glutathione cycle is required for HMP shunt stimulation by hydrogen peroxide.

The idea that the HMP shunt is activated during phagocytosis both for the generation of reducing equivalents for superoxide production in the phagosomes and for the detoxification of hydrogen peroxide in the cytosol, was also substantiated by our experiments with GSSG reductase-deficient leukocytes. As Figure 18.5 shows, the HMP shunt activity in these cells is stimulated to a much lesser extent than in normal cells. Knowing that the reaction of H_2O_2 with GSH cannot lead to HMP shunt activation in the

Glucose-1-^{14}C oxidation

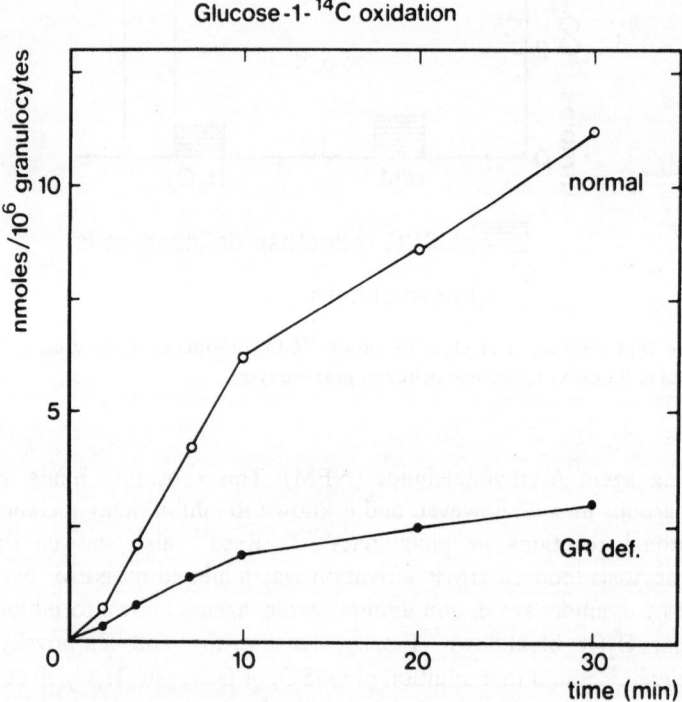

Figure 18.5 HMP shunt activity of normal and GSSG reductase-deficient granulocytes during phagocytosis

patient's cells, we have to conclude that in these cells the superoxide generation as such causes the shunt to be accelerated independently of the glutathione cycle. Our results indicate that less NADPH is needed for oxygen reduction alone than for the combination of oxygen reduction and H_2O_2 detoxification.

An alternative function for the glutathione system in phagocytic leukocytes has been proposed by Strauss et al.[25] From their observation that the activity of GSSG reductase increased two to three times within 15 s after addition of particles to cells, at a time when the NADPH oxidase activity had not yet increased, these authors drew the conclusion that the formation of hydrogen peroxide might depend on a preceding reduction of GSSG. The following order of reactions was proposed:

(a) $\quad GSSG + NADPH + H^+ \xrightarrow{\text{GSSG reductase}} 2\,GSH + NADP^+$

(b) $\quad 2\,NADP^+ + \text{glucose-6-PO}_4 \xrightarrow{\text{G6PD}} 2\,NADPH + 2\,H^+ + CO_2 +$ ribulose-5-PO_4

(c) $\quad NADPH + H^+ + O_2 \xrightarrow{\text{NADPH oxidase}} H_2O_2 + NADP^+$

(d) $\quad 2\,GSH + H_2O_2 \xrightarrow{\text{GSH peroxidase}} GSSG + 2\,H_2O$

Several points of criticism of this hypothesis are possible. Firstly, the reported activation of GSSG reductase at the start of phagocytosis has never been confirmed by other workers[75]. Secondly, as in erythrocytes, the ratio of GSSG:GSH in granulocytes is very low[76], in the order of 1:100. It is not clear, therefore, how and why this ratio should be decreased even more to start the formation of H_2O_2. The resulting increase in $NADP^+$ can hardly be expected to stimulate substantially the glucose-6-PO_4 dehydrogenase reaction. And finally, this set of reactions implies that all hydrogen peroxide must react with GSH, since GSSG is needed again in reaction (a) above. This would leave no H_2O_2 available for bactericidal reactions, a conclusion which is in conflict with the overwhelming evidence that H_2O_2 is directly involved in this function. Moreover, what would be the sense of this set of reactions if it is not to produce H_2O_2?

Glutathione peroxidase deficiency

Nevertheless, the theory of Strauss et al.[25] has been used to explain the curious observation that phagocytic leukocytes which lack glutathione peroxidase activity do not produce H_2O_2 during phagocytosis[73]. In 1968 Quie et al.[77] described for the first time two (unrelated) female CGD patients. Later, many more have been found[78-80]. In 1970, however, Holmes et al.[73] discovered that glutathione peroxidase activity in the leuko-cytes of the first two female CGD patients was depressed. This GSH peroxidase deficiency proved not to be a general property of female CGD phagocytes: subsequently discovered cases showed no abnormality in this respect[79,80]. Moreover, Malawista and Gifford[81] reported a partial defi-ciency of GSH peroxidase in the cells of a brother of one of the two patients described by Quie et al.[77] and Holmes et al.[73], and Matsuda[82] did likewise with another, unrelated, male CGD patient.

From these observations and from the fact that deficient selenium intake leads to depression of GSH peroxidase together with a killing deficiency toward *Candida albicans*[83], it follows that this enzyme is essential for proper bactericidal activity of phagocytic leukocytes. From the scheme shown in Figure 18.3, however, it is not clear why GSH peroxidase-deficient cells should not generate H_2O_2 in normal amounts. Therefore, the theory of Strauss et al.[25] has been used to explain this phenomenon[73,82]. As indicated above, this theory is hardly acceptable. Alternatively, cell damage caused by H_2O_2 (or superoxide) in the cytosol could play a role, since a proper functioning glutathione system might well be essential for leukocyte integrity[73,76,83]. With the cells from the family with glutathione reductase deficiency we have been able to distinguish between the two possible roles for glutathione in phagocytic cells only for or also for pro-tection against oxidative damage (Reed[67]), the other is for the generation of hydrogen peroxide (Strauss et al.[25]).

Glutathione reductase deficiency

Table 18.3 shows that a GSSG reductase deficiency of 85–90% is present both in the leukocytes and in the purified granulocytes of all three children in this family. Figure 18.6 shows that the oxygen consumption of these granulocytes followed a peculiar pattern: after 5–10 min of stimulation, the reaction stopped, in contrast to normal cells which continued at a high res-piratory rate for much longer periods. Figure 18.7 shows the same to be true for the H_2O_2 generation. In Figure 18.5 a similar pattern can be observed in HMP shunt activity, although it should be noted that this parameter

TABLE 18.3   Glutathione reductase activity* in the leukocytes and purified granulocytes of family M

Subjects	Leukocytes	Granulocytes
Father	178	nt
Mother	187	nt
Brother	41	23
Patient	38	27
Sister	37	19
10 normals	205–353	189–350

* GSSG reductase activity in μmol/min/10^{11} cells at 25 °C
nt = not tested

was already decreased at the onset of phagocytosis. As mentioned above, the latter phenomenon may be explained by an HMP shunt stimulation to provide reducing equivalents for O_2^- generation only, not for H_2O_2 detoxification (which is impossible in these cells).

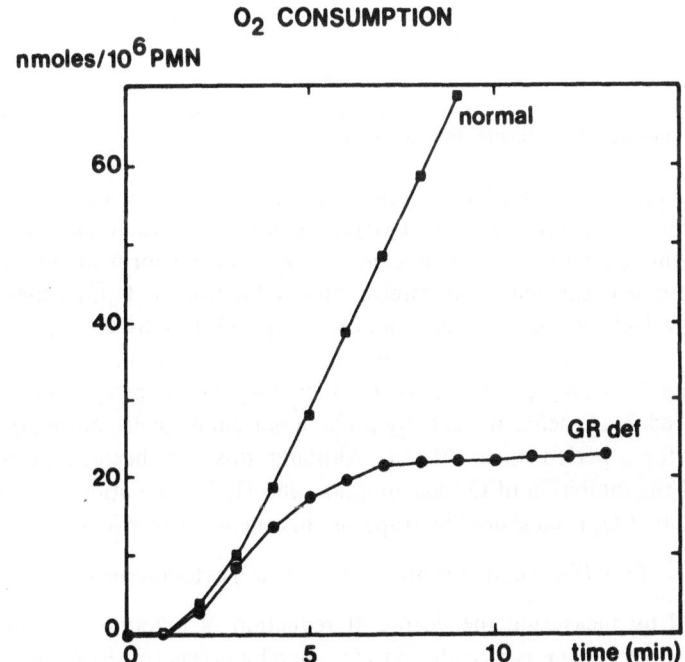

Figure 18.6   Oxygen consumption of normal and GSSG reductase deficient granulocytes during phagocytosis (reproduced with publisher's permission from reference 85)

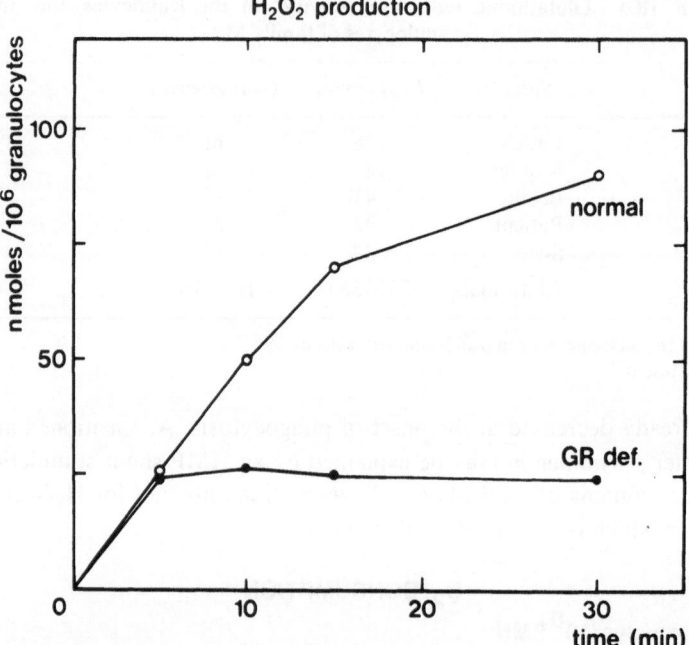

Figure 18.7 Hydrogen peroxide formation by normal and GSSG reductase-deficient granulocytes during phagocytosis

This unique metabolic behaviour provides no clue, however, to which mechanism is operating in phagocytic leukocytes. Assuming that after 5–10 min, glutathione is completely in the oxidized form in the GSSG reductase-deficient cells, this might cause inhibition of H_2O_2 generation either by lack of substrate in reaction (d) (p. 273) or by damage to the cells in the absence of detoxification in the glutathione cycle.

Figure 18.8 provides the answer. Measuring the O_2^- production of the GSSG reductase-deficient cells, we found a normal response during phagocytosis for a period up to 30 min. Although this is rather unexpected in view of the inhibition of O_2 consumption and H_2O_2 generation, it must be realized that O_2^- is measured by trapping this agent with ferricytochrome c:

$$O_2^- + (Fe^{3+}) \text{ cytochrome } c \rightarrow O_2 + (Fe^{2+}) \text{ cytochrome } c,$$

followed by measuring the degree of reduction of cytochrome c at 550 nm[84]. As a result, O_2^- is reoxidized to O_2, thereby preventing its dismutation to H_2O_2. Thus, under the conditions of this experiment, the GSSG reductase-deficient cells are protected against damage by H_2O_2, in contrast to the experiments shown in Figures 18.5, 18.6 and 18.7. This explains

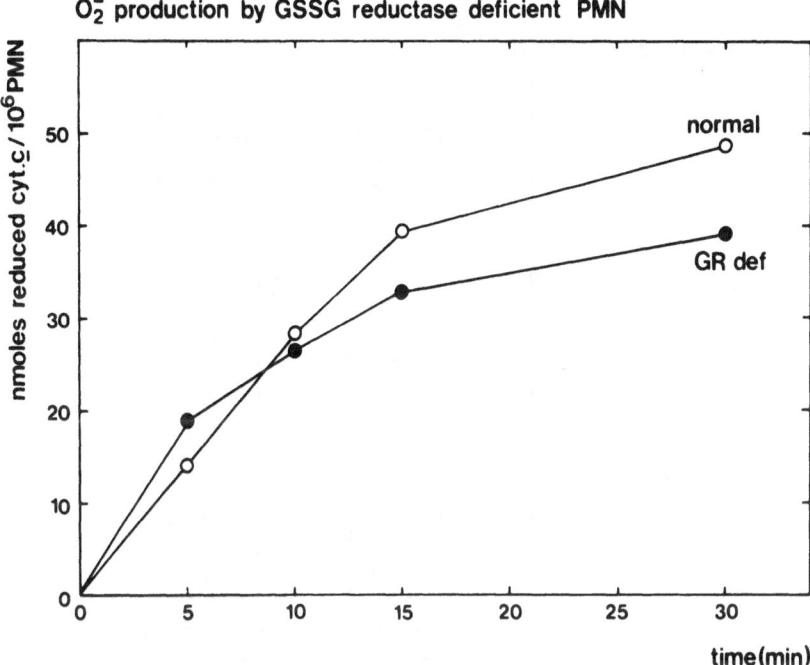

Figure 18.8   Cytochrome *c* reduction by normal and GSSG reductase-deficient granulocytes during phagocytosis (reproduced with publisher's permission from reference 85)

why the patient's cells remain metabolically active in the presence of cytochrome *c*, and provides a strong argument for the protective role of the glutathione system in normal cells. Moreover, the result shown in Figure 18.8 also indicates that GSSG reductase-deficient cells *are* able to generate normal amounts of superoxide, in spite of the absence of a functionally active glutathione cycle. This virtually excludes the validity of the mechanism proposed by Strauss *et al*.[25].

Finally, we have also been able to show the increased sensitivity of the GSSG reductase-deficient leukocytes towards oxidative stress. Figure 18.9 shows that these cells show a short, but normal oxygen consumption when challenged with ingestible particles. If, however, such cells are pretreated for 10 min with a H_2O_2-generating system, the oxidative response is practically absent, in contrast to normal cells. These experiments show that the glutathione system is of vital importance for the proper functioning of phagocytic leukocytes.

The three children in the family with glutathione reductase deficiency are not abnormally susceptible to infections[46]. In accordance, we found a

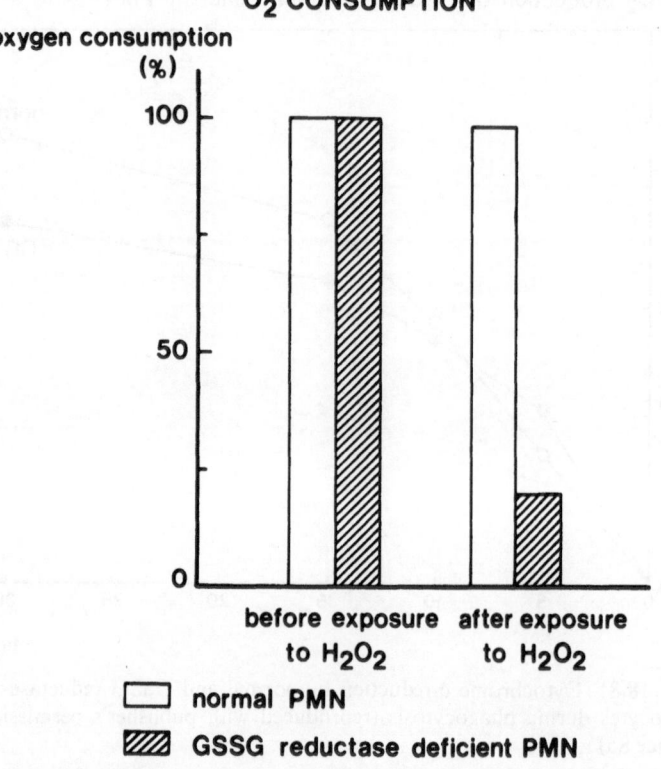

Figure 18.9 Susceptibility to oxidative stress of normal and GSSG reductase-deficient granulocytes during phagocytosis. Oxygen consumption was measured at 4 min after starting phagocytosis, both before and after exposing cells to a H_2O_2-generating system (glucose + glucose oxidase), followed by washing (reproduced with publisher's permission from reference 85)

normal *in vitro* chemotaxis toward casein, normal *in vitro* phagocytosis of *Staphylococcus aureus* and normal *in vitro* killing of these bacteria[85]. Obviously, the short metabolic burst of which these cells are capable suffices for adequate bacterial killing. The problem remains, however, why such a big difference of phagocyte function *in vivo* and *in vitro* exists between patients with GSH peroxidase deficiency and those with GSSG reductase deficiency. The explanation might be that in the GSSG reductase deficiency, GSH may serve to detoxify oxidative agents and repair oxidative damage (see the introduction to this chapter) until all glutathione is in the oxidized form. Such a period may be long enough to allow effective bacteria killing. This possibility is absent in GSH peroxidase-deficient granulocytes.

Glutathione synthetase deficiency

One more deficiency of the glutathione system has been found to affect phagocyte function: GSH synthetase deficiency. Spielberg et al.[35] have examined the leukocytes of a boy with oxoprolinuria, containing less than 4% of normal GSH synthetase activity and less than 25% of normal glutathione levels. They found that the phagocytizing leukocytes accumulated twice the amount of H_2O_2 as normal cells do and showed impaired killing of ingested bacteria[86]. Neutropenia was observed during infection in the patient. Again, this may be explained by oxidative damage in the cytosol of such cells. It should be mentioned that GSH synthetase deficiency will not always lead to defects in phagocyte function; in a case in which GSH levels in erythrocytes was less than 5% of normal[27], GSH in the granulocytes was half normal and no abnormality in granulocyte function or metabolism could be observed[88]. Perhaps only in oxoprolinuria, in which the GSH synthetase deficiency seems to be generalized, phagocyte function is affected.

Protection by glutathione

One target for oxidative damage in the phagocytic leukocytes, which is protected by glutathione, is the microtubule system. Oliver and colleagues[71] have studied the movement of surface-bound Con-A on these cells. They found that capping of Con-A and inhibition of microtubule assembly occur only when GSH levels in the cell are decreased by 30–70%. Recent work by Oliver et al.[76,87] indicates that not GSH as such, but especially the levels of GSSG, or mixed disulphides between GSSG and protein-thiol groups (GSSR), are responsible for tubulin depolymerization and inhibition of microtubule assembly. The impairment of other cell functions in phagocytic cells with a defect in glutathione metabolism (GSH peroxidase, GSSG reductase and GSH synthetase) indicates that tubulin is probably one of many targets for oxidative damage in such cells.

Finally, from these observations we may conclude that the glutathione system is essential for effective phagocyte host-defence. Apparently, this system is more important in maintaining the reducing environment of the cytosol than is catalase. Although both catalase and the glutathione system are able to detoxify hydrogen peroxide, acatalasaemic patients do not suffer from an increased incidence of infections and their phagocytes show a normal in vitro response toward micro-organisms[89]. Probably, catalase removes H_2O_2 only efficiently at high concentrations. Moreover, in contrast to catalase, the fact that the glutathione system is not only able to *prevent* oxidative damage in trapping radicals and peroxides, but also able to *repair* such damage by reducing S–S bridges, makes this system more important than catalase in maintaining cell integrity.

CONCLUSIONS

In erythrocytes, as well as in eye lens cells and phagocytic leukocytes, the glutathione system offers protection against oxidative stress. Deficiencies in this system, either in the glutathione cycle itself, in the synthesis of glutathione, or in the system to keep glutathione in the reduced form, may lead to serious clinical disorders, such as haemolytic anaemia, severe recurrent infections and/or cataracts. The glutathione system is not involved in the generation of bactericidal oxygen products in phagocytic leukocytes.

References

1. Kossower, E. M. (1976). Chemical properties of glutathione. In I. M. Arias and W. B. Jakoby (eds.). *Glutathione, Metabolism and Function*, p. 1 (New York: Raven Press)
2. Flohé, L. and Günzler, W. A. (1974). Glutathione peroxidase. In L. Flohé, H. Ch. Benöhr, H. Sies, H. D. Waller and A. Wendel (eds.). *Glutathione*. Proc. 16th Conf. German Soc. Biol. Chem., p. 132. (Stuttgart: Georg Thieme Publishers)
3. Flohé, L. and Günzler, W. A. (1976). Glutathione-dependent enzymatic oxido-reduction reactions. In I. M. Arias and W. B. Jakoby (eds.). *Glutathione, Metabolism and Function*, p. 17. (New York: Raven Press)
4. Hartter, P. and Weber, U. (1974). The thiol-disulfide exchange reactions of asymmetric disulfides of cysteine and cyclic cysteine peptides with G–SH. In L. Flohé, H. Ch. Benöhr, H. Sies, H. D. Waller and A. Wendel (eds.). *Glutathione*. Proc. 16th Conf. German Soc. Biol. Chem., p. 29. (Stuttgart: Georg Thieme Publishers)
5. Beutler, E. and Srivastava, S. K. (1974). G–SH metabolism of the lens. In L. Flohé, H. Ch. Benöhr, H. Sies, H. D. Waller and A. Wendel (eds.). *Glutathione*. Proc. 16th Conf. German Soc. Biol. Chem., p. 201. (Stuttgart: Georg Thieme Publishers)
6. Srivastava, S. K. and Beutler, E. (1970). Glutathione metabolism of the erythrocyte. The enzymic cleavage of glutathione-haemoglobin preparations by glutathione reductase. *Biochem. J.*, **119**, 353
7. Beutler, E. (1974). Glutathione reductase. In L. Flohé, H. Ch. Benöhr, H. Sies, H. D. Waller and A. Wendel (eds.). *Glutathione*. Proc. 16th Conf. German Soc. Biol. Chem., p. 109. (Stuttgart: Georg Thieme Publishers)
8. Kossower, E. M. and Kossower, N. S. (1976). Chemical basis of the perturbation of glutathione–glutathione disulfide status of biological systems by diazenes. In I. M. Arias and W. B. Jakoby (eds.). *Glutathione, Metabolism and Function*, p. 139. (New York: Raven Press)

9. Kossower, E. M. and Kossower, N. S. (1974). Manifestations of changes in the G–SH – G–S–S–G status of biological systems. In L. Flohé, H. Ch. Benöhr, H. Sies, H. D. Waller and A. Wendel (eds.). *Glutathione*. Proc. 16th Conf. German Soc. Biol. Chem., p. 287. (Stuttgart: Georg Thieme Publishers)

10. Hochberg, A., Rigby, M. and Dimant, E. (1961). The incorporation *in vitro* of glycine and L-glutamic acid into glutathione of human erythrocytes. *Biochim. Biophys. Acta*, **90**, 464

11. Boivin, P. and Galand, C. (1965). La synthèse du glutathion au cours de l'anémie hémolytique congénitale avec déficit en glutathion réduit. Déficit congénital en glutathion synthétase érythrocytaire? *Nouv. Rev. Franç Hématol.*, **5**, 707

12. Meister, A. (1974). Biosynthesis and utilization of glutathione; the γ-glutamyl cycle and its function in amino acid transport. In L. Flohé, H. Ch. Benöhr, H. Sies, H. D. Waller and A. Wendel (eds.). *Glutathione*. Proc. 16th Conf. German Soc. Biol. Chem., p. 56. (Stuttgart: Georg Thieme Publishers)

13. Meister, A. (1976). Glutathione and the γ-glutamyl cycle. In I. M. Arias and W. B. Jakoby (eds.). *Glutathione, Metabolism and Function*, p. 35. (New York: Raven Press)

14. Chasseaud, L. F. (1974). Glutathione S-transferases. In L. Flohé, H. Ch. Benöhr, H. Sies, H. D. Waller and A. Wendel (eds.). *Glutathione*. Proc. 16th Conf. German Soc. Biol. Chem., p. 90. (Stuttgart: Georg Thieme Publishers)

15. Chasseaud, L. F. (1976). Conjugation with glutathione and mercapturic acid excretion. In I. M. Arias and W. B. Jakoby (eds.). *Glutathione, Metabolism and Function*, p. 77. (New York: Raven Press)

16. Srivastava, S. K. and Beutler, E. (1969). The transport of oxidized glutathione from human erythrocytes. *J. Biol. Chem.*, **244**, 9

17. Srivastava, S. K. and Beutler, E. (1969). Cataract produced by tyrosinase and tyrosine systems in rabbit lens *in vitro*. *Biochem. J.*, **112**, 421

18. Sies, H., Gerstenecker, C., Menzel, H. and Flohé, L. (1972). Oxidation in the NADP system and release of GSSG from hemoglobin-free perfused rat liver during peroxidatic oxidation of glutathione by hydroperoxides. *FEBS Lett.*, **27**, 171

19. Smith, J. E. (1974). Relationship of *in vivo* erythrocyte glutathione flux to the oxidized glutathione transport system. *J. Lab. Clin. Med.*, **83**, 444

20. Misra, H. P. and Fridovich, I. (1972). The generation of superoxide radical during the autoxidation of hemoglobin. *J. Biol. Chem.*, **247**, 6960

21. Jacob, H. S., Ingbar, S. H. and Jandl, H. S. (1965). Oxidative hemolysis and erythrocyte metabolism in hereditary acatalasia. *J. Clin. Invest.*, **44**, 1187

22. Aebi, H. and Suter, H. (1974). Protective function of reduced glutathione (G–SH) against the effect of prooxidative substances and of irradiation in the red cell. In L. Flohé, H. Ch. Benöhr, H. Sies, H. D. Waller and A. Wendel (eds.). *Glutathione*. Proc. 16th Conf. German Soc. Biol. Chem., p. 192. (Stuttgart: Georg Thieme Publishers)

23. Gross, R. T., Bracci, R., Rudolph, N., Schroeder, E. and Kochen, J. A. (1967). Hydrogen peroxide toxicity and detoxification in the erythrocytes of newborn infants. *Blood*, **29**, 481

24. Zeller, E. A. (1953). Contribution to the enzymology of the normal and cataractous lens. III. On the catalase of the crystalline lens. *Am. J. Ophthalmol.*, **36**, 51

25. Strauss, R. R., Paul, B. B., Jacobs, A. A. and Sbarra, A. J. (1969). The role of the phagocyte in host–parasite interactions. XIX. Leukocytic glutathione reductase and its involvement in phagocytosis. *Arch. Biochem. Biophys.*, **135**, 265

26. Konrad, P. N., Richards, F., Valentine, W. N. and Paglia, D. E. (1972). γ-Glutamyl cysteine synthetase deficiency; a cause of hereditary hemolytic anemia. *N. Engl. J. Med.*, **286**, 557

27. Oort, M., Loos, J. A. and Prins, H. K. (1961). Hereditary absence of reduced glutathione in the erythrocytes. A new clinical and biochemical entity. *Vox Sang.*, **6**, 370

28. Prins, H. K., Oort, M., Loos, J. A., Zürcher, C. and Beckers, T. A. (1966). Congenital non-spherocytic hemolytic anaemia associated with glutathione deficiency of the erythrocytes. Hematologic, biochemical and genetic studies. *Blood*, **27**, 145

29. Boivin, P., Galand, C., André, R. and Debray, J. (1966). Anémies hémolytiques congénitales avec déficit isolé en glutathion réduit par déficit en glutathion synthétase. *Nouv. Rev. Franç. Hématol.*, **6**, 859

30. Boivin, P., Galand, C. and Bernard, J. F. (1974). Deficiencies in G–SH biosynthesis. In L. Flohé, H. Ch. Benöhr, H. Sies, H. D. Waller and A. Wendel (eds.). *Glutathione*. Proc. 16th Conf. German Soc. Biol. Chem., p. 146. (Stuttgart: Georg Thieme Publishers)

31. Mohler, D. N., Majerus, P. W., Minnich, V., Hess, C. E. and Garrick, M. D. (1970). Glutathione synthetase deficiency as a cause of hereditary hemolytic disease. *N. Engl. J. Med.*, **283**, 1253

32. Larsson, A., Zetterström, R., Hagenfeldt, L., Andersson, R., Dreborg, S. and Hornell, H. (1974). Pyroglutamic aciduria (5-oxoprolinuria), an inborn error of glutathione metabolism. *Pediatr. Res.*, **8**, 852

33. Larsson, A., Zetterström, R., Hörnell, H. and Porath, U. (1976). Erythrocyte glutathione synthetase in 5-oxoprolinuria: Kinetic studies of the mutant enzyme and detection of heterozygotes. *Clin. Chim. Acta*, **73**, 19

34. Marstein, S., Jellum, E., Halpern, B., Eldjarn, L. and Perry, T. L. (1976). Biochemical studies of erythrocytes in a patient with pyroglutamic acidemia (5-oxoprolinemia). *N. Engl. J. Med.*, **295**, 406

35. Spielberg, S. P., Kramer, L. I., Goodman, S. I., Butler, J., Tietze, F., Quinn, P. and Schulman, J. D. (1977). 5-Oxoprolinuria: biochemical observations and case report. *J. Pediatr.*, **91**, 237

36. Necheles, T. F., Maldonado, N., Barquet-Chediak, A. and Allen, D. M. (1969). Homozygous erythrocyte glutathione-peroxidase deficiency: clinical and biochemical studies. *Blood*, **33**, 164

37. Necheles, T. F. (1974). The clinical spectrum of glutathione-peroxidase deficiency. In L. Flohé, H. Ch. Benöhr, H. Sies, H. D. Waller and A. Wendel (eds.). *Glutathione*. Proc. 16th Conf. German Soc. Biol. Chem., p. 173. (Stuttgart: Georg Thieme Publishers)

38. Necheles, T. F., Boles, T. A. and Allen, D. M. (1968). Erythrocyte glutathione peroxidase deficiency and hemolytic disease of the newborn infant. *J. Pediatr.*, **72**, 319

39. Boivin, P., Galand, C., Hakim, J. and Guéroult, N. (1969). Anémie hémolytique avec déficit en glutathione peroxydase chez un adulte. *Enzym. Biol. Clin.*, **10**, 68

40. Boivin, P., Galand, C., Hakim, J. and Blery, M. (1970). Déficit en glutathion-peroxidase érythrocytaire et anémie hémolitique médicamenteuse. *Presse Med.*, **78**, 171

41. Benedetti, P. (1966). Glutathione peroxidase deficiency. *Symposium on Problems of Fetal Distress.* (Siena, Italy)

42. Beutler, E. (1971). Abnormalities of the hexose monophosphate shunt. *Semin. Hematol.*, **8**, 311

43. Beutler, E. (1969). Effect of flavin compounds on glutathione reductase activity: *in vivo* and *in vitro* studies. *J. Clin. Invest.*, **48**, 1957

44. Löhr, G. W., Blume, K. G., Rüdiger, H. W. and Arnold, H. (1974). Genetic variability in the enzymatic reduction of oxidized glutathione. In L. Flohé, H. Ch. Benöhr, H. Sies, H. D. Waller, and A. Wendel (eds.). *Glutathione.* Proc. 16th Conf. German Soc. Biol. Chem., p. 165. (Stuttgart: Georg Thieme Publishers)

45. Staal, G. E. J., Helleman, P. W., de Wael, J. and Veeger, C. (1969). Purification and properties of an abnormal glutathione reductase from human erythrocytes. *Biochim. Biophys. Acta*, **185**, 39

46. Loos, J. A., Roos, D., Weening, R. S. and Houwerzijl, J. (1976). Familial deficiency of glutathione reductase in human blood cells. *Blood*, **48**, 53

47. Brewer, G. J. (1969). 6-Phosphogluconate dehydrogenase and glutathione reductase. In J. J. Yunis (ed.). *Biochemical Methods in Red Cell Genetics*, p. 139. (New York and London: Academic Press)

48. Lausecker, C., Heidt, P., Fischer, D., Hartleyb, H. and Löhr, G. W. (1965). Anémie hémolytique constitutionnelle avec déficit en 6-phosphogluconate deshydrogénase. *Arch. Franç. Pediatr.*, **22**, 789

49. Scialom, C., Najean, Y. and Bernard, J. (1966). Anémie hémolytique congénital non-sphérocytaire avec déficit incomplet en 6-phosphogluconate deshydrogénase. *Nouv. Rev. Franç. Hématol.*, **6**, 452

50. Dern, R. J., Brewer, G. J., Tashian, R. E. and Shows, T. B. (1966). Hereditary variation of erythrocytic 6-phosphogluconate dehydrogenase. *J. Lab. Clin. Med.*, **67**, 255

51. Kinoshita, J. H. and Merola, L. O. (1973). Oxidation of thiol groups of the human lens. In *The Human Lens – in Relation to Cataract.* Ciba Foundation Symposium 19 (new series), p. 173. (Amsterdam: Associated Scientific Publishers)

52. Truscott, R. J. W. and Augusteyn, R. C. (1977). Oxidative changes in human lens proteins during senile nuclear cataract formation. *Biochim. Biophys. Acta*, **492**, 43

53. Zinkham, W. H. (1961). A deficiency of glucose-6-phosphate dehydrogenase activity in lens from individuals with primaquine-sensitive erythrocytes. *Bull. Johns Hopkins Hosp.*, **109**, 206

54. Westring, D. W. and Pisciotta, A. V. (1966). Anemia, cataracts, and seizures in patients with glucose-6-phosphate dehydrogenase deficiency. *Arch. Intern. Med.*, **118**, 385

55. Helge, H. and Borner, K. (1966). Kongenitale nichtsphärozytäre hämolytische Anämie, Kataract und Glukose-6-phosphat-dehydrogenase Mangel. *Deutsch. Med. Wochenschr.*, **91**, 1584

56. Cooper, M. R., De Chatelet, L. R., McCall, C. E., La Via, M. F., Spurr, C. L. and Baehner, R. L. (1972). Complete deficiency of leukocyte glucose-6-phosphate dehydrogenase with defective bactericidal activity. *J. Clin. Invest.*, 51, 769

57. Johnston, R. B., Jr. and Baehner, R. L. (1970). Improvement of leukocyte bactericidal activity in chronic granulomatous disease. *Blood*, 35, 350

58. Patriarca, P., Cramer, R., Moncalvo, S., Rossi, F. and Romeo, D. (1971). Enzymatic basis of metabolic stimulation in leukocytes during phagocytosis: The role of activated NADPH oxidase. *Arch. Biochem. Biophys.*, 145, 255

59. Hohn, D. C. and Lehrer, R. I. (1975). NADPH oxidase deficiency in X-linked chronic granulomatous disease. *J. Clin. Invest.*, 55, 707

60. Curnutte, J. T., Kipnes, R. S. and Babior, B. M. (1975). Defect in pyridine nucleotide dependent superoxide production by a particulate fraction from the granulocytes of patients with chronic granulomatous disease. *N. Engl. J. Med.*, 293, 628

61. Segal, A. W. and Peters, T. J. (1976). Characterisation of the enzyme defect in chronic granulomatous disease. *Lancet*, i, 1363

62. Briggs, R. T., Karnovsky, M. L. and Karnovsky, M. J. (1977). Hydrogen peroxide production in chronic granulomatous disease. A cytochemical study of reduced pyridine nucleotide oxidase. *J. Clin. Invest.*, 59, 1088

63. Baehner, R. L., Johnston, R. B., Jr. and Nathan, D. G. (1972). Comparative study of the metabolic and bactericidal characteristics of severely glucose-6-phosphate dehydrogenase-deficient polymorphonuclear leukocytes and leukocytes from children with chronic granulomatous disease. *J. Reticuloendothel. Soc.*, 12, 150

64. Gray, G. R., Klebanoff, S. J., Stamatoyannopoulos, G., Austin, T., Naiman, S. C., Yoshida, A., Kliman, M. R. and Robinson, G. S. F. (1973). Neutrophil dysfunction, chronic granulomatous disease and nonspherocytic haemolytic anaemia caused by complete deficiency of glucose-6-phosphate dehydrogenase. *Lancet*, ii, 530

65. Rodey, G. E., Jacob, H. S., Holmes, B., McArthur, J. R. and Good, R. A. (1970). Leucocyte G-6-PD levels and bactericidal activity. *Lancet*, i, 355

66. Holmes-Gray, B. and Good, R. A. (1971). Chronic granulomatous disease of childhood. In R. A. Good and D. W. Fisher (eds.). *Immunobiology, Current Knowledge of Basic Concepts in Immunology and their Clinical Applications*, p. 55. (Stanford: Sinauer Associates, Inc.)

67. Reed, P. W. (1969). Glutathione and the hexose monophosphate shunt in phagocytizing and hydrogen peroxide-treated rat leukocytes. *J. Biol. Chem.*, 244, 2459

68. Noseworthy, J. Jr. and Karnovsky, M. L. (1972). Role of peroxide in the stimulation of the hexose monophosphate shunt during phagocytosis by polymorphonuclear leukocytes. *Enzyme*, 13, 110

69. Vogt, M. T., Thomas, C., Vassallo, C. L., Basford, R. E. and Gee, J. B. L. (1971). Glutathione-dependent peroxidative metabolism in the alveolar macrophage. *J. Clin. Invest.*, 50, 401

70. Mandell, G. L. (1972). Functional and metabolic derangements in human neutrophils induced by a glutathione antagonist. *J. Reticuloendothel. Soc.*, 11, 129

71. Oliver, J. M., Albertini, D. F. and Berlin, R. D. (1976). Effects of glutathione-

oxidizing agents on microtubule assembly and microtubule-dependent surface properties of human neutrophils. *J. Cell. Biol.*, **71**, 921

72. Holmes-Gray, B., Haseman, J., Buron, S., Saccoccia, P. and Good, R. A. (1971). The relationship of glutathione levels and metabolism of human leukocytes. *Fed. Proc.*, **30**, 693Abs.

73. Holmes, B., Park, B. H., Malawista, S. E., Quie, P. G., Nelson, D. L. and Good, R. A. (1970). Chronic granulomatous disease in females. A deficiency of leukocyte glutathione peroxidase. *N. Engl. J. Med.*, **283**, 217

74. Baehner, R. L., Gilman, N. and Karnovsky, M. L. (1970). Respiration and glucose oxidation in human and guinea-pig leukocytes: comparative studies. *J. Clin. Invest.*, **49**, 692

75. Rossi, F., Romeo, D. and Patriarca, P. (1972). Mechanism of phagocytosis-associated oxidative metabolism in polymorphonuclear leukocytes and macrophages. *J. Reticuloendothel. Soc.*, **12**, 127

76. Burchill, B. R., Oliver, J. M., Pearson, C. B., Leinbach, E. D. and Berlin, R. D. (1977). Microtubule dynamics and glutathione metabolism in phagocytizing human polymorphonuclear leukocytes. *J. Cell. Biol.*, **76**, 439

77. Quie, P. G., Kaplan, E. L., Page, A. R., Gruskay, F. L. and Malawista, S. E. (1968). Defective polymorphonuclear leukocyte function and chronic granulomatous disease in two female children. *N. Engl. J. Med.*, **278**, 976

78. Johnston, R. B. Jr. and Newman, S. L. (1977). Chronic granulomatous disease. In *The Pediatric Clinics of North America, Vol. 24.* p. 365. (Philadelphia: W. B. Saunders)

79. Windhorst, D. B. and Katz, E. D. (1972). Normal enzyme activities in chronic granulomatous disease leukocytes. *J. Reticuloendothel. Soc.*, **11**, 400

80. De Chatelet, L. R., Shirley, P. S. and McPhail, L. C. (1976). Normal leukocyte glutathione peroxidase activity in patients with chronic granulomatous disease. *J. Pediatr.*, **89**, 598

81. Malawista, S. E. and Gifford, R. H. (1975). Chronic granulomatous disease of childhood (GCD) with leukocyte glutathione peroxidase (LPG) deficiency in a brother and sister: a likely autosomal recessive inheritance. *Clin. Res.*, **23**, 416Abs

82. Matsuda, I., Oka, Y., Taniguchi, N., Furuyama, M., Kodama, S., Arashima, S. and Mitsuyama, T. (1976). Leukocyte glutathione peroxidase deficiency in a male patient with chronic granulomatous disease. *J. Pediatr.*, **88**, 581

83. Serfass, R. E. and Ganther, H. E. (1975). Defective microbicidal activity in glutathione peroxidase-deficient neutrophils of selenium-deficient rats. *Nature (London)*, **255**, 640

84. Babior, B. M., Kipnes, R. S. and Curnutte, J. T. (1973). Biological defense mechanisms. The production by leukocytes of superoxide, a potential bactericidal agent. *J. Clin. Invest.*, **52**, 741

85. Weening, R. S., Roos, D., Van Schaik, M. L. J., Voetman, A. A., De Boer, M. and Loos, J. A. (1978). The role of glutathione in the oxidative metabolism of phagocytic leukocytes. Studies in a family with glutathione reductase deficiency. In F. Rossi, P. L. Patriarca and D. Romeo (eds.). *Movement, Metabolism and Bactericidal Mechanisms of Phagocytes*, p. 277. (Padova: Piccin Medical Books)

86. Spielberg, S. P., Boxer, L. A., Oliver, J. M., Butler, E. J. and Schulman, J. D. (1977). Altered phagocytosis and microtubule function in leukocytes from

a patient with severe glutathione synthetase deficiency (5-oxoprolinuria). In *Proc. Intern. Symp. Inborn Errors of Metabolism in Man.* (Basel: S. Karger) (In press)

87. Oliver, J. M., Spielberg, S. P., Pearson, C. B. and Schulman, J. D. (1978). Microtubule assembly and function in normal and glutathione synthetase-deficient polymorphonuclear leukocytes. *J. Immunol.*, **120**, 1131

88. Roos, D. Unpublished observations

89. Aebi, H. and Suter, H. (1969). Catalase. In J. J. Yunis (ed.). *Biochemical Methods in Red Cell Genetics*, p. 255. (New York: Academic Press)

19

Defective initiation of the metabolic stimulation in phagocytizing granulocytes

R. S. Weening, D. Roos and
Margriet L. J. van Schaik

INTRODUCTION

Peripheral blood phagocytes. i.e. monocytes and granulocytes. are of crucial importance in the elimination of invading micro-organisms. These cells perform their task by migrating in a gradient of humoral stimuli towards the infected area (chemotaxis). recognizing and ingesting the invaders (phagocytosis). and subsequently by killing and degrading such organisms. Obviously, defects in any of these functions will lead to severe recurrent bacterial and fungal infections.

For an effective killing of micro-organisms by human phagocytes the production of several oxidative products during the formation of the phagosome (part of the plasma membrane which envelops the particles) is critical. During ingestion of particles. the oxygen uptake by phagocytes increases more than 15-fold[1,2]. Figure 19.1 shows that these cells reduce oxygen to superoxide radicals (O_2^-)[3] (reaction 2), which then combine with protons to hydrogen peroxide. The reducing equivalents for this reaction are provided by glucose through its oxidation in the hexose monophosphate (HMP) shunt (reaction 1)[1]. From the study of chronic granulomatous disease (CGD) we know that a defect in either the superoxide-producing system or in the hexose monophosphate shunt will lead to defective bacterial killing.

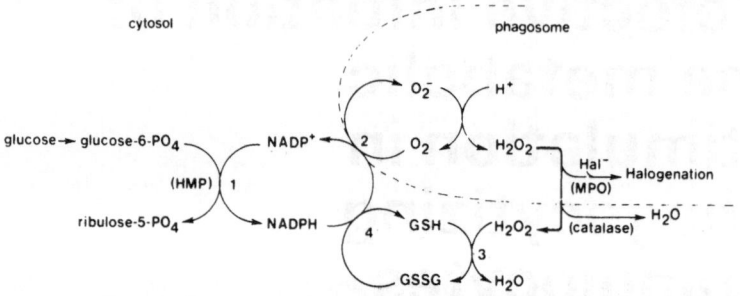

Figure 19.1 Schematic representation of the oxidative metabolism of PMN; (1) glucose-6-phosphate dehydrogenase + 6-phosphogluconate dehydrogenase; (2) NADPH oxidase; (3) glutathione peroxidase; (4) glutathione reductase; MPO, myeloperoxidase

The bactericidal activity of superoxide and hydrogen peroxide is increased by the liberation of the lysosomal enzyme myeloperoxidase into the phagosomes. Together with a halide, these agents provide a very effective antimicrobial system[4]. Excess hydrogen peroxide, leaking into the cytoplasm of the phagocytes, is detoxified by catalase and/or the glutathione cycle (Figure 19.1, reactions 3 and 4)[5].

From studies with soluble stimulators of granulocyte metabolism it has become evident that phagocytosis is no prerequisite for the generation of oxygen metabolites by these cells. The same conclusion has been reached from experiments with cells treated with inhibitors of phagocytosis: under such conditions attachment of particles to the cells provides sufficient stimulus for oxidative activation[6]. Therefore, it is now generally accepted that perturbation of the plasma membrane, either by soluble activators or by particle binding, triggers the one-electron reduction of oxygen to superoxide.

During investigation of granulocytes from TB and SB (brother and sister) with CGD-like symptoms, we discovered that these cells had a normal activity of all enzymes known to be required for oxidative killing reactions. Nevertheless, an ineffective *in vitro* killing of *Staphylococcus aureus* bacteria was found. Moreover, certain poorly opsonized particles were normally ingested but did not cause metabolic activation of the granulocytes of these patients (in contrast to normal cells). Other, more densely opsonized particles, caused a normal oxidative reaction. We conclude that a defective triggering of the oxidative metabolism is the cause of this unique dysfunction. From these studies it also appears that binding and subsequent phagocytosis of particles are not sufficient for metabolic stimulation. Since ingestion was not an adequate stimulus of metabolism, it follows that only adherence is a necessary, though not sufficient, event in the initiation of the oxidative metabolism of phagocytes.

RESULTS AND DISCUSSION

The chemotactic responsiveness as well as the uptake of *Staphylococcus aureus* bacteria by the granulocytes of patients TB and SB is normal[7,8]. However, the intracellular killing of this strain of bacteria is diminished[7]. Since humoral and cellular immunity is unaffected, the observed killing defect most likely causes the severe clinical symptoms in these patients.

Stimulation of oxygen consumption, superoxide generation, and hexose monophosphate shunt activity was strongly diminished during incubation with latex particles in the presence of human AB serum (Table 19.1). So far, this is exactly what is found in chronic granulomatous disease. For comparison, values found with CGD granulocytes (six males, four females) have been included in Table 19.1. In sharp contrast to the findings in CGD we find that incubation of the cells from TB and SB with immunoglobulin-G (IgG)-coated latex results in normal metabolic stimulation (Table 19.1).

Similar results were obtained with IgG aggregates[8]. Although the granulocytes of SB produce somewhat less H_2O_2 than normal, possibly due to the corticosteroid treatment she received during these investigations, it is obvious that her granulocytes *are able* to generate considerable amounts of H_2O_2. Therefore, TB and SB do not suffer from the classic form of CGD. Moreover, the normal metabolic stimulation after ingestion of IgG latex excludes any enzyme deficiency in this pathway.

To investigate the possibility that the patients' cells ingest latex in the presence of serum to a lesser degree than IgG-coated latex, we compared the uptake of these two different particles by the granulocytes of patient TB. As shown in Table 19.2 it is clear that after 15 min of incubation, serum-opsonized latex particles were taken up to a normal extent. We conclude, therefore, that the absent respiratory burst during phagocytosis of serum-opsonized latex by the patients' granulocytes must be due to a defect in the initial steps of cell activation. Although it has been suggested that

TABLE 19.1 Respiratory burst in patients' granulocytes

Parameter	Additions	Controls	TB (♂)	SB (♀)	CGD
Oxygen consumption	none	0.6– 3.1 (n=24)	0– 0.6 (n=2)	0 (n=3)	0–1.3 (n=10)
	latex + serum	15.1–29.7 (n=24)	1.1– 1.6 (n=2)	0.8– 2.0 (n=3)	0–1.4 (n=10)
	IgG-latex	19.6–20.7 (n=3)	20.9–21.1 (n=3)	6.6 (n=1)	nt
Superoxide generation	none	0.7– 1.3 (n=13)	0– 0.2 (n=3)	0 (n=2)	0–0.2 (n=6)
	latex + serum	4.2–11.1 (n=13)	0– 0.3 (n=3)	0– 0.1 (n=2)	0–0.1 (n=6)
	IgG-latex	6.2–17.9 (n=3)	9.3–12.2 (n=2)	8.7 (n=1)	nt
Hydrogen peroxide production	none	0– 0.2 (n=10)	0– 0.4 (n=3)	0.2– 0.3 (n=2)	0 (n=10)
	IgG-latex	13.1–21.0 (n=10)	6.9–24.7 (n=3)	10–12.3 (n=2)	0 (n=10)
HMP shunt activity	none	0.1– 0.2 (n=5)	0 (n=1)	0.2 (n=1)	0 (n=6)
	latex + serum	1.3– 2.7 (n=8)	0.4 (n=1)	0.3 (n=1)	0–0.2 (n=6)
	IgG-latex	1.4– 5.8 (n=4)	1.5– 4.5 (n=2)	2.4 (n=1)	nt

Oxygen consumption was measured with an oxygen electrode[2]; superoxide generation by reduction of cytochrome c[14], hydrogen peroxide production with a fluorimetric method[15], and HMP shunt activity by liberation of $^{14}CO_2$ from l-[^{14}C]glucose[8]. Results are expressed in nmol/10^6 granulocytes/10 min (range)
nt = not tested

TABLE 19.2   Phagocytosis of latex and IgG latex by granulocytes from patient TB

	Cells which had taken up particles (%)	Mean number of particles per cell
Latex + serum	96	8
IgG-latex	96	6

Numbers given were obtained by twice counting 200 cells in electron microscopic pictures

in CGD a defective *activation* of NADPH oxidase could be a cause of the absent respiratory burst, no clear evidence of this theory has been presented so far[9].

For activation of phagocyte metabolism, binding of particles to the cells by means of opsonins is needed. These opsonins are immunoglobulin G (IgG) antibodies, which bind with their F_C part to the cell membrane, and the complement component C_3, which binds to the C_3 receptor of the plasma membrane. (Although the existence of discrete structures in the plasma membrane of granulocytes with high binding affinity for F_C or C_3 and mediating biological activation of these cells have not with certainty been recognized, the term 'receptor' is nevertheless used in this article for the sake of simplicity.) Since only IgG-coated latex caused metabolic stimulation of the patients' cells, we investigated the opsonins present on both serum-opsonized and IgG-coated latex. Table 19.3 shows

TABLE 19.3   Immunoglobulin G on latex particles

	IgG_1*	IgG_2*	IgG_3*	IgG_4*
Serum-treated latex	32	2	32	0
IgG-coated latex	128	> 128	256	> 128

* Dilution of latex which still gave visible agglutination with rabbit antisera specific for human IgG subclasses

that IgG-coated latex contains more IgG of all subclasses than serum-opsonized latex does. This suggests that the patients' granulocytes, in contrast to normal granulocytes, are not stimulated by serum-opsonized latex due to some abnormality in the F_C receptors on the patients' cells. On the other hand, from the fact that serum-opsonized zymosan, which contains mainly C_3, is not iodinated by the patients' cells (Table 19.4), it follows that the C_3 receptor on the patients' granulocytes must also be affected.

TABLE 19.4   Iodination of zymosan particles by PMN of family B

	Mean*	Range*	n†
TB	1	0–2	3
SB	2	1–2	2
Father	12	9–14	2
Mother	15	11–22	3
Sister	13	9–17	2
Three brothers	26	21–34	1
Eleven normals	32	19–52	1

* μmol/10^{10} PMN per hour
† number of tests per individual

From Table 19.4 it may also be inferred that the abnormality is probably inherited in an autosomal recessive way. Both (healthy) parents and a sister showed intermediate iodination values on at least two different occasions. With other parameters, however, no heterozygosity could be detected.

Trying to elucidate the actual defect of the patients' cells, we tested whether F_c and C_3 receptors were present at all on the surface of these cells. This was done by measuring rosette formation between patients' granulocytes and red blood cells coated with either human IgG antibodies alone (which bind to the F_c receptor of the granulocytes) or with IgM antibodies + complement (which bind to the C_3 receptor of the granulocytes). As shown in Table 19.5, the granulocytes of TB and SB form normal rosettes with both types of opsonized erythrocytes. These experiments indicate the presence of F_c and C_3 receptors on the patients' cells. but give no information as to the amount of these receptors.

Relatively little is known about the mechanism of metabolic stimulation of phagocytes. Under conditions of adherence without ingestion (e.g. adhesion of cells to a non-phagocytosable surface[10]. inhibition of phago-

TABLE 19.5   Rosette formation by PMN*

	Controls			TB	SB
	Mean	Range	n		
EA	58	46–70	15	88	69
EAC	60	54–73	6	83	nt

* Percentage of PMN forming rosettes with opsonized erythrocytes
nt = not tested
EA = IgG-coated erythrocytes
EAC = IgM + complement-coated erythrocytes

cytosis by cytochalasin B[11]) normal metabolic stimulation is possible. Therefore. phagocytosis is no prerequisite for this activation. From the results obtained with the granulocytes of patients TB and SB. it follows that even particle attachment (followed by ingestion) is not sufficient for the activation of the oxidative metabolism.

From observations of phagocyte stimulation by soluble activators. such as phorbol myristate acetate[12], complement component C_5a[11], or the calcium ionophore A23187[13], it has been concluded that either membrane perturbation as such, or an increased influx of calcium ions, might be the actual triggering signal for the activation of the oxidative metabolism. Figure 19.2 shows schematically some of these ideas. Whether calcium influx is indeed necessary and. if so. whether this acts by activation of the cyclic nucleotide system is still much in debate.

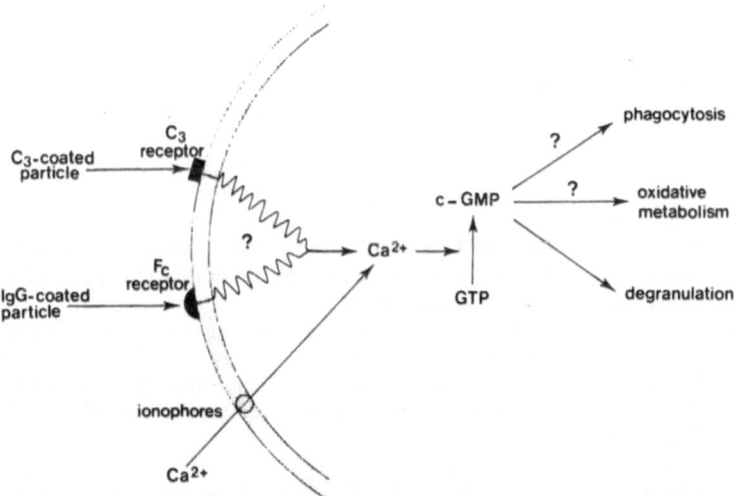

Figure 19.2   The possible role of the cyclic nucleotide system in the stimulation of several cell functions after binding of opsonized particles. After binding of particles, Ca^{2+} fluxes may stimulate cyclic nucleotide synthesis. Although it has been shown that these nucleotides regulate lysosomal enzyme release, their role, if any, in phagocytosis and metabolic stimulation is less defined

The actual defect in the patients' cells may be an insufficient number of receptors on the surface, or an abnormal quality of these receptors. In the former case, possibly enough bonds are formed between particles and cells to activate the process of phagocytosis, but not enough to activate the oxidative metabolism. Alternatively, a normal amount of receptors may be present on the patients' cells, but metabolic stimulation may require an abnormal high amount of receptors to be bound. This latter possibility could be caused by an insufficient influx of calcium ions after receptor binding. Further experiments are needed, therefore, to elucidate the molecular defect in this abnormality.

Acknowledgements

We thank Dr C. M. R. Weemaes and the family B for their kind co-operation and Dr J. A. Loos for many fruitful discussions. This study was supported by financial aid from the Netherlands Organization for the Advancement of Pure Research (ZWO). The Hague, The Netherlands (grant no. 91-5).

References

1. Sbarra, A. J. and Karnovsky, M. L. (1959). The biochemical basis of phago-cytosis. I. Metabolic changes during the ingestion of particles by polymorpho-nuclear leukocytes. *J. Biol. Chem.*, **234**, 1355
2. Weening, R. S., Roos, D. and Loos, J. A. (1974). Oxygen consumption of phagocytizing cells in human leukocyte and granulocyte preparations: A comparative study. *J. Lab. Clin. Med.*, **83**, 570
3. Babior, B. M., Kipnes, R. S. and Curnutte, J. T. (1973). Biological defense mechanisms. The production by leukocytes of superoxide. a potential bac-tericidal agent. *J. Clin. Invest.*, **52**, 741
4. Klebanoff, S. J. (1967). A peroxidase-mediated antimicrobial system in leukocytes. *J. Clin. Invest.*, **46**, 1078
5. Reed, P. W. (1969). Glutathione and the hexose monophosphate shunt in phagocytizing and hydrogen peroxide-treated rat leukocytes. *J. Biol. Chem.*, **244**, 2459
6. Cheson, B. D., Curnutte, J. T. and Babior, B. M. (1977). The oxidative killing mechanisms of the neutrophil. In R. S. Schwartz (ed.). *Progress in Clinical Immunology*, *Vol. 3*, 8
7. Van der Meer, J. W. M., Van Zwet, T. L., Van Furth, R. and Weemaes, C. M. R. (1975). New familial defect in microbicidal function of polymor-phonuclear leukocytes. *Lancet*, ii, 630
8. Weening, R. S., Roos, D., Weemaes, C. M. R., Homan-Müller, J. W. T. and Van Schaik, M. L. J. (1976). Defective initiation of the metabolic stimu-lation in phagocytizing granulocytes: a new congenital defect. *J. Lab. Clin. Med.*, **88**, 757
9. Curnutte, J. T., Kipnes, R. S. and Babior, B. M. (1975). Defect in pyridine nucleotide-dependent superoxide production by a particulate fraction from the granulocytes of patients with chronic granulomatous disease. *N. Engl. J. Med.*, **293**, 628
10. Johnston, R. B. Jr., Lehmeyer, J. E. and Guthrie, L. A. (1976). Generation of superoxide and chemiluminescence by human monocytes during phago-

cytosis and on contact with surface-bound immunoglobulin G. *J. Exp. Med.,* **143,** 1551

11.   Goldstein, I. M., Roos, D., Kaplan, H. B. and Weismann, G. (1975). Complement and immunoglobulins stimulate superoxide production by human leukocytes independently of phagocytosis. *J. Clin. Invest.,* **56,** 1155

12.   Repine, J. E., White, J. G., Clawson, C. C. and Holmes, B. H. (1974). The influence of phorbol myristate acetate on oxygen consumption by polymorphonuclear leukocytes. *J. Lab. Clin. Med.,* **83,** 911

13.   Romeo, D., Zabucchi, G., Miani, N. and Rossi, F. (1975). Ion movement across leukocyte plasma membrane and excitation of their metabolism. *Nature (London),* **253,** 542

14.   Weening, R. S., Wever, R. and Roos, D. (1975). Quantitative aspects of the production of superoxide radicals by phagocytizing human granulocytes. *J. Lab. Clin. Med.,* **85,** 245

15.   Homan-Müller, J. W. T., Weening, R. S. and Roos, D. (1975). Production of hydrogen peroxide by phagocytizing human granulocytes. *J. Lab. Clin. Med.,* **85,** 198

20

Modification of genetic expression in phagocytes
R. A. Harkness, M. Grant and S. M. Cockle

INTRODUCTION

That cells interact with their environment and that such interactions can include changes in enzyme activities seem obvious. In complex organisms changes in the internal environment especially in the endocrine system are potent causes of cellular change. This review attempts to summarize some of the available evidence on known controls of intracellular activities and sites of action of such controls with special emphasis on the phagocytic polymorphonuclear neutrophil leukocyte, PMNL. Since the steroid hormones or their analogues are widely used in therapeutics, emphasis has been placed on the steroids which are known to act through modification of genetic expression. So where evidence is available this outline is concerned with the influence of steroid hormones and related compounds on enzyme activities in phagocytes.

The modulation of enzyme activities within phagocytes provides a problem in the diagnosis of genetic defects; reductions due to 'environmental' controls could be confused with genetic defects. Such modulation also provides an opportunity for treatment which has so far been little deliberately used.

The inborn errors of metabolism offer an opportunity to test this approach which appears to work in the endocrine system itself. Marked physiological ACTH stimulation of a defective adrenal cortex can produce a normal basal steroid output which is inadequate only when the patients were stressed[1]. One limitation is that experimentally hormonal stimulation may only produce a 2-fold increase in an enzyme activity. But such an increase may be enough to avoid the biological consequences of a defect, provided that activities are raised to more than about 10% of normal or control mean activities. No clinical effects are regularly seen in the hetero- zygotes for many serious, even fatal, defects in whom enzyme activities are about 50% of the normal mean. In the phagocyte 25% of control mean glucose-6-phosphate dehydrogenase activity is enough for normal intra- cellular killing[2], whereas less than 10% is not[3]. In intermittent and in less severe maple syrup urine disease activities of the relevant enzyme are generally higher than in the severe condition[4], although studies in individual families may not always show this correlation[5].

ALKALINE PHOSPHATASE

Alkaline phosphatase has been the subject of intensive study which has included investigation of its hormonal control. High activities are present in the particulate fraction of phagocytes[6]. There is also a good correlation between histochemical and spectrophotometric estimates of activity in phagocytes[7]. As a consequence of this it has been possible to show that alkaline phosphatase activity of a leukocyte or LAP falls with its age from a score of 83.8 ± 4.5 in cells with a simple ring nuclei to 48.0 ± 1.2 in older cells with complex nuclei; the correlation of age with nuclear morphology was checked with tritiated thymidine[8]. Such findings may explain the raised LAP found in myeloid metaplasia and polycythaemia vera.

Evidence of endocrine control is clear; women of reproductive age (19– 48 years) have significantly higher LAP than men but after the menopause activities in women fall to approach those in men. In children there are high activities in newborn and a steady fall with age. Both girls and boys have similar activities in the upper half of the range found in adult females of reproductive age[9]. LAP activity increases 2- to 3-fold in normal preg- nancy. Activities are low in missed abortion and show a rapid rise followed by a marked fall to subnormal levels on fetal death. Similar changes occur during the induction of labour with hypertonic saline[10]. Those changes are like the changes which have been described in oestrogen output in these obstetric conditions. In serial studies of LAP during the menstrual cycle there is a rise in the middle of the cycle corresponding to a rise in oestrogen production at this time. From the above evidence it seems probable that oestrogen increases LAP.

Studies of the *in vitro* effects of steroid hormones on alkaline phosphatase have been mainly concerned with the stimulatory effects of glucocorticoids in cultured cells[11]. Later studies have used more physiological concentrations (1 μmol/l) to produce increased activity[12]. Early *in vivo* studies showed that glucocorticoids stimulated LAP[9] and that the normal increase in serum activity produced by cortisone is not detectable in hypophosphatasia[13]. Alkaline phosphatase activity in intestine is also increased by cortisone[14]. It may, however, not be justifiable to conclude that cortisone acts directly on the bone, liver, kidney and on the 'intestine' genetic loci (see below).

Total alkaline phosphatase activity may be derived from a wide variety of enzyme proteins. In man, at least three main structural genes are responsible for alkaline phosphatase; one is active in liver, bone and kidney, one in intestine and another in placentae. In pregnancy, placental activity is controlled by the fetus although in certain tumours there may be reactivation of the placental locus. This locus and the others show genetic polymorphism; there are at least three common autosomal alleles controlling the placental enzyme[15]. Unfortunately the three genetic loci appear to produce alkaline phosphatases of roughly the same molecular weight of $1.2–1.4 \times 10^5$ daltons[16,17]. Although antibodies readily distinguish the liver, kidney and bone enzyme structure from the intestinal and placental types of structure, the two latter show cross-reactions[16].

In phagocytes it is not clear which structural locus or loci are active in addition to that responsible for the enzyme in bone, liver and kidney. The early evidence from hypophosphatasia in which the enzyme is very low in bone, liver and kidney was of a virtual absence of activity in leukocytes by both histochemical[13] and spectrophotometric methods[18]. Later studies have generally not confirmed this and shown results at the lower end of the normal range[19]. Two cases of hypophosphatasia studied recently have shown LAP activities in a severely affected child of 6 months, of 6 in contrast to 2 and 4 μmol/l/min per mg protein in two samples from an adult with only dental changes. These results are within the normal range although at its lower end[20].

After synthesis in the ribosomes, alkaline phosphatase may be associated into an active dimer with zinc at the active site in leukocytes[21] and other tissues[22]. Experimental zinc deficiency can lower tissue alkaline phosphatase activity[23]. The importance of such changes in human disease is not clear, because clinically the disease states associated with zinc deficiency can be improved without raising zinc concentrations in body fluids[24]. The iron-containing proteins also do appear to be susceptible to nutritional deficiency and this is relevant to human disease as shown by iron deficiency anaemia. Iron deficiency may be a factor in the control of the haem enzyme, myeloperoxidase, in phagocytes.

Breakdown of the enzyme within the cell appears to be different in bone and liver since electrophoresis will separate 'bone' and 'liver' forms of the enzyme[25, 26] despite their common origin from the same structural gene as shown by their absence in hypophosphatasia. Tissue-specific processing offers another control point.

The release of enzyme from the cell is another control point; the secretion of alkaline phosphatase from the intestine is partly linked with fat ingestion as well as secretor status and ABO blood group[27]. Such secretion or membrane transfer may be related to the degree of glycosylation, largely with N-acetylneuraminic acid[28].

From the evidence available on alkaline phosphatase in man control of enzyme activities within human cells can occur at many points. The evidence for multiple sites of control for some other enzymes in the rat has been reviewed by Schimke[29] and Schimke and Doyle[30].

PEROXIDASE

The haem enzyme myeloperoxidase, or MPO, is a major component of the polymorphonuclear neutrophil leukocyte and is a component of the granules of this cell. Its activity can be measured with a variety of chromogenic substrates although the relationship of this activity to the amount of enzymic protein present can be complicated especially by the existence of alternative reaction pathways[31]. MPO is involved in the killing of ingested micro-organisms using the H_2O_2 produced during the metabolic burst which follows phagocytosis (see the chapters by Baehner, Romeo and Segal, respectively in this volume). The activity of this enzyme in phagocytes is highly variable and as a consequence diagnosis of a genetic cause of deficiency is difficult[32].

One of the more understandable reductions in MPO activity is produced by ampicillin. The usual therapeutic dose of 500 mg producing a mean fall ($\pm$ SEM) in activity to $70 \pm 7.8\%$ and $81 \pm 27\%$ of control values 1 and 2 h after the dose. Activities returned to control values the next day. Such reductions were not due to a circadian variation. Further details and the relevant *in vitro* reduction have already been given[33]. Haem enzymes are also inhibited by sulphonamides[34, 35] which can also inhibit candidacidal activity[36].

Although it is difficult to demonstrate significant amounts of penicillin inside cells[37], there is much evidence to show that penicillins cross cell membranes, including the gut wall and placenta[38]. Penicillins are detectable in cultured cells[39, 40]. In man, inhibitory effects are demonstrable on cytochrome P_{450}-dependent systems[41, 42]. *In vitro* studies are difficult due to the instability of the penicillins in solution and the slow reactions of penicillins with haem enzymes[43] and with other proteins[44]. Such short-term disturbances of MPO or other enzyme activities should not be confused with genetic defects if repeat samples are taken after the end of drug treatment. Repeat samples are necessary because phagocytes cannot be stored nor can they be established in cell culture.

There is a growing list of causes of reversible defects in the biological activity closely related to MPO activity, intracellular microbial killing in phagocytes; this includes virus infection in children[45], undernutrition[46], and iron deficiency[47] which are associated with a wide variety of enzymic changes in phagocytes[48].

ALTERATIONS IN PATHOLOGICAL CONDITIONS

A 'normal' range of leukocyte MPO activities is shown in Figure 20.1 for adults and children. Results from children with recurrent urinary tract

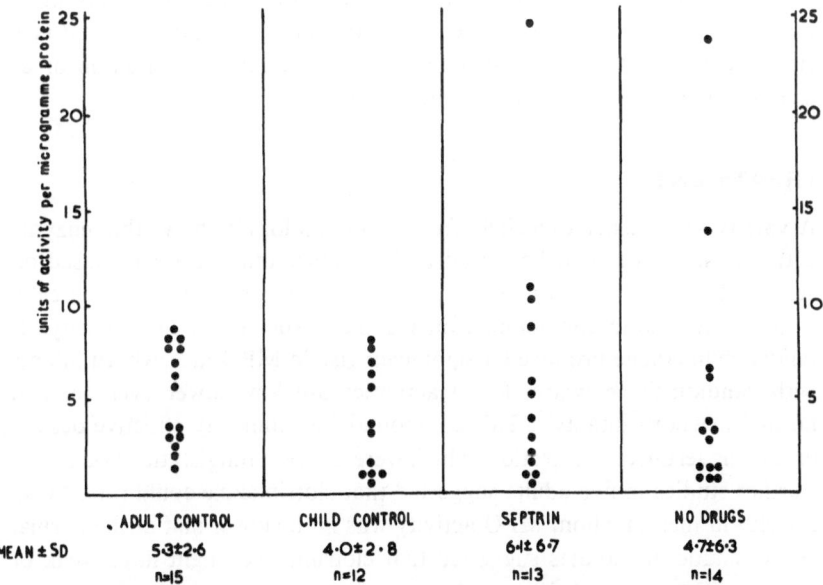

Figure 20.1 Polymorphonuclear neutrophil leukocyte (PMNL) myeloperoxidase activity in normal adults and children. Children with recurrent urinary tract infection with 'Septrin' treatment and untreated (no drugs) have mean activities which are not significantly different from either other children or adults using *t* and *u* tests. Methods as described by Renz *et al.*[53]

infection with and without treatment with trimethoprim and sulpha-methoxazole (Septrin, Burroughs Wellcome, UK) are shown. From the results in Figure 20.1 there appears to be no alteration in MPO activity from inflammation in the urinary tract. However, there are differences in some form of inflammatory bowel disease. In 20 patients with ulcerative colitis the distribution of MPO activities was different from that in 17 normal controls which was similar to that in 16 patients with Crohn's disease ($0.025 < p < 0.05$: Kolmorgorov–Smirnov test). This reduction was due to a predominance of patients with total colonic disease in the 15 patients with low MPO activities; four of the five patients with high MPO activities had limited disease. Only four of the low MPO activities were associated with low serum iron concentrations; 18 patients who had under-gone total colectomy for ulcerative colitis had normal activities[49]. This undue susceptibility of MPO activities to reduction is not a normal response to inflammation (Figure 20.1) and may be involved in the pathogenesis of the disease. Somewhat similar conclusions were reached by Stendahl *et al.*[50] in their studies on reduced MPO activity in a patient with pustular psoriasis.

It is difficult to determine whether the patient with an intermittent bactericidal defect studied by Drutz and Cline[51] should be tentatively classified as an alteration associated with a pathological condition or as an effect of extensive drug treatment, or as both.

TREATMENT

A variety of evidence especially from endocrinology[52] shows that enzyme activities in tissues can be raised and therefore that treatment based on such findings may sometimes be possible. For example, the systematically active, antimycotic compound clotrimazole, bisphenyl-(2-chlorophenyl)-l-imidazolylmethane produced a significant rise in MPO in newborn infants with candidiasis in whom MPO activities are low, lower even than in normal newborn infants[53]. This compound was clinically effective despite producing serum concentrations which were not even fungistatic *in vitro*[54,55]. Further studies in five adults suggested that clotrimazole could raise MPO activity in men in whom MPO activity was in the lower half of the normal range; endocrine studies suggested that clotrimazole might have weak or anti-oestrogenic activity[56].

In vitro incubation of clotrimazole with phagocytes and with horse-radish peroxidase showed no effect on peroxidase activity. The results suggested that clotrimazole was only effective in raising MPO activity *in vivo* and thus might have stimulated the synthesis of MPO.

In view of the above results, the weak or anti-oestrogen clomiphene was given to four normal men. One normal therapeutic dose of 50 mg produced approximately 2-fold rises in MPO activity in all four men (Figure 20.2). Catalase activity in the phagocytes was not regularly increased which

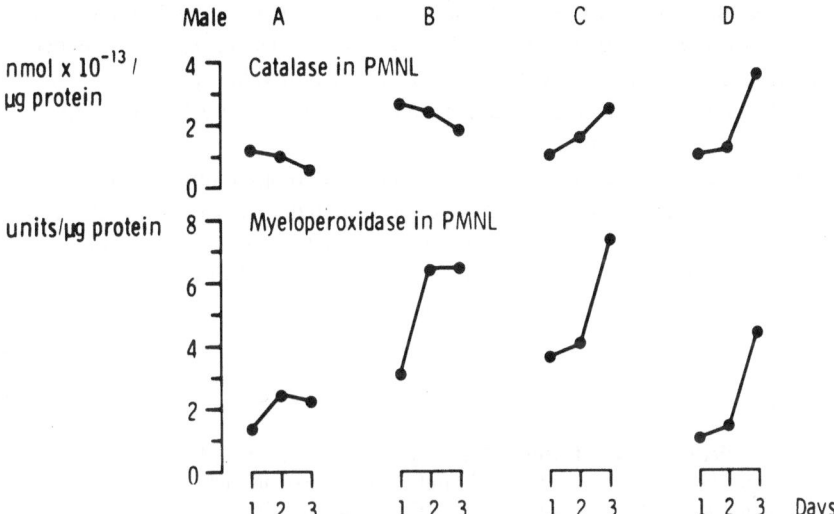

Figure 20.2   Effect of clomiphene, 50 mg on day 2, on polymorphonuclear neutrophil leukocyte (PMNL) myeloperoxidase and catalase activities in four normal males A, B, C and D. Methods as described by Renz et al.[53]

suggested that there was no generalized increase in the specific activity of haemoproteins. It may be relevant that the increased susceptibility of the male to infections[57] may have, at least in part, a hormonal basis. In addition 'physiological' doses of oestrogen induce a peroxidase in rat uterus[58] and endogenous peroxidase appears in other oestrogen target tissues on stimulation with strong and weak oestrogens[59].

Oestrogens can stimulate 'granulopoiesis' in mice[60] and tissue culture[61]. Despite the relatively large amounts of oestrogen used in the latter two sets of experiments, the results are consistent with a peak in polymorphonuclear neutrophil leukocytes (PMNL) found 1 to 2 days after the oestrogen peaks of the human menstrual cycle[62]. The increases shown in Figure 20.2 in peroxidase activity may be linked to the above increased number of PMNL but since specific activity rises in a fraction which consists of 95% or more PMNL such rises are not secondary to an increase in the number of PMNL.

Stimulation of the activity of other particulate enzymes present in

PMNL, especially the acid hydrolases, might be of therapeutic interest. Only some tentative generalizations may be suggested from a lengthy and widely scattered literature. Many early studies showed increases in a variety of acid hydrolase activities after steroid hormones[63], sometimes in large amounts. If there were concerted increases in protein synthesis in a tissue acid, hydrolases could be part of that increase. For example, acid phosphatase and arylsulphatase A and B activities increase in the cervix after oestradiol-17β administration, as does alkaline phosphatase activity[64]. It is not yet clear whether such rises are closely linked to those found for peroxidase activity.

In conclusion, evidence in man shows that there are a number of control points for alkaline phosphatase in cells and that at least one of these is sensitive to steroid hormones. Peroxidase activity would also appear to be oestrogen sensitive. Further evidence is needed to decide whether such stimulation is directly useful in treatment.

References

1. Thistlethwaite, D., Darling, J. A. B., Fraser, R., Mason, P. A., Rees, L. H. and Harkness, R. A. (1975). Familial glucocorticoid deficiency. Studies of diagnosis and pathogenesis. *Arch. Dis. Child.*, **50**, 291

2. Rodey, G. E., Jacob, H. S., Holmes, B., McArthur, J. R. and Good, R. A. (1970). Leucocyte G-6-PD levels and bactericidal activity. *Lancet*, **i, 355**

3. Cooper, M. R., De Châtelet, L. R., McCall, C. E., Lavia, M. F., Spurr, C. L. and Baehner, R. L. (1970). Leucocyte G-6-PD deficiency. *Lancet*, **ii,** 110

4. Dancis, J., Hutzler, J., Snyderman, S. E. and Cox, R. P. (1972). Enzyme activity in classical and variant forms of maple syrup urine disease. *J. Pediatr.*, **81,** 312

5. Valman, H. B., Patrick, A. D., Seakins, J. W. T., Platt, J. W. and Gompertz, D. (1973). Family with intermittent maple syrup urine disease. *Arch. Dis. Child.*, **48,** 225

6. Michell, R. H., Karnovsky, M. J. and Karnovsky, M. L. (1970). The distribution of some granule associated enzymes in guinea-pig polymorphonuclear leucocytes. *Biochem. J.*, **116,** 207

7. Diamant, Y. Z., Sadovsky, E. and Gal, A. (1971). Evaluation of the leukocyte alkaline phosphatase activity. Comparison of the biochemical and cytochemical assay. *Clin. Chim. Acta*, **34,** 73

8. Williams, D. M. (1975). Leucocyte alkaline phosphatase as a marker of cell maturity: a quantitative, cytochemical and autoradiographic study. *Brit. J. Haematol.*, **31,** 371

9. Rosner, F. and Lee, S. L. (1965). Endocrine relationships of leukocyte alkaline phosphatase. *Blood*, **25,** 356

10. Sadovsky, E., Zuckerman, H., Diamant, Y. Z. and Polishuk, W. Z. (1970). Leukocyte alkaline phosphatase and fetal prognosis in placental dysfunction. *Am. J. Obstet. Gynecol.*, **108,** 979

11. Cox, R. P. and MacLeod, C. M. (1964). Regulation of alkaline phosphatase in human cell cultures. *Cold Spring Harbor Symp. Quant. Biol.*, **29**, 233

12. Waters, M. D. and Summer, G. K. (1969). Prednisolone induction of alkaline phosphatase in human skin fibroblasts. *Biochim. Biophys. Acta*, **177**, 650

13. Beisel, W. R., Benjamin, N. and Austen, J. G. (1959). Absence of leucocyte alkaline phosphatase activity in hypophosphatasia. *Blood*, **14**, 975

14. Verzar, F., Sailer, E. and Richterrich, R. (1952). Einfluss der Nebennieren-rinde auf die alkalische Phosphatase der Dünndarmschleimhaut. *Helv. Physiol. Pharm. Acta*, **10**, 231

15. Robson, E. B. and Harris, H. (1965). Genetics of alkaline phosphatase polymorphism of human placenta. *Nature (London)*, **207**, 1257

16. Boyer, S. H. (1963). Human organ alkaline phosphatases: Discrimination by several means including starch gel electrophoresis of antienzyme-enzyme supernatant fluids. *Ann. N. Y. Acad. Sci.*, **103**, 938

17. Fosset, M., Chappelet-Tordo, D. and Lazdunsku, M. (1974). Intestinal alkaline phosphatase. Physical properties and quaternary structure. *Biochemistry*, **13**, 1783

18. Kretchmer, N., Stone, C. and Bauer, C. (1958). Hereditary enzyme defects as illustrated by hypophosphatasia. *Ann. N. Y. Acad. Sci.*, **75**, 279

19. Rubecz, I., Mehes, K., Klujber, L., Bozzay, L., Weissenbach, J. and Fenyvesi, J. (1974). Hypophosphatasia: screening and family investigation. *Clin. Gen.*, **6**, 155

20. Brydon, W. G., Crofton, P. M., Smith, A. F., Barr, D. G. D. and Harkness, R. A. (1975). Hypophosphatasia: enzyme studies in cultured cells and tissues. *Biochem. Soc. Trans.*, **3**, 927

21. Trubowitz, S., Feldman, D., Morgenstern, S. W. and Hunt, V. M. (1961). The isolation, purification and some properties of the alkaline phosphatase of human leucocytes. *Biochem. J.*, **80**, 369

22. Hiwada, K. and Wachsmith, E. D. (1974a). Catalytic properties of alkaline phosphatase from pig kidney. *Biochem. J.*, **141**, 283

23. Prasad, A. S., Oberleas, D., Wolf, P. and Horowitz, J. P. (1967). Studies on zinc deficiency: changes in trace elements and enzyme activities in tissues of zinc deficient rats. *J. Clin. Invest.*, **46**, 549

24. Mikac-Devic, D. (1970). Methodology of zinc determinations and the role of zinc in biochemical processes. *Adv. Clin. Chem.*, **13**, 271

25. Fishman, W. H. and Ghosh, N. K. (1967). Isoenzymes of human alkaline phosphatase. *Adv. Clin. Chem.*, **10**, 255

26. Fishman, W. H. (1974). Perspective on alkaline phosphatase isoenzymes. *Am. J. Med.*, **56**, 617

27. Langman, M. J. S., Leuthold, E., Robson, E. B., Harris, J., Luffman, J. E. and Harris, H. (1966). Influence of diet on the intestinal component of serum alkaline phosphatase in people of different ABO blood groups and secretor status. *Nature (London)*, **212**, 41

28. Hiwada, K. and Wachsmith, E. D. (1974b). Alkaline phosphatase from pig kidney. Microheterogenecity and the role of neuraminic acid. *Biochem. J.*, **131**, 293

29. Schimke, R. T. (1969). On the role of synthesis and degradation in regulation of enzyme levels in animal tissues. *Current Topics in Cellular Regulation*, **1**, 77 (London: Academic Press)

30. Schimke, R. T. and Doyle, D. (1970). Control of enzyme levels in animal tissues. *Ann. Rev. Biochem.*, **39**, 929

31. Childs, R. E. and Bardsley, W. G. (1975). The steady state kinetics of peroxidase with 2.2'-azino-di-(3-ethyl-benzthiazoline-6-sulphonic acid) as a chromogen. *Biochem. J.*, **145**, 93

32. Harkness, R. A. (1977). A comparison of leucocytes and cultured fibroblasts in diagnosis. In R. A. Harkness and F. Cockburn (eds.). *The Cultured Cell and Inherited Metabolic Disease*, pp. 90–104. (Lancaster: MTP Press)

33. Harkness, R. A. and Grant, M. (1977). Pharmacological and other controls of enzyme activities in polymorphonuclear phagocytes. *Proceedings of the First European Conference on Phagocytic Leucocytes*. pp. 399–406. (Padova: Piccin Medical Books)

34. Main, E. R., Shinn, L. E. and Mellon, R. R. (1939). Anticatalase activity of sulphanilamide and related compounds. IV. Peroxide accumulation and growth inhibition of pneumococcus. *Proc. Soc. Exp. Biol. Med.*, **42**, 115

35. Lipmann, F. (1941). The oxidation of *p*-aminobenzole acid catalyzed by peroxidase and its inhibition by sulphanilamide. *J. Biol. Chem.*, **139**, 977

36. Lehrer, R. I. (1971). Inhibition by sulfonamides of the candidacidal activity of human neutrophils. *J. Clin. Invest.*, **50**, 2498

37. Mandell, G. L. (1973). Interaction of intraleukocytic bacteria and antibiotics *J. Clin. Invest.*, **52**, 1673

38. Boreus, L. O. (1971). Placental transfer of ampicillin in man. *Acta Pharmacol. Toxicol.*, **29**, Suppl. 3, 250

39. Eagle, H. (1954). The binding of penicillin in relation to its cytotoxic action. III. The binding of penicillin by mammalian cells in tissue culture *J. Exp. Med.*, **100**, 117

40. Showacre, J. L., Hopps, H. E., du Buy, H. G. and Smadel, J. E. (1961). Effects of antibiotics on intracellular *Salmonella typhosa*. 1. Demonstration by phase microscopy of prompt inhibition of intracellular multiplication. *J. Immunol.*, **87**, 153

41. Willman, R. and Pulkinen, M. O. (1971). Reduced maternal plasma and urinary oestriol during ampicillin treatment. *Am. J. Obstet. Gynecol.*, **109**, 873

42. Harkness, R. A., Scott, R. D. M. and Strong, J. A. (1974). Physiological and pharmacological factors affecting the 6β-hydroxylation and 17-epimerisation of methandrostenolone. *Biochem. Soc. Trans.*, **2**, 119

43. Renz, M., Nicol, A. D. and Harkness, R. A. (1972). Drugs as inhibitors of catalase and peroxidase. In: T. MacPhee (ed.). *Host Resistance to Commensal Bacteria*, p. 209. (London, Edinburgh: Churchill Livingstone)

44. Corran, P. H. and Waley, S. G. (1975). The reaction of penicillin with proteins. *Biochem. J.*, **149**, 357

45. Craft, A. W., Reid, M. M. and Low, W. T. (1976). Effects of virus infections on polymorph function in children. *Br. Med. J.*, **1**, 1570

46. Gotch, F. M., Spry, C. J. F., Mowat, A. G., Beeson, P. B. and MacLennan, I. C. M. (1975). Reversible granulocyte killing defect in anorexia nervosa. *Clin. Exp. Immunol.*, **21**, 244

47. Chandra, R. K. (1973). Reduced bactericidal activity of polymorphs in iron deficiency. *Arch. Dis. Child.*, **48**, 864

48. Avila, J. L., Velazquez, G., Correa, A. C., Correa, C., Castillo, C. and

Convit, J. (1973). Leucocytic enzyme differences between the clinical forms of malnutrition. *Clin. Chim. Acta*, **49**, 5

49. Renz, M., Ward, M., Eastwood, M. A. and Harkness, R. A. (1976). Neutrophil function and myeloperoxidase activity in inflammatory bowel disease. *Lancet*, ii, 584

50. Stendahl, O., Hed, J. and Molin, L. (1978). Lack of myeloperoxidase-mediated iodination in granulocytes from a patient with pustular psoriasis. This volume Ch. 24, pp. 331–339.

51. Drutz, D. J. and Cline, M. J. (1975). Intermittent neutrophil–monocyte bactericidal defects in a patient with sarcoidosis. *Am. Rev. Resp. Dis.*, 112, 387

52. Pitot, H. C. and Yatvin, M. B. (1973). Interrelationships of mammalian hormones and enzyme levels *in vivo*. *Physiol. Rev.*,53, 228

53. Renz, M., Cohen, M., Farquhar, J. W. and Harkness, R. A. (1974). Elevation of myeloperoxidase activity in infants with oral candidiasis treated with clotrimazole. *Postgrad. Med. J.*, 50, (Suppl. 1) 20

54. Holt, R. J. and Newman, R. L. (1972). Laboratory assessment of the antimycotic drug, clotrimazole. *J. Clin. Pathol.*, 25, 1089

55. Milner, L. J. R. (1974). Mycological studies in the use of clotrimazole in bronchopulmonary aspergillosis and neonatal and vaginal candidiasis. *Postgrad. Med. J.*, 50, (Suppl. 1) 20

56. Harkness, R. A. and Renz, M. (1974). Endocrine effects of the antimycotic compound clotrimazole, and its related effects on enzymic activities in leucocytes. *Br. J. Clin. Pharmacol.*, 1, 342P

57. Washburn, T. C., Medearis, D. N. and Childs, B. (1965). Sex differences in susceptibility to infections. *Pediatrics*, 35, 57

58. McNabb, T. and Jellineck, P. H. (1975). Purification and properties of oestrogen-induced uterine peroxidase. *Biochem. J.*, 151, 275

59. Anderson, W. A., Kang, Y. H. and De Sombre, E. R. (1975). Endogenous peroxidase: specific marker for tissues displaying growth dependency on oestrogen. *J. Cell. Biol.*, 64, 668

60. Fox, L. E. (1961). Action of estrogens on bone marrow. *J. Pharmacol. Sci.*, 50, 436

61. Reisner, E. H. (1966). Tissue culture of bone marrow. II. Effect of steroid hormones on haematopoiesis *in vitro*. *Blood*, 27, 260

62. Bain, B. J. and England, J. H. (1975). Variations in leucocyte count during the menstrual cycle. *Br. Med. J.*, 2, 473

63. Kerr, L. M. H., Campbell, J. G. and Levvy, G. A. (1950). Further observations on the changes in β-glucuronidase activity in the mouse. *Biochem. J.*, 46, 278

64. Zachariah, E. and Moudgal, N. R. (1977). Enzyme changes in the cervix of the rat and hamster during the oestrous cycle. *J. Endocrinol.*, 72, 153

21

Neutrophil granulocyte chemotaxis in a reversible Boyden chamber

N. H. Valerius

The most widely used technique for measuring leukocyte chemotaxis *in vitro* is some modification of the method introduced by Boyden[1]. This technique uses a chamber that is divided into two compartments by a membrane filter, the upper compartment containing the cells and the lower one containing the chemotactic agents. A concentration gradient is thus formed across the thickness of the membrane filter. The pore size of this filter is sufficiently small to prevent the cells from dropping through the filter, usually between 3 and 8 microns depending on the type of cells to be tested. During the incubation period the leukocytes migrate through the filter. The chemotactic activity can then be expressed either by the distance moved into the filter by the front line of cells or by the number of cells that have passed all the way through the filter and are lying on its attractant opposite surface. This method, however, has been reported to be inaccurate[2], since an unpredictable number of cells may detach from the filter after their arrival at its attractant surface. They will thus elude enumeration and the result will be falsely low.

In the following it will be shown that this source of error can be eliminated by reversing the chemotaxis chambers during the incubation. The cells arriving at the attractant surface after the reversing of the chambers will now remain on this surface, and also many of the cells that have already fallen off the filter may return. It will further be shown that the number of cells that fall off the filter surface after migration depends upon the chemotactic agent used. This finding may explain some of the often very conflicting results that have been reported in studies on leukocyte chemotaxis in various clinical disorders[3-6].

The neutrophil chemotactic activity was determined as previously described[7]. Briefly, leukocytes were isolated from peripheral blood, and the

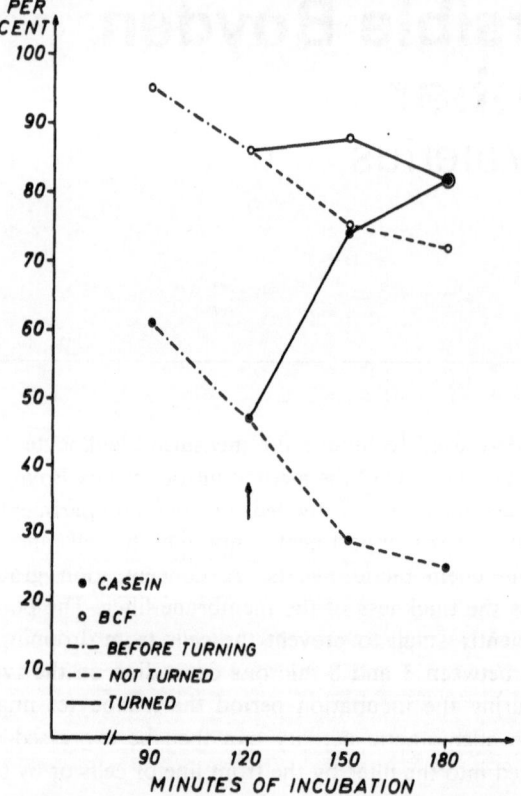

Figure 21.1 Number of cells adhering to the attractant surface of the filter as percentage of the total number of cells migrating through the filter on attraction with casein and BCF at varying incubation times. The chambers were either turned upside down (——) or left without being reversed (————) after 2 h incubation (arrow). Automatic counting. Mean of two experiments. Reproduced with permission from *Acta Pathol. Microbiol. Scand.*[7]

concentration of polymorphonuclear cells was adjusted at 10^6 per ml. The chemotactic factors used were casein 5 mg/ml and a bacterial chemotactic factor (BCF), which was a culture filtrate of *Escherichia coli*. The standard incubation time was 3 h, and the chemotaxis chambers were turned upside down after 2 h of incubation. Counting of the cells was performed either by direct microscopy, the results being expressed as the number of cells per field of vision, or counting was performed using an automatic image analysis system (Classimat, Leitz, Germany), in which the microscopic image was reproduced by a television camera on a monitor screen, and the video signal subsequently evaluated electronically, giving the number of cells per screen field.

Figure 21.1 shows the number of cells lying on the filter as percentage of the total number of migrating cells. This was determined as the number of cells on the filter surface plus those that had fallen off. The cells were attracted by either casein or BCF, and the chambers were incubated for

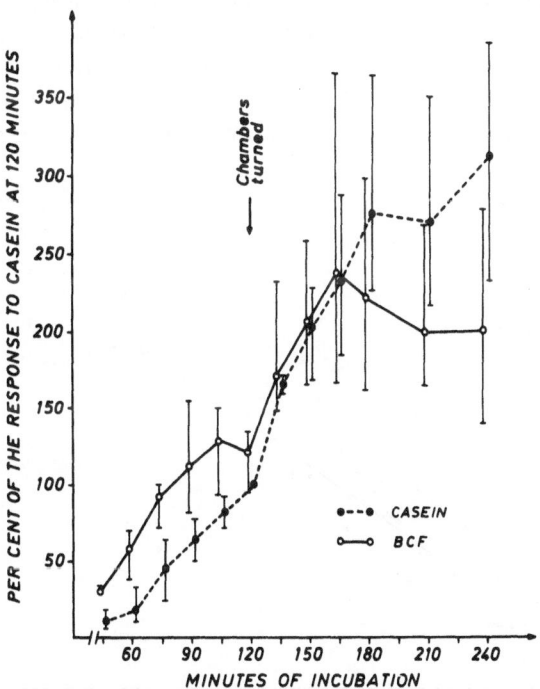

Figure 21.2 Time-course of neutrophil granulocyte chemotaxis to casein and BCF. The results are expressed as the number of cells on the attractant surface of the filter as percentage of the number at 2 h using casein as attractant. Automatic counting. Mean and range of three experiments. Reproduced with permission from *Acta Pathol. Microbiol. Scand.*[7]

varying periods of time. The chambers which were incubated for more than 2 h were either reversed at this time or left unreversed. It is seen that the percentage of cells remaining on the filter surface is much lower on attraction with casein than with BCF in the unreversed chambers. This means that the loss of cells from the filter surface is proportionately much higher using casein than BCF. On the other hand, in the chambers which were reversed at 2 h it is seen that the percentage of the total number of migrating cells, which were found to adhere to the filter surface, was the same in casein-stimulated and BCF-stimulated chambers. This means that the different loss of cells from the filter surface induced by different chemotactic factors can be eliminated by reversing the chambers during the incubation.

Figure 21.2 shows the number of cells on the filter surface at varying times on attraction with casein and with BCF. The results are expressed as percentage of the number of cells at 2 h on attraction with casein. The chemotactic activity to casein was found to increase throughout an incubation period of 4 h, while a peak activity to BCF occurred at $2\frac{1}{2}$ h to $2\frac{3}{4}$ h of incubation. However, the initial migration was far stronger on attraction with BCF than with casein. This difference was larger than could be ascribed to the different loss of cells shown in Figure 21.1. The observation

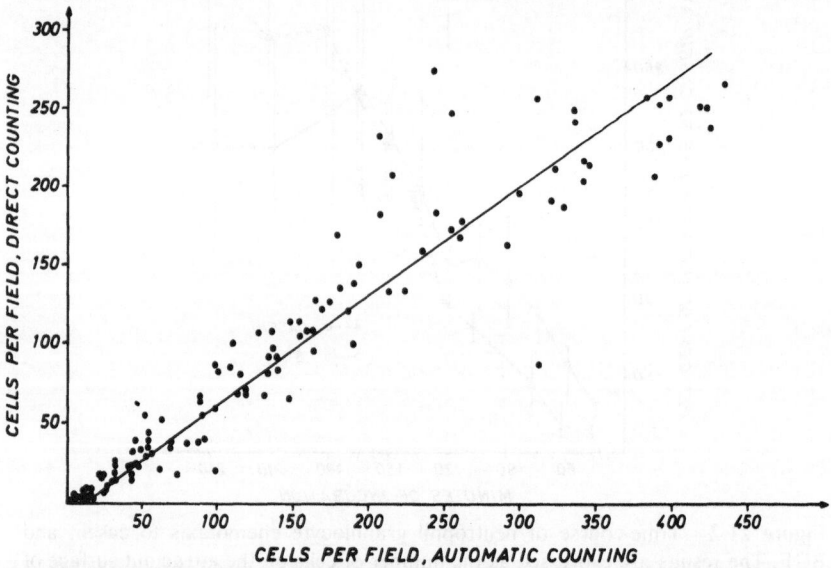

Figure 21.3 Relationship between the results by direct and automatic counting of 134 filters ($r=0.98$), calculated from logarithmic values. Reproduced with permission from *Acta Pathol. Microbiol. Scand.*[7]

of this different kinetic behaviour of neutrophils on attraction with casein or BCF may suggest that BCF has a stronger attracting effect on a relatively small proportion of neutrophils, whereas casein exerts a weaker effect on a larger proportion of cells.

Figure 21.3 shows the relationship between the results from direct and automatic counting of 134 filters. The figures obtained were higher using automatic counting than direct counting in spite of a smaller field of vision. This was due mainly to the registration in automatic counting, also of some of the cells that were lying immediately below the filter surface and, to a lesser extent, to the registration of occasional impurities of the filter. However, the good correlation seems to show that these sources of error are of minor importance. Automatic counting permits evaluation of a far larger area of the filter than it is possible to do in practice by direct counting. Automatic counting may therefore perhaps give a better assessment of the chemotactic activity in filters in which the cells are unevenly distributed. The major advantage of the automatic counting is that it is quick, the major drawback that it is expensive.

CONCLUSIONS

It has been the intention to show that it is important when measuring leukocyte chemotaxis using a Boyden chamber technique to prevent loss of cells from the filter surface and that reversing of the chambers during the incubation is one way to do this. Also that a different neutrophil kinetic behaviour to casein and to BCF may suggest the presence of neutrophils with different affinities. The introduction of an automatic counting system may avoid the most tedious and time-consuming part of chemotaxis experiments.

Acknowledgements

This work was supported by the Danish Medical Research Council. Thanks are due to Mrs Annette Winkel and Mrs Hanne Tamstorf for excellent technical assistance.

References

1. Boyden, S. (1962). The chemotactic effect of mixtures of antibody and antigen on polymorphonuclear leucocytes. *J. Exper. Med.*, **115**, 453
2. Keller, H. U., Borel, J. F., Wilkinson, P. C., Hess, M. W. and Cottier, H. (1972). Re-assessment of Boyden's technique for measuring chemotaxis. *J. Immunol. Meth.*, **1**, 165

3. Fikrig, S. M., Reddy, C. M., Orti, E., Herod, L. and Suntharalingam, K. (1977). Diabetes and neutrophil chemotaxis. *Diabetes*, **26**, 466

4. Hill, H. R., Warwick, W. J., Dettloff, J. and Quie, P. G. (1974). Neutrophil granulocyte function in patients with pulmonary infections. *J. Pediatr.*, **84**, 55

5. McCall, C. E., Caves, J., Cooper, R. and de Châtelet, L. (1971). Functional characteristics of human toxic neutrophils. *J. Infect. Dis.*, **124**, 68

6. Mowat, A. G. and Baum, J. (1971). Chemotaxis of polymorphonuclear leucocytes from patients with diabetes mellitus. *N. Engl. J. Med.*, **284**, 621

7. Valerius, N. H. (1977). Neutrophil granulocyte chemotaxis *in vitro*. Comparison of the response to casein and a bacterial chemotactic factor, and evaluation of an automatic method for counting cells on a membrane filter surface. *Acta Path. Microbiol. Scand. Sect. C*, **85**, 289

22

Simplified tests of leukocytic function
S. Olling, R. Hultborn and
I. Mattsby-Baltzer

INTRODUCTION

Disturbed leukocyte bactericidal function has been described in many patients suffering from increased frequency of infections[1]. A multitude of methods have been used, including cytochemical and functional tests for screening patients and for differentiating various deficiencies. Frequently used functional tests are modifications of the Maaløe technique[2] where the bactericidal activity for *Staphylococcus aureus* is determined by sampling and plating from a mixture of leukocytes, serum and bacteria before and after incubation.

Because of the inherent variation of plate counts and possible variation due to bacterial agglutination when quantitating bacteria, Muschel and Treffers[3] developed a photometric growth assay for the bactericidal activity of serum. Stimulated by satisfactory results with our simplified test for *serum* bactericidal activity, based on photometry of reference samples containing 50%, 10% and 1% of the initial bacterial concentration[4], we have developed an analogous test for *phagocytic* bactericidal capacity (FBC).

A phagocytic bactericidal test is a functional one whilst the nitroblue tetrazolium (NBT) reduction test[5] and analysis of the 'respiratory burst'[6] are analysing basic biochemical activities. The FBC test will be described together with a semiquantitative NBT test and a respirometric procedure previously presented by Hultborn and Olling[7] for screening of leukocytes showing dysphagocytosis.

MATERIALS AND METHODS

Biological material

Blood donors from the adjoining hospital were used as reference group. One of these was tested ten times and another four times in the course of 1 year.

One family, parents with five children, three of whom suffered from chronic granulomatous disease (CGD) and a 68-year old male suffering from chronic mucocutaneous candidiasis, thymoma and myasthenia gravis constituted the patient group. Clinical and laboratory details on these patients are published elsewhere[8, 9].

Blood was taken in heparinized plastic tubes (final concentration of heparin 25/ml) and was analysed within 2 h. Leukocyte suspension in autologous plasma was prepared by use of methylcellulose-sodium metrizoate sedimentation[10]. From 20 ml blood about 8 ml leukocyte suspension was obtained. The number of granulocytes was determined by microscopy, but the concentration was *not* standardized. The concentration of granulocytes was usually $1-10 \times 10^6$/ml.

A serum-resistant *Escherichia coli* strain and a *Staphylococcus aureus* Oxford 502A strain were used in the FBC test. From a 16 h brain heart infusion (BHI) broth (Difco lab.) of each strain, dilutions in Hank's solution to 10^{-4}, 10^{-5} and 10^{-6} were prepared. A 16 h culture of *Escherichia coli* contained $1-7 \times 10^9$ bacteria/ml and of *Staphylococcus aureus* $1-5 \times 10^9$ bacteria/ml. To the Hank's solution used in the FBS test 10 I.E. heparin was added per ml solution.

Serum from ten AB Rh(+) blood donors were pooled and stored in aliquots at $-70\,°C$. Dilution to $\frac{1}{3}$ in Hank's solution was made prior to the FBC testing.

Phagocytic bactericidal capacity (FBC) test

A leukocyte suspension (4 ml) was rinsed twice in Hank's solution and resuspended to a volume of 2 ml. According to the scheme in Table 22.1, leukocytes, serum and *Staphylococcus aureus* were added in various

TABLE 22.1 The scheme for the phagocytic bactericidal capacity (FBC) test. To six tubes (a–f) were added leukocytes, serum and bacteria in various amounts. The bacterial suspensions were 1/10 000, 1/100 000 and 1/1 000 000 dilutions of a 16 h broth culture. After appropriate incubation (2 h or none, with tumbling or without), water was added to lyse the leukocytes followed by addition of concentrated broth.

| | Tube no. | | | | | |
	a	b	c	d	e	f
Content, 0.1 ml of:						
leukocytes	+	+		+	+	+
serum	+	+	+	+	+	+
bacteria 1/10 000	+	+	+	+		
bacteria 1/100 000					+	
bacteria 1/1 000 000						+
Hank's solution			+			
Incubation at 37 °C:						
time hours	2	2	2	0	0	0
tumbling	yes	no	yes			

amounts to six tubes (a–f) to a final volume of 0.3 ml in each tube. In another set of six tubes leukocytes, serum and *Escherichia coli* were mixed.

Tubes (a) and (c) were incubated with, and tube (b) without, tumbling at 37 °C for 2 h. During this time phagocytosis and intracellular bacterial killing is supposed to take place in tube (a). To exclude the possibility of bactericidal activity not due to phagocytosis, tubes (b) and (c) were included. Leukocytes, serum and bacteria incubated without tumbling (b) should give no bacterial reduction[11] as should serum and bacteria tumbled without leukocytes (c).

Distilled water, 6 ml (+4 °C) was then added to each tube. The tubes were left for 5 min, during which time the leukocytes lysed due to the hypotonicity, and phagocytosed bacteria were liberated. Then 1.5 ml concentrated BHI broth was added to each tube. The concentrated BHI broth was prepared by dissolving the BHI powder in $\frac{1}{5}$ of the volume of water recommended by the manufacturer, i.e. the broth was concentrated five times. Tubes (a), (b) and (c) were then placed in a refrigerator at +4 °C.

To the reference tubes – (d), (e) and (f) (Table 22.1) – thus containing leukocytes, serum and 1/1, 1/10 and 1/100 of the bacterial inoculum, water was directly added, followed by concentrated broth. Tubes (d), (e) and (f) were placed without previous incubation at +4 °C.

All tubes were stored at +4 °C overnight. The following day the tubes were incubated at +37 °C for growth. After 5–6 h the tubes were shaken several times, placed in the beam of a photometer (Vitatron) and the absorbance, E, of the content in each tube registered.

By comparison with the reference tubes the bactericidal activity due to phagocytosis in tube (a) was classified:

$\leqslant 50\%$ bacteria killed   (E of tube (a) greater than half the E of tube (d))
51–90% bacteria killed   (E of tube (a) less than half the E of tube (d) or the same E as reference tube (e))
91–98% bacteria killed   (E of tube (a) between E of tubes (e) and (f))
$\geqslant 99\%$ bacteria killed   (E of tube (a) the same or less than tube (f))

Nitroblue tetrazolium (NBT) test

This was done according to Hultborn and Olling[7]. To each of four plastic tubes containing 0.4 ml NBT solution (100 mg NBT in 100 ml Hank's solution) was added 0.5 ml of the leukocyte suspension to be tested. Two of these tubes also contained 0.05 ml latex suspension for phagocytic stimulation. The two pairs of stimulated/non-stimulated samples were incubated for 5 and 15 min in a shaking water-bath at $+37\,^{\circ}C$.

Further reduction of NBT was interrupted by adding 5 ml 0.5 N HCl. After centrifugation the amount of insoluble reduced NBT in the pellet was estimated by visual inspection.

The results were classified as:

low activity – none or barely visible reduced NBT even after phagocytosis;
normal activity – NBT reduction without phagocytosis and increase after phagocytosis;
high activity – NBT reduction without phagocytosis and no or little increase after phagocytosis

Differential spectrophotorespirometry (DSR) test

This was done according to Hultborn and Olling[7]. Oxyhaemoglobin was added to a 1 ml leukocyte suspension, which was divided into two samples. To one sample was added endotoxin. The samples were placed in two airtight cuvettes which were put in the sample and reference beams of a spectrophotometer (Zeiss DMR–21) at $+37\,^{\circ}C$. Any difference in respiratory rate resulted in different reduction rates of the haemoglobin which in turn caused a difference in absorbance of the two samples at 435 nm.

The results were divided into:

normal activity—increase upon stimulation with endotoxin;
pathological activity—no increase upon stimulation with endotoxin.

RESULTS

Blood donors

In the FBC test a wide range of killing capacity was obtained when analysing 100 consecutive blood donors, as can be seen in Table 22.2. More
than 90% killing of the *Escherichia coli* was obtained in 87 experiments.
In six cases 50% or less killing was obtained. Five of these six killed 50% or
less of the *Staphylococcus aureus* inoculum as well. More than 90% killing
of *Staphylococcus aureus* occurred in 70 cases and 50% or less killing in
11 cases.

TABLE 22.2   FBC tests on 100 consecutive blood donors

Per cent bacteria killed	Escherichia coli	Staphylococcus aureus
≤ 50	6	11
51–90	7	19
91–98	43	52
≥ 99	44	18
Total	100	100

One of the blood donors, a male aged 26 years, with less than 50% killing of both bacterial strains, was tested four times. In none of these tests
was 50% or more bactericidal activity reached. He was in excellent health
and had normal routine laboratory tests, including leukocyte count. NBT
test was normal but DSR test was not performed. In ten consecutive tests
on another blood donor only one step difference between the results was
recorded, as seen in Table 22.3.

With the NBT test 230 consecutive blood donors gave normal activity
in 207 cases (90%) and high activity in 23 (10%). None showed low

TABLE 22.3   Ten consecutive FBC tests on one healthy person

Per cent bacteria killed	Escherichia coli	Staphylococcus aureus
≤ 50		
51–90		3
91–98	5	7
≥ 99	5	
Total	10	10

TABLE 22.4   Simplified leukocyte function tests performed on a family with three members suffering from chronic granulomatous disease (CGD)

| | Parents | | Siblings | | | | |
			1	2	3	4	5
Sex	M	F	F	M	F	M	F
CGD	no	no	yes	yes	no	no	yes
NBT test	normal	normal	low	low	normal	normal	low
DSR test	normal	pathol.	pathol.	pathol.	normal	pathol.	pathol.
FBC test:*							
Staphylococcus aureus	80	0	0	0	0	20	0
Escherichia coli	90	50	70	70	20	50	40

* Per cent bacteria killed estimated with a crude intrapolation

activity. With the DSR test 20 consecutive leukocyte samples from blood donors were analysed. In all, a normal increase in oxygen consumption occurred upon endotoxin stimulation.

Patients

The result of the phagocytic tests on a family with three siblings suffering from CGD are presented in Table 22.4. The FBC tests were only performed once on each patient, while DSR and NBT tests were done at least twice. The three siblings with clinical evidence of CGD gave low NBT activity and the others normal activity. The leukocytes from the father and one daughter responded normally with increase in oxygen consumption in the DSR test, but they did not in the rest of the family. In the FBC test only the sample from the father showed good bactericidal activity for both *Staphylococcus aureus* and *Escherichia coli*.

A patient with chronic mucocutaneous candidiasis did not kill *Staphylococcus aureus* but *Escherichia coli* was killed (95%, 90% and 95%) in three experiments.

DISCUSSION

In the present study three tests on leukocyte function were used: phagocytic bactericidal capacity (FBC), nitroblue tetrazolium reduction (NBT) and differential spectrophotometry (DSR). As the last two have been presented elsewhere, the discussion will mainly be confined to the FBC test.

The ratio of granulocytes to bacteria is known to be of importance for the outcome of phagocytosis[12]. In most tests the ratio is adjusted to 1:1 or more bacteria than granulocytes. In the FBC test, on the other hand, the phagocytes were not standardized with regard to the number but with regard to the volume blood from which they were obtained. The 0.1 ml rinsed leukocyte suspension in each tube originated from about 0.5 ml heparinized blood. This gives usually a ratio of at least 1 to 10 granulocytes per bacteria.

Another main difference from most bactericidal tests is the use of the weak hypotonic solution in which the granulocytes are lysed after the incubation for phagocytosis. That is, addition of 6 ml water to 0.3 ml leukocyte–serum–bacteria mixture, a dilution of 1:20. The leukocytes were exposed to the hypotonic solution for 5 min during which time leukocytes were destroyed. This could be verified by light microscopy. Living bacteria, on the other hand, are supposed not to be affected. It is, however, possible that bacteria with a partly destroyed cell wall are lysed and killed. The stronger and longer time the osmotic forces are acting, the less destruction of the bacterial cell wall due to phagocytosis may be needed for bacterial lysis, as indicated by preliminary electron microscopy studies[13].

The 'phagocytic' bacterial killing in a test may thus be due both to an intracellular granulocytic bactericidal effect and also to killing due to osmotic lysis. We assume that the latter type of killing is less expressed in the FBC test than in traditional tests, due to the weak hypotonicity used.

A disadvantage of the FBC test is that it is not possible to differentiate extracellular from intracellular surviving bacteria. The use of antibiotics or gradient-centrifugation is needed for that distinction. Another drawback is that the exact figures for bacterial killing cannot be obtained with the technique employed. By including more reference tubes with varying percentages of the bacterial inoculum and by using 30 and 60 min incubation periods it is possible to analyse further the phagocytic activity.

Serum has a pronounced bactericidal activity against many strains while others are serum-resistant. When tumbling serum and 'serum-resistant' bacteria, a weak but significant bacterial killing starts in some cases after half an hour's incubation[13]. This is in contrast to ordinary serum bactericidal activity which does not need tumbling and which starts within minutes. Some Gram-negative bacilli may be sensitive to this kind of tumbling-dependent serum bactericidal activity. This is the reason for always including tube (c) in the FBC test.

No major difference was obtained in the FBC test when retesting two blood donors. The CGD patients which had suffered from several severe infections with *Staphylococcus aureus*, were not able to kill this organism *in vitro*. The patient with mucocutaneous candidiasis performed good phagocyte killing of *Escherichia coli* but not of *Staphylococcus aureus*.

However, he never suffered from any severe *Staphylococcus aureus* infection. His granulocytes were able to reduce NBT but the granulocytes from the CGD patients were not.

The biological significance of these abnormalities in FBC tests are mainly unknown. Together with other tests on phagocytic function, for example chemotaxis, it may be possible to evaluate phagocytic function in patients with increased frequency of infections.

Acknowledgements

The skilful technical assistance of Mrs. I. Engberg, L. Johansson, A.-M. Jonsson and H. Kanu is greatly appreciated. Thanks are due also to Drs B. Elgefors, H. Mobacken and H. Peterson for their co-operation in the study of the patients. This work was supported by grants from the Medical Faculty, University of Göteborg.

References

1. Stossel, T. P. (1974). Phagocytosis. *N. Engl. J. Med.*, **290**, 717
2. Maaløe, O. (1946). *On the Relation between Alexin and Opsonin.* (Copenhagen: Munksgaard)
3. Muschel, L. H. and Treffers, H. P. (1956). Quantitative studies on the bactericidal actions of serum and complement. *J. Immunol.*, **76**, 1
4. Olling, S., Hanson, L. Å., Holmgren, J., Jodal, U., Lincoln, K. and Lindberg, V. (1973). The bactericidal effect of normal human serum on *E. coli* strains from normals and from patients with urinary tract infections. *Infection*, **1**, 24
5. Baehner, R. L. and Nathan, D. G. (1968). Quantitative nitroblue tetrazolium test in chronic granulomatous disease. *N. Engl. J. Med.*, **278**, 971
6. Holmes, B. and Good, R. A. (1972). Laboratory models of chronic granulomatous disease. *Res. J. Reticuloendothel. Soc.*, **12**, 216
7. Hultborn, R. and Olling, S. (1973). Studies on leucocyte function by measuring respiration and nitroblue tetrazolium reduction by simplified methods. *Scand. J. Clin. Lab. Invest.*, **32**, 297
8. Lindholm, L., Mobacken, H. and Olling, S. (1977). Deficient neutrophil function in a patient with chronic mucocutaneous canditiasis, thymoma and myasthenia gravis. *Acta Dermatovenereol.*, **57**, 335
9. Eljetors, B., Olling, S. and Peterson, H. (1978). Chronic granulomatous disease in three siblings. *Scand. J. Infect. Dis.* (in press)
10. Bøyum, A. (1968). Separation of leucocytes from blood and bone marrow. *Scand. J. Clin. Lab. Invest.*, **21**, (Suppl.) 28
11. Hirsch, J. G. and Strauss, B. (1964). Studies on heat-labile opsonic or rabbit serum. *J. Immunol.*, **92**, 145
12. Clauson, C. C., Repine, J. E. and Kunce, J. (1976). Quantitation of maximal bactericidal capacity in human neutrophils. *J. Lab. Clin. Med.*, **88**, 316
13. Olling, S. Unpublished observations

23

Antigen-induced neutrophil dysfunction in a patient with chronic eczema, recurrent 'cold' staphylococcal infections and hyperimmuno-globulinaemia E
K. Schopfer and K. Baerlocher

INTRODUCTION

In 1966 Davis et al.[1] reported two girls with chronic eczema and recurrent 'cold' staphylococcal infections. The authors suggested that these patients may have a defect in local resistance to staphylococcal infections, related to an abnormality of the mediators of the acute inflammatory response. These and other patients with comparable clinical findings have subsequently been studied by Hill et al.[2] who found hyperimmunoglobulinaemia E and impaired chemotaxis of polymorphonuclear leukocytes (PMN) in *vitro* as the particular immunological features of this clinical syndrome. A substantial number of patients has since been reported with similar clinical and immunological characteristics[3-12]. The mechanisms leading to granulocyte dysfunction *in vitro* and the relationship to the recurrent, atypical staphylococcal infections *in vivo*, however, are not yet understood. There is some evidence that immediate-type hypersensitivity reactions and impaired PMN function *in vitro* may be related. We have observed in recent years three patients with chronic eczema, recurrent 'cold' staphylococcal infections and hyperimmunoglobulinaemia E. One patient has been studied more extensively and the preliminary data obtained suggest that the diminished PMN chemotaxis *in vitro* is probably not due to an intrinsic cellular defect but results from antigen-induced and IgE mediated hypersensitivity reaction interfering with normal local neutrophil function.

CASE REPORT

The male patient FH, born 9 May 1962, has suffered since his third week of life from severe chronic eczema and atypical staphylococcal infections. The eczema was most severe in his first years of life and involved almost 100% of the body surface. The history of infectious disease requiring hospitalization is summarized in Figure 23.1. A severe staphylococcal pneumonia with extensive bullae formation in 1967 could only be controlled by pulmonary surgery. In 1969–70 he was hospitalized for 6 months because of meningoencephalitis due to *Cryptococcus neoformans* infection.

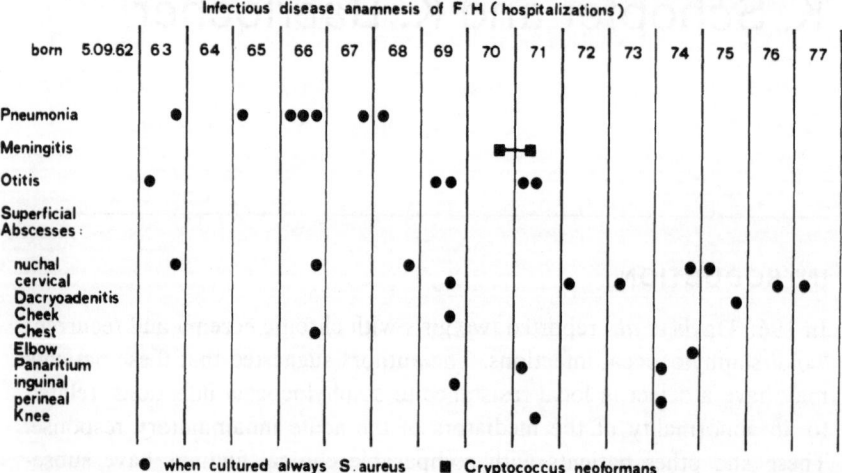

Figure 23.1 History of infectious diseases requiring the hospitalization of FH are indicated. Frequent infections occurred between the hospitalizations

Residual epilepsy still requires phenobarbital treatment. Between the hospitalizations the patient frequently suffered from infectious disease, mainly recurrent bronchitis, middle ear and skin infections up to his eighth year of life, and later mainly skin infections. He has now been kept free from infections for almost a year by sustained antibiotic prophylaxis. He has never had signs of systemic infections (no hepatosplenomegaly), and he has never suffered from gastrointestinal infections. The course of the usual viral infections during childhood was uneventful, there were no complications. He was vaccinated according to the local policy, and he expressed normal delayed-type hypersensitivity after intradermal PPD testing because of BCG vaccination. FH has three healthy siblings; the mother has contact dermatitis upon exposure to detergents, and she also reports a few asthmatic episodes. One brother of the patient's mother was hospitalized twice for surgical drainage of cervical staphylococcal infection.

CLINICAL AND IMMUNOLOGICAL STUDIES

The clinical course of the patient's staphylococcal infections shows some striking features. There was never fever during infections and, locally, there were no classical signs of inflammation, although the skin abscesses usually were very extensive (up to 500 ml could repeatedly be evacuated from the abscess cavity). The abscess formation goes on clinically silent, painless, over a prolonged period of time, and generally the patient's well-being is hardly affected. The abscesses contain necrotic, bloodstained material; typical pus production is lacking. There is no neutrophilic response in the peripheral blood, but significant eosinophilia can be observed, which disappears in the intervals between the clinically overt infections (Figure 23.2). Furthermore, a remarkable 'switch' of the site of the main infections from the lungs and middle ears to the skin can be observed with increasing age of the patient (Figure 23.1). *In vivo* and *in vitro* evaluation of specific humoral and cellular immunity as well as of the complement system by classical methods revealed no abnormality. Hyperimmunoglobulinaemia E was first detected in 1970 (around 7000 IU/ml during the last year). Specific IgE against egg white and cow's milk were found by radioallergosorbent test (RAST, Pharmacia). *In vitro* tests of PMN function included chemotaxis, phagocytosis, killing experiments with *Staphylococcus aureus* and *Candida albicans* as well as metabolic studies (NBT reduction, hexose monophosphate shunt activity and iodination in resting and phagocytozing PMNs). No significant differences from simultaneously conducted control experiments were observed.

For further studies the clinical and immunological features of the disease

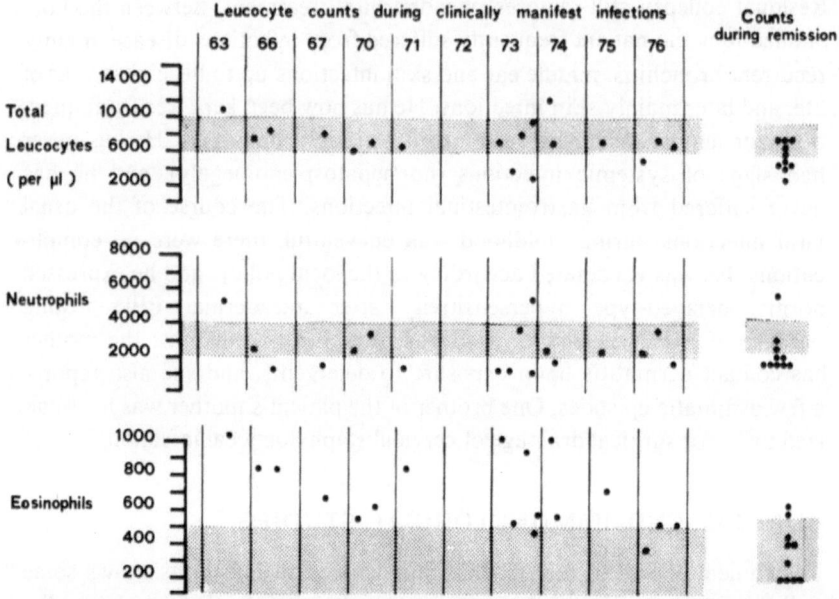

Figure 23.2 Leukocyte counts in the peripheral blood during the episodes of infectious disease necessitating hospitalization. The patient's own normal values in the intervals between severe infections are plotted on the right

were re-evaluated and the following characteristics were in particular considered: (1) the site of the infectious disease, mainly lungs and skin; (2) the lack of recurrence of lung infections with ageing, the skin remaining the main site of infections in the older patient; (3) no systemic infections due to *Staphylococcus aureus* or other bacterial pathogens; (4) *Staphylococcus aureus* being the only agent responsible for recurrence of infections; (5) the atypical systemic and local inflammatory response; and (6) the hyper-immunoglobulinaemia E.

The following preliminary experiments were designed to test if *in vitro* PMN function could be impaired by the interaction of a possible antigen with specific IgE and target cells. Chemotaxis of washed PMN was always normal; however, if chemotactic response of PMNs was assayed in the presence of ovalbumin, severe inhibition of migration could be observed. The inhibition was most pronounced if the cells were pre-incubated with autologous, not heat-inactivated serum (Figure 23.3).

However, the significance of these *in vitro* observations to explain the clinical situation is not clear. Therefore, the possibility was examined as to whether antistaphylococcal antibodies of the IgE class could be responsible for mediating PMN dysfunction locally upon contact with

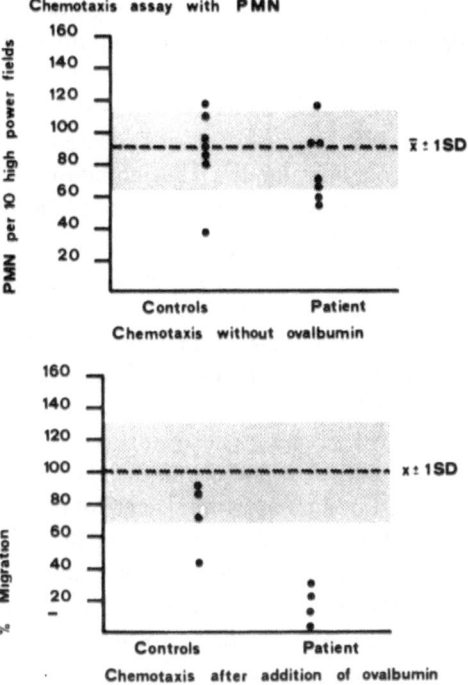

Figure 23.3 Results of the chemotaxis assays with PMNs. The shadowed area indicates our laboratory normal range. In the lower graph the values are related to the control experiment with washed PMNs without the addition of ovalbumin. This value is taken as 100%, percentage migration is then calculated. Each dot represents the mean value of triplicate assays

invading staphylococcal antigens. Preliminary data show that antistaphylococcal antibodies of the IgE class may indeed be present and chemotactic response of PMNs *in vitro* is diminished when incubated together with *Staphylococcus aureus*, whereas inhibition in control experiments is not significant.

COMMENT

Chronic eczema, recurrent 'cold' staphylococcal infections mainly of the skin and the lungs with atypical signs of the inflammatory response, as well as hyperimmunoglobulinaemia E and chemotactic dysfunction of PMNs *in vitro*, seem to be pathogenetically linked. The data of our *in vitro* studies demonstrate that chemotactic migration of PMNs is inhibited upon interaction of an antigen with specific IgE incubated together in the PMN preparation. The number of basophils in our preparation varied from 0.5 to 2% (2500 to 10 000 cells in the final incubation mixture). Basophils are known to degranulate if bridging of membrane-bound IgE by an antigen occurs[13]. Histamine, one of the mediators released[14], has been shown to inhibit PMN chemotaxis *in vitro*[15-19], as well as degranulation of lysosomal enzymes into the surrounding fluid[15]. The inhibition of these events is probably mediated by an increase of intracellular cyclic AMP[15-17]. In our present study, as well, PMN migration may be due to the action of histamine released from the basophils present in the PMN population. We cannot yet exclude the possibility that other factors which may interact with PMN migration *in vitro* might be present, for example factors produced by mononuclear cells after interaction with antigen. However, the short incubation time (2 h) and the low degree of contamination (always less than 5%) by mononuclear cells argue against such a possibility.

The relevance of these *in vitro* findings to the clinical situation remains unclear. The basic defect of immunity in this patient may be the formation of antistaphylococcal IgE antibodies. Mediators of the immediate-type hypersensitivity reaction are then released upon interaction of antigens with specific IgE bound to mast cells in lungs and skin[13] and thus interfere locally with normal neutrophil function. Locally induced failure of degranulation and release of lysosomal enzymes from neutrophils could result in defective handling of the invading antigen and of impaired inflammatory response. No systemic infection would result, since systemic phagocyte function is normal. Thus, formation of recurrent staphylococcal abscesses may be the clinical expression of an imbalance between normal systemic and impaired local host defence mechanisms. Furthermore, the possible development of blocking antibodies, e.g. in bronchial secretion, might abolish the antigen-induced and IgE-mediated adverse effect on neutrophil function. This could explain the lack of pulmonary infections in the grown-up patient FH. The skin remains especially susceptible since it lacks mechanical integrity due to chronic eczema; furthermore, the half-life of receptor-bound IgE to mast cells in the skin is about five times longer than of circulating IgE[13].

More studies are needed to clarify the pathogenetic links between chronic eczema, recurrent, atypical staphylococcal infections, hyperimmunoglobulinaemia E and impaired chemotaxis of PMNs *in vitro*. Also, the therapeutical possibility of induction of blocking antibodies in such situations or of histamine receptor blocking agents on PMNs should be considered.

Acknowledgement

We are indebted to Annemarie Smulders, who gave excellent technical assistance.

References

1. Davis, S. D., Schaller, J. and Wedgewood, R. J. (1966). Job's syndrome, recurrent, 'cold', staphylococcal abscesses. *Lancet*, **i**, 1013
2. Hill, H. R., Quie, P. G., Pabst, H. F., Ochs, H. D., Clark, R. A., Klebanoff, S. J. and Wedgewood, R. J. (1974). Defect in neutrophil granulocyte chemotaxis in Job's syndrome of recurrent, 'cold' staphylococcal abscesses. *Lancet*, **ii**, 617
3. Hill, H. R. and Quie, P. G. (1974). Raised serum-IgE levels and defective neutrophil chemotaxis in three children with eczema and recurrent bacterial infections. *Lancet*, **i**, 183
4. Van Scoy, R. E., Hill, H. R., Ritts, R. E. and Quie, P. G. (1975). Familial neutrophil chemotaxis defect, recurrent bacterial infections, mucocutaneous candidiasis and hyperimmunoglobulinemia E. *Ann. Intern. Med.*, **82**, 766
5. Pincus, S. H., Thomas, I. T., Clark, R. A. and Ochs, H. D. (1975). Defective neutrophil chemotaxis with variant ichthyosis hyperimmunoglobulinemia E, and recurrent infections. *J. Pediatr.*, **87**, Part I, 908
6. Hill, H. R., Williams, P. B., Krueger, G. G. and Janis, B. (1976). Recurrent staphylococcal abscesses associated with defective neutrophil chemotaxis and allergic rhinitis. *Ann. Intern. Med.*, **85**, 39
7. Fontan, G., Lorente, F., Rodriguez, M. C. G. and Ojeda, J. A. (1976). Defective neutrophil chemotaxis and hyperimmunoglobulinemia E – a reversible defect? *Acta Paediatr. Scand.*, **65**, 509
8. Church, J. A., Frenkel, L. D., Wright, D. G. and Bellanti, J. A. (1976). T lymphocyte dysfunction, hyperimmunoglobulinemia E, recurrent bacterial infections, and defective neutrophil chemotaxis in a Negro child. *J. Pediatr.*, **88**, 982
9. Rogge, J. L. and Hanifin, J. M. (1976). Immunodeficiencies in severe atopic dermatitis. Depressed chemotaxis and lymphocyte transformation. *Arch. Dermatol.*, **112**, 1391
10. Dahl, M. V., Greene, W. H. and Quie, P. G. (1976). Infection, dermatitis, increases IgE, and impaired neutrophil chemotaxis. A possible relationship. *Arch. Dermatol.*, **112**, 1387
11. Blum, R., Geller, G. and Fisch, L. A. (1977). Recurrent severe staphylococcal infections, eczematoid rash, extreme elevations of IgE, eosinophilia and divergent chemotactic responses in two generations. *J. Pediatr.*, **90**, 607
12. Jacobs, J. C. and Norman, M. E. (1977). A familial defect of neutrophil chemotaxis with asthma, eczema, and recurrent skin infections. *Pediatr. Res.*, **11**, 732
13. Ishizaka, K. and Ishizaka, T. (1971). Mechanisms of reaginic hypersensitivity. A review. *Clin. Allergy*, **1**, 9
14. Lichtenstein, L. M. and Osler, A. G. (1964). Studies on the mechanisms of hypersensitivity phenomena. *J. Exp. Med.*, **120**, 507

15. Zurier, R. B., Weissmann, G., Hoffstein, S., Kammerman, S. and Tai, H. H.
     (1974). Mechanisms of lysosomal enzyme release from human leukocytes.
     II. Effects from cAMP and cGMP, autonomic agonists, and agents which
     affect microtubule function. *J. Clin. Invest.*, 53, 297
16. Rivkin, I., Rosenblatt, J. and Becker, E. L. (1975). The role of cyclic AMP
     in the chemotactic responsiveness and spontaneous motility of rabbit peri-
     toneal neutrophils. The inhibition of neutrophil movement and the elevation
     of cyclic AMP levels by catecholamines, prostaglandins, theophylline and
     cholera toxin. *J. Immunol.*, 115, 1126
17. Hill, H. R., Estensen, R. D., Quie, P. G., Hogan, N. A. and Goldberg, N. D.
     (1975). Modulation of human neutrophil chemotactic responses by cyclic
     3',5'-guanosine monophosphate and cyclic 3',5'-adenosine monophos-
     phates. *Metabolism*, 24, 447
18. Clark, R. A. F., Sandler, J. A., Gallin, J. I. and Kaplan, A. P. (1977).
     Histamine modulation of eosinophil migration. *J. Immunol.*, 118, 137
19. Lett-Brown, M. A. and Leonard, E. J. (1977). Histamine-induced inhibition
     of normal human basophil chemotaxis to C5a. *J. Immunol.*, 118, 815

24

Lack of myeloperoxidase-mediated iodination in granulocytes from a patient with generalized pustular psoriasis

O. Stendahl, C. Dahlgren,
J. Hed and L. Molin

INTRODUCTION

For effective killing of micro-organisms by granulocytes, the production of one or more oxidative metabolites is essential. During phagocytosis, a considerable increase in oxygen consumption[1], superoxide radical formation[2] and hydrogen peroxide generation[3] is observed. Although superoxide radicals seem to be intermediates in the hydrogen peroxide production[4], both products have microbicidal properties. The microbicidal activity of hydrogen peroxide is greatly enhanced by a halide and the granule associated enzyme myeloperoxidase[5]. In addition to these oxygen-dependent systems, several other granule associated microbicidal agents[6-9] may be active within the phagolysosome.

The relative importance of these different microbicidal systems in relation to the inflammatory response is not clarified. Although the MPO–H_2O_2–halide system is considered to be the major antimicrobial system in normal human polymorphonuclear leukocytes (PMNL), lack of MPO[10] in contrast to lack of NADPH oxidase in chronic granulomatous disease (CGD)[11], gives rise only to discrete clinical symptoms. In view of these facts the present report concerning a patient with generalized pustular psoriasis (GPP), the granulocytes of whom exhibit defective iodination of ingested yeast particles due to lack of MPO, may shed light on the relative role of MPO. Since pustular psoriasis is characterized by acute recurrent exacerbations with fever, leukocytosis and development of subcorneal sterile pustules containing PMNL, the linkage between MPO deficiency and development of the pustular disease in this patient is hard to overlook. Biochemical and functional studies were performed to elucidate the metabolic and genetic nature of the defect, and whether alternative functional properties leading to intraphagocytic killing are operative within the phagocytic cells.

LACK OF MYELOPEROXIDASE-MEDIATED IODINATION

During the investigation of PMNL function in patients with generalized pustular psoriasis[12], one patient (EÅ) was found to have a pronounced decrease in the iodination of ingested yeast particles (Table 24.1)[13]. None of the other GPP patients showed diminished iodination activity, although some were more severely ill than EÅ. Since phagocytic uptake of fluores-

TABLE 24.1   Iodination and oxidative metabolism in granulocytes from a patient (EÅ) with generalized pustular psoriasis compared to different control groups

Granulocytes from	Iodination*	HMS†	Superoxide production‡
Controls	$0.91 \pm 0.10(15)$§	$3683 \pm 660(15)$§	$21 \pm 6(3)$§
GPP	$0.84 \pm 0.06(11)$§	$4577 \pm 620(11)$§	—
Bacterial infection	$0.76 \pm 0.12(12)$§	$3950 \pm 730(12)$§	—
EÅ (blood)	0.08 ± 0.01 (5)§	6250 (3)§	$26 \pm 4(3)$§
EÅ (pustules)	0.09 (2)	—	—

* MPO-mediated iodination, in nmol $I/10^6$ granulocytes/30 min, was assayed as the amount of TCA-precipitable iodination during phagocytosis of yeast cells[20]

† Hexose monophosphate shunt activity, in cpm of $^{14}CO_2$ released/5×10^6 granulocytes/60 min, was assayed as the amount of $^{14}CO_2$ released from glucose-^{14}C-1 during phagocytosis of yeast cells[20]

‡ Superoxide production, in nmol reduced cytochrome $c/5 \times 10^6$ PMNs/30 min, was assayed as the amount of O_2^--dependent cytochrome c reduced during phagocytosis of STZ[2]

§ Mean ± SEM. Number of experiments within parentheses.

cent yeast cells and the oxidative metabolism, superoxide production and hexose monophosphate activity (Table 24.1), were not reduced, the lack of iodination would be due to reduced MPO activity within the phagocytic cell.

TABLE 24.2 Contents of lysosomal enzymes in leukocytes isolated from a patient (EÅ) with deficient MPO-mediated iodination and from his relatives

Patient	MPO (Guiacol units/10^6 granulo- cytes)	Lysozyme ($\mu g/10^6$ granulocytes)	N-acetyl-β- glucosaminidase (nmol substrate hydrolysed/10^6 granulocytes/min)	β-Glucuronidase (nmol substrate hydrolysed/10^6 granulocytes/min)
Controls (n = 5)	240 ± 33*	3.3 ± 0.7*	3.01 ± 0.46*	0.38 ± 0.08*
EÅ	36	2.6	2.9	0.32
PÅ	150	3.0	2.2	0.30
E-LÅ	180	2.8	2.4	0.25
LÅ	250	2.8	2.5	—
Mother Å	190	3.3	2.6	0.21
Father Å	230	2.8	2.5	0.41

* Mean ± SD

Biochemical analysis for the granule contents of MPO, lysozyme, N-acetyl-β-glucosaminidase and β-glucuronidase, revealed a selective reduction of MPO (Table 24.2), whereas all the other enzymes were within our normal range. Immunochemical analysis by Dr I. Olsson, University of Lund, of MPO and other granule-associated proteins (lactoferrin, elastase, collagenase and basic proteins) showed that only MPO was reduced, being less than 1% of normal values.

MICROBICIDAL ACTIVITY

The earlier investigation of PMNs from GPP[12] showed diminished microbicidal activity towards Escherichia coli. The MPO-deficient PMNL exhibits a more pronounced impairment of microbicidal activity against Escherichia coli (Figure 24.1) and Candida albicans (Figure 24.2).

The normal MPO-mediated microbicidal activity of PMN is inhibited by azide and cyanide compounds[14]. The effect of these compounds on normal and MPO-deficient PMNL is shown in Figure 24.3. The residual microbicidal activity of the MPO-deficient PMNL is not inhibited to the

TABLE 24.3 Iodination activity in granulocytes from a patient (EÅ) with GPP and from his relatives

Granulocytes from	Iodination (nmol I/10⁶ granulocytes/30 min)
EÅ	0.08 ± 0.01^5
PÅ	0.81^2
E-LÅ	1.09^2
LÅ	0.92^2
Mother Å	0.82^2
Father Å	0.98^2

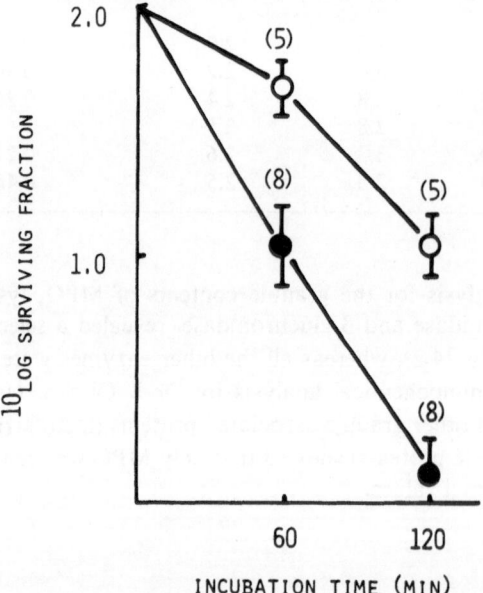

Figure 24.1 The bactericidal activity of leukocytes isolated from the patient (EÅ) (O) and from controls (●) on *Escherichia coli* 0111. Vertical bars represent SEM. Number of experiments within parentheses (from reference[13])

same extent (50–52%) as that of normal cells (90–98%). These data suggest that the microbicidal systems of MPO-deficient PMNL possess alternative, compensatory mechanisms. Since the oxidative metabolism is increased and the other granule constituents are within normal range, several compensatory systems would be at hand.

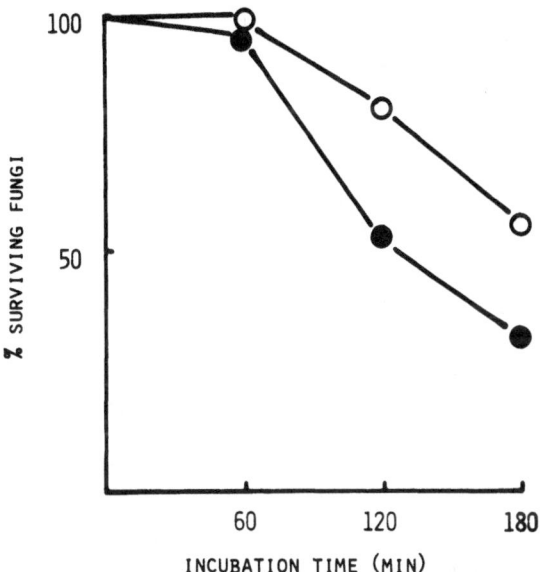

Figure 24.2 The fungicidal activity of leukocytes isolated from a patient (EÅ) (O) and from controls (●) on *Candida albicans*. The values represent the mean of three experiments (from reference[13])

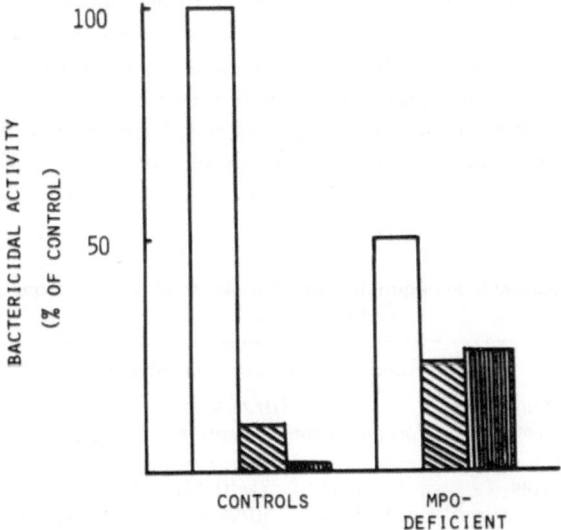

Figure 24.3 The inhibitory effect of $10^{-3}M$ azide (▨) and $10^{-3}M$ cyanide (▥) on the bactericidal activity of normal and MPO-deficient leukocytes. The values represent the mean of two experiments. Incubation time 2 h (from reference[13])

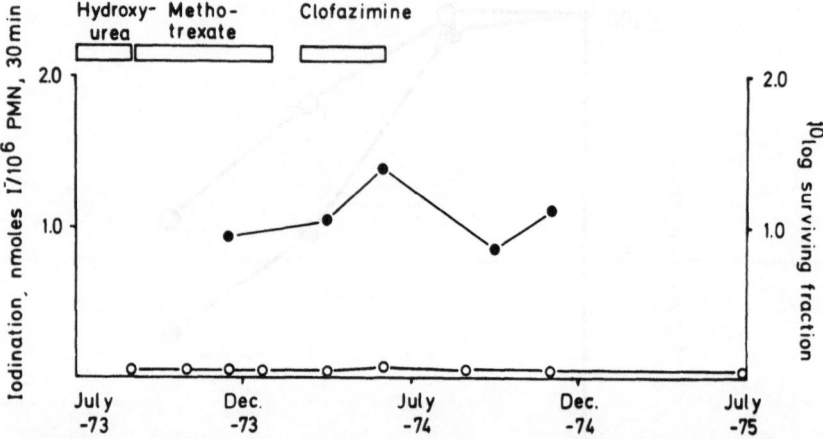

Figure 24.4   The relation of bactericidal activity (2 h) (●) and MPO-mediated iodination (○) to treatment with various drugs and to the course of the disease (from reference[13])

RANDOM LOCOMOTION AND CHEMOTAXIS

During the course of investigation there was little variation in the function of the leukocytes (Figure 24.4). Periodic chemotherapy and folic acid deficiency did not seem to influence the cells. However, when the leukocytes were tested for random locomotion and chemotaxis there was a marked decrease in random locomotion but the chemotaxis was normal (Table 24.4). Since the motility properties have not been assayed in the other GPP patients and at different stages of the disease, we can however not yet evaluate whether this abnormality preceded the pustular disease or was due to longstanding leukocytosis. Morphologically, no immature or toxic leukocytes were observed. The cause and role of this decreased motility is presently being investigated.

TABLE 24.4   Random locomotion and chemotaxis of PMNL from a patient (EA) with GPP

| | *Random locomotion and chemotaxis** | | |
| | | *Attractant:* | |
Granulocytes from	*Normal serum*	*EÅ serum*	*Gey's*
Controls	52/96(4)	51/104(4)	53/53(4)
EÅ	22/78(4)	20/98(4)	25/26(4)

* Random motility and chemotaxis were assayed using an agarose method after modification from Nelson *et al.*[21]. The numbers express in arbitrary units the motility distance towards control (Gey's) and attractant. The difference expresses the chemotactic activity.

HEREDITARY STUDIES

Studying the genetic nature of the observed iodination deficiency, no apparent hereditary transmission was observed although a deceased identical twin also suffered from psoriasis. All the relatives (parents and three children) exhibited normal iodination activity and normal levels of lysosomal enzymes (Table 24.2) – except MPO in PÅ which was reduced to 63%.

CONCLUSION

Although the pathogenesis of pustular psoriasis is still unknown, certain facts are known. Neutrophils accumulate rapidly to form subcorneal pustules during exacerbations. This could be due to activation of chemotactic factors, such as immunoglobulins and C_3, since these have been detected in pustules[15]. Furthermore, in pustulosis palmoplantaris and certain other dermatoses the leukocytes show impaired phagocytic uptake[16]. In the present case, impaired motility and microbicidal activity may enhance the seriousness of the disease. Although micro-organisms have never been isolated from pustules, aerobic as well as anaerobic microbes cannot be completely ruled out as the cause of pustular development, since the disease is often precipitated by infections such as respiratory diseases[17]. Leukocytes isolated from pustules showed activity similar to blood leukocytes *in vitro*. However, when accumulating in the pustules, where the oxygen tension is lowered, the leukocytes may exhibit a further impairment of the phagocytic activity. This would ultimately lead to requirements for more cells and development of more pustules. In no patient with GPP was the opsonizing activity of serum diminished[12], and the immunoglobulin levels were also normal in this patient.

Patients with myeloperoxidase-deficient leukocytes may not be too rare, and could be found during screening of larger patient groups. The detected MPO deficiency generally has little clinical significance, but when suffering from certain other disorders, such as allergic reactions, dermatosis, surgical trauma, where the leukocyte function is heavily challenged, these patients may develop symptoms related to this immunodeficiency. Thus, the observation of impaired MPO activity should not be overlooked. Since the molecular basis of the triggering mechanisms for the respiratory burst, and the relative contributions of the various bactericidal agents (H_2O_2, superoxide anions, singlet oxygen, hydroxyl radicals, phospholipase A_2, lactoferrin and cationic proteins) remain to be clarified, no well-documented conclusion can yet be drawn about the alternative mechanisms activated in MPO-deficient leukocytes. Futhermore, the MPO deficiency might have relevance to the development of an inflammatory reaction since the MPO system in PMNL has recently been shown to have cytotoxic activity against other mammalian cells[18] (e.g. tumour cells and leukocytes). This mechanism could normally function as a modulator of the inflammatory response[19].

Acknowledgements

The technical assistance of Ellinor Granström is gratefully acknowledged. This study was in part supported by grants from E. Welanders Stiftelse and Svenska Läkaresällskapets forskningsråd.

References

1. Sbarra, A. J. and Karnovsky, M. L. (1959). The biochemical basis of phagocytosis. I. Metabolic changes during the ingestion of particles by polymorphonuclear leukocytes. *J. Biol. Chem.*, **234**, 1355
2. Curnutte, J. T. and Babior, B. M. (1974). Biological defence mechanisms. The effect of bacteria and serum or superoxide production by granulocytes. *J. Clin. Invest.*, **53**, 1662
3. Iyer, G. Y. N., Islam, M. F. and Quastel, J. H. (1961). Biochemical aspects of phagocytosis. *Nature (London)*, **192**, 535
4. Klebanoff, S. J. (1974). Role of the superoxide anion in the myeloperoxidase mediated antimicrobial system. *J. Biol. Chem.*, **249**, 3724
5. Klebanoff, S. J. (1972). Role of myeloperoxidase-mediated antimicrobial systems in intact leukocytes. *J. Reticuloendothel. Soc.*, **12**, 170
6. Wilson, L. A. and Spitznagel, J. K. (1968). Molecular and structural damage to *Escherichia coli* produced by antibody, complement and lysosome systems. *J. Bacteriol.*, **96**, 1339
7. Baggiolini, M., de Duve, C. and Mason, P. L. (1970). Association of lactoferrin with specific granules in rabbit heterophil leukocytes. *J. Exp. Med.*, **131**, 559
8. Odeberg, H., Olsson, I. and Wenge, P. (1975). Cationic proteins in human granulocytes. IV. Esterase activity. *Lab. Invest.*, **32**, 86
9. Weiss, J., Franson, R. C., Beckendite, Susan, Schmeidler, Katherine and Elsbach, P. (1975). Partial characterization and purification of a rabbit granulocyte factor that increases permeability of *E. coli. J. Clin. Invest.*, **55**, 33
10. Lehrer, R. I. and Cline, M. J. (1969). Leukocyte myeloperoxidase deficiency and disseminated candidiasis: the role of myeloperoxidase in resistance to *Candida* infection. *J. Clin. Invest.*, **48**, 1479
11. Quie, P. G. (1977). Disorder of phagocyte function: Biochemical aspects. In T. J. Greenwalt and G. A. Jamieson (eds.). *The Granulocyte: Function and Clinical Utilization*, p. 157. (New York: Alan R. Liss, Inc.)

12. Lindgren, S. and Stendahl, O. (1975). Phagocytic activity of polymorphonuclear leukocytes in GPP. *Acta Dermatovenereol.*, **56**, 229

13. Stendahl, O. and Lindgren, S. (1976). Function of granulocytes with deficient myeloperoxidase-mediated iodination in a patient with generalized pustular psoriasis. *Scand. J. Haematol.*, **16**, 144

14. Klebanoff, S. J. (1970). Myeloperoxidase: Contribution to the microbicidal activity of intact leukocytes. *Science*, **169**, 1095

15. Husby, G., Rajka, G. and Eeg Larsen, T. (1973) Immunofluorescence studies in pustulosis palmo-plantaris. *Acta Dermatovenereol.*, **53**, 123

16. Molin, L. and Rajka, G. (1971). Phagocytic activity of neutrophil leukocytes in pustulosis palmo-plantaris, chronic discoid lupus erythematosus and erysipelas. *Acta Dermatovenereol.*, **51**, 138

17. Lindgren, S. and Groth, O. (1975). Generalized pustular psoriasis. A report on thirteen cases. *Acta Dermatovenereol.*

18. Clark, R. A., Klebanoff, S. J., Einstein, A. B. and Fefer, A. (1975). Peroxidase-H_2O_2-halide system: Cytotoxic effect on mammalian tumour cells. *Blood*, **45**, 161

19. Edelson, P. J. and Cohn, Z. A. (1973). Peroxidase-mediated mammalian cell cytotoxicity. *J. Exp. Med.*, **138**, 318

20. Bröte, L. and Stendahl, O. (1975). The function of polymorphonuclear leukocytes after surgical trauma. *Acta Chir. Scand.*, **141**, 565

21. Nelson, R. D., Quie, P. G. and Simmons, R. L. (1975). Chemotaxis under agarose: A new and simple method for measuring chemotaxis and spontaneous migration of human polymorphonuclear leukocytes and monocytes. *J. Immunol.*, **115**, 1650

25

Functional characteristics of neutrophil granulocytes from children with recurrent respiratory infections
J. H. Wandall, V. Binder, B. Friis and B. Bech

INTRODUCTION

Impaired function of polymorphonuclear neutrophil granulocytes (PMN) is associated with recurrent bacterial infections. Inherited defects in the chemotactic response[1] and in different microbicidal enzymes have been described[2]. It is however unclear to what extent the granulocyte function in patients with a history of recurrent infections is impaired.

The aim of this investigation is to study the function of granulocytes from children with recurrent respiratory infections without other predisposing disease, for example, cystic fibrosis, asthma and α_1-antitrypsin deficiency.

MATERIAL AND METHODS

Fifteen patients (nine boys, six girls, aged 2–19 years, median age 10 years) with history of recurrent respiratory bacterial infections since early childhood were studied when fit. All patients had pulmonary changes verified by X-ray examination and reduced pulmonary function as demonstrated by spirometry.

Criteria for exclusion were a history of cystic fibrosis, allergic asthma, α-l-antitrypsin deficiency or respiratory disease in the neonatal period.

Control groups:

1. Thirty-three blood donors (17 males, 16 females, aged 23–68 years, median age 33 years) with no history of chronic or recent disease.

2. Twelve healthy children (nine boys, three girls, aged 2–10 years, median age 6 years) admitted to hospital for minor surgery, for example, inguinal hernia or phimosis.

Leukocyte spontaneous and chemotactic migration, serum-independent and -dependent phagocytosis, the spontaneous and stimulated nitroblue tetrazolium (NBT) reduction to formazan were determined *in vitro*. Briefly the procedures were as described below.

Chemotactic response

Heparinized blood (10 units/ml) was withdrawn and erythrocytes sedimented with methylcellulose 150. The leukocyte-rich plasma was used directly and as washed with Hank's balanced salt solution (HBSS) – pH 7.3 – before use. Leukocytes were then layered on a cellulose-ester filter (Millipore, pore size 3 μm) in a cytocentrifuge at 22 g_{max} for 5 min. Filters were placed in chemotactic chambers at 37 °C for 3 h using HBSS with casein (Merck) 5 mg/ml as attractant. The chemotactic migration was quantitated as a chemotactic index expressing the proportion of cells migrating 50 μm down into the filter in a given area. Further, the migration was quantitated by the leading front method, that is the maximal distance in μm migrated by at least two cells per high-power field.

Phagocytosis and NBT reduction

Blood was withdrawn with ACD (N.I.H. form. A) mixed with $\frac{1}{4}$ vol. dextran 250 and erythrocytes sedimented. The leukocyte-rich plasma was centrifuged for 10 min, 80 g_{av} at 4°C and the leukocytes washed in phosphate buffered saline three times before resuspension in Krebs–Henseleit bicarbonate buffer (KHBB) – pH 7.2 – with calcium 0.9 mM/e/1 and magnesium 1.27 mM/e/1. This final cell suspension contained $4-12 \times 10^6$ leukocytes, 65–95% being phagocytes (PMN, monocytes and eosinophilic granulocytes).

The initial rate of phagocytosis of oil red O coloured paraffin oil was determined according to Stossel[3] with certain modifications. Serum-independent phagocytosis was determined as uptake of bovine serum albumin (BSA, Armour), emulsion and serum-dependent phagocytosis from the uptake of opsonized lipopolysaccharide from *Escherichia coli* 026B6 (Difco Lab., USA, Boivin method) emulsion. Opsonization was done with an equal volume autolgous serum for 15 min at 37 °C. For simultaneous determination of initial rate of phagocytosis and NBT reduction to formazan the following procedure was used:

Into 15 ml centrifuge tubes were pipetted 10 μl KCN 0.1 M. 250 μl KHBB or 250 μ. NBT 1 mg/ml in KHBB (Sigma gr. III, completely soluble) and 250 μl leukocyte suspension, and the tubes were placed in a reciprocating bath at 37 °C and shaken at 120 strokes/min. After 4 min prewarmed emulsion (100 μl BSA emulsion or 250 μl opsonized LPS emulsion) was added. After a further 4 min the reaction was stopped by addition of 10 ml 1 mM N-ethylmaleimide in sodium chloride 0.148 M. Uningested emulsion was discarded by centrifugation at 500 g_{av} for 20 min. After one wash the walls of the tubes were cleaned by dioxan-moistened tissue and the cell pellet extracted with *p*-dioxan (Merck) 1 ml. The extracts were clarified by centrifugation (1000 g, 10 min) and read in a Zeiss spectrophotometer at 525 nm and 580 nm in a 1 cm light path cell. All samples were analysed in duplicate. Differences between duplicate incubations were normally less than 8%, and always less than 15%. From the absorbance the amount of ingested paraffin oil and the generation of formazan were calculated.

Serum lysozyme was determined by rocket immunoelectrophoresis in agarose 1% (L'Industrie Biologie Française, A–37) using Tris-veronal buffer pH 8.6, ionic strength 0.075, with human lysozyme as standard.

Blood smears, coverslips, leukocyte counts and nuclear segmentation of PMNs were performed after staining with May–Grünwald–Giemsa stain and at least 200 cells counted.

RESULTS

Children with recurrent respiratory infections had neutrophil counts, mean nuclear segmentation and serum lysozyme values as presented in Table 25.1.

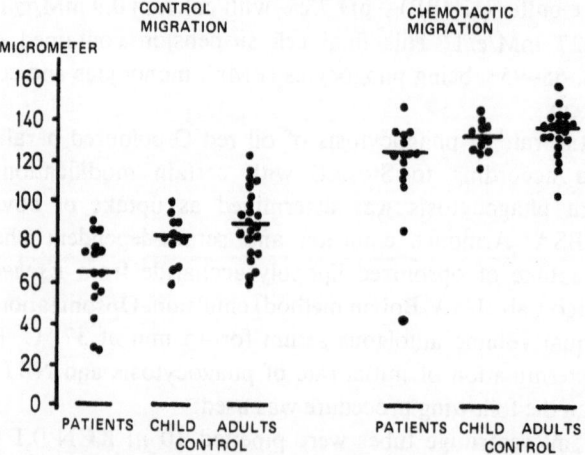

Figure 25.1 The spontaneous and chemotactic migration as measured by the leading front in patients with recurrent respiratory infections and in adult and child controls. The bars represent the medians

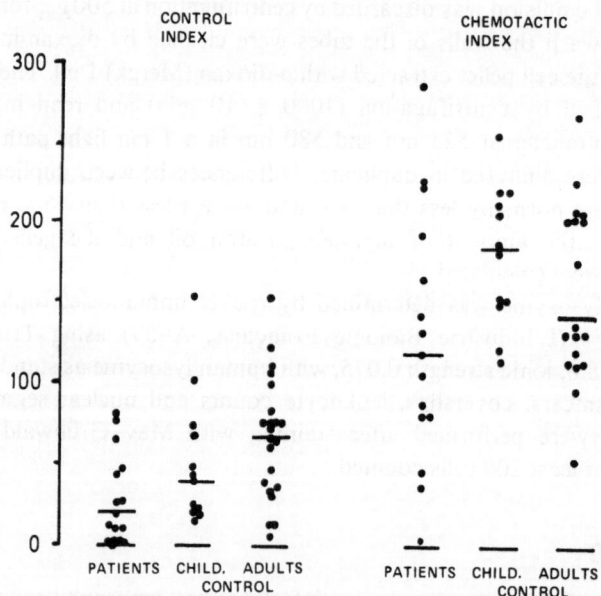

Figure 25.2 The spontaneous and chemotactic migration expressed as the chemotactic index. Values observed in the group of patients with recurrent respiratory infections and of controls. The bar represents the median

TABLE 25.1 Neutrophil counts, mean nuclear segmentation and serum lysozyme as observed in patients with recurrent respiratory infections and in healthy controls

	Neutrophil count per μl		Mean nuclear segmentation		Serum lysosyme mg/l	
	median	*range*	*median*	*range*	*median*	*range*
Patients	2265	351–8398	2.6	1.7–3.4	1.6	1.3–2.3
Controls						
children	2546	1386–3952	2.3	1.9–3.3	——	——
adults	3594	1593–6125	2.6	2.2–3.3	2.5	1.5–4.3

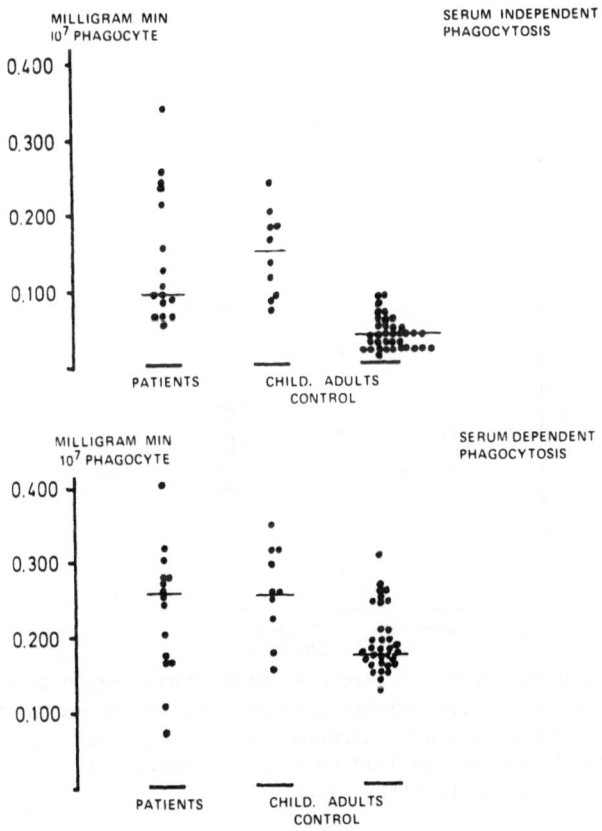

Figure 25.3 Initial rate of phagocytosis of bovine serum albumin emulsion (serum-independent) and of opsonized LPS emulsion (serum-dependent) in children with recurrent respiratory infections and in adult and child controls. The bars represent the median values

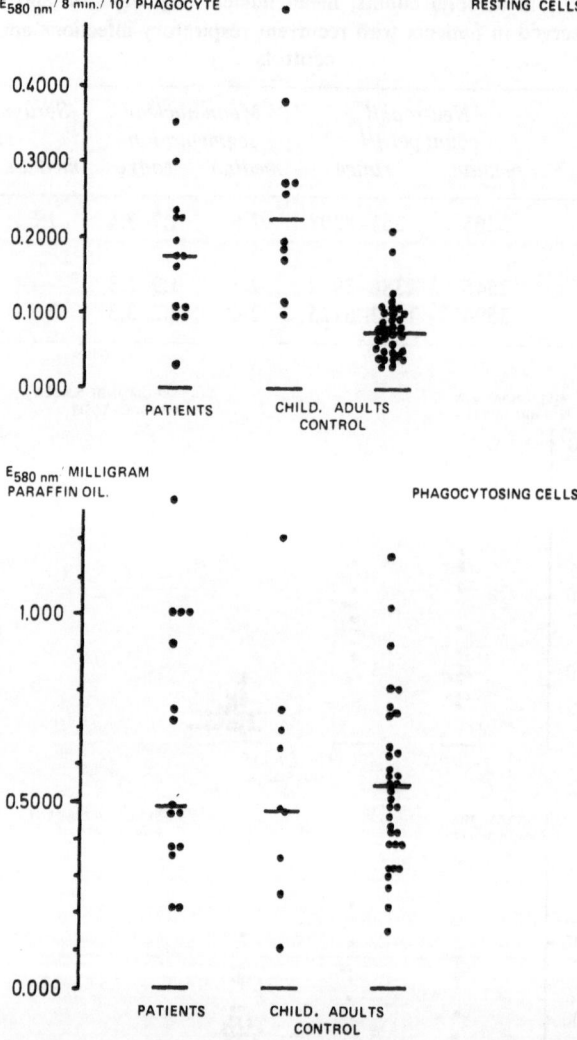

Figure 25.4   Reduction of NBT to formazan expressed as change in absorbance at 580 nm. Values of the spontaneous and stimulated test are presented from children with recurrent respiratory infections and from adult and child controls. Stimulated values have been corrected for spontaneous reduction of NBT and for ingestion. The bars represent the median values

The observed values of spontaneous and chemotactic migration are depicted in Figures 25.1 and 25.2. A decreased spontaneous and chemotactic motility was observed of leukocytes from three patients. The control indices of these patients were as low as 0–1.4 with a decreased chemotactic response of 1.7–48 in contrast to normal children 124–254. This low motility was evident by the leading front method as well. The chemotactic function of leukocytes from these patients could not be restored by removal of plasma. Phagocytosis and NBT reduction of leukocytes from these patients were normal. One of these patients was found to have nuclear segmentation of 1.7, being lower than any of the controls but with a normal neutrophil count.

The initial rate of phagocytosis of BSA emulsion (Figure 25.3) was normal in all patients indicating normal ingestion. Two patients showed normal ingestion of BSA emulsion but decreased ingestion of serum-treated LPS emulsion. One of these patients showed a value for serum-dependent phagocytosis which was below that for serum-independent phagocytosis.

The reduction of NBT to formazan by resting as well as phagocytosing cells was in no instance impaired (Figure 25.4).

An unexpected observation was that healthy children exhibited significantly higher phagocytosis of BSA emulsion and of opsonized LPS emulsion than leukocytes from healthy adult donors ($p < 0.01$, Wilcoxon test for random samples). The spontaneous reduction of NBT was similarly increased.

DISCUSSION

The present investigation is an evaluation of neutrophil function in a group of children with recurrrent severe bacterial infections since early childhood. During the period of investigation a diagnosis of cystic fibrosis was considered in one of the patients but not established with certainty. This patient showed decreased chemotactic function and had a low mean nuclear segmentation of neutrophils which may explain the observed decreased chemotactic function. Another two patients were shown to have decreased chemotactic function. In these two patients the defect must reside within the cell itself since removal of plasma did not restore the chemotactic response to casein. There was no correlation between the maturity of PMN as evaluated by the segmentation and the decreased chemotactic function.

The possible defect in opsonins in the two patients with decreased ingestion of serum-treated LPS emulsion but normal ingestion of BSA emulsion is not readily explained. The most probable explanation is an acute episode, as transient low levels of unspecific opsonins are known to occur during the acute phase of the inflammatory response[4].

As shown by our investigation, three children were found to have decreased chemotactic function and the other two children to have reduced serum opsonins. These results in a limited group of patients encourage 'screening' of granulocyte functions in patients with recurrent bacterial infections.

CONCLUSIONS

1. Impaired chemotactic responses to casein were found in leukocytes from three out of 15 children with recurrent bacterial respiratory infections.

2. Impaired unspecific serum opsonins were found in two out of 15 children with recurrent respiratory infections.

3. Leukocytes from healthy children exhibited significantly higher phagocytosis and greater spontaneous NBT reduction than leukocytes from healthy adults.

References

1. Miller, M. E., Oski, F. A. and Harris, M. B. (1971). Lazy leucocyte syndrome. *Lancet*, i, 665
2. Klebanoff, S. J. (1971). Intraleukocytic microbicidal defects. *Ann. Rev. Med.*, 22, 39
3. Stossel, Th. (1973). Evaluation of opsonic and leukocyte function with a new spectrophotometric test in patients with infection and with phagocytic disorders. *Blood*, 42, 121
4. Schutte, M., DiCamelli, R., Murphy, P., Sadove, M. and Gewurz, H. (1975). Effects of anæsthesia, surgery and inflammation upon host defense mechanisms. I. Effects upon complement systems. *Int. Arch. Allergy Appl. Immunol.*, 48, 706

26

Pneumocystis carinii infection in a girl with chronic granulomatous disease treated with transfusions of granulocytes

F. Karup Pedersen, K. S. Johansen, J. Rosenkvist, I. Tygstrup and N. H. Valerius

CASE HISTORY

The patient was 11 years old when first seen at the University Clinic of Paediatrics in Copenhagen. She is the middle child in a family with three siblings; her two sisters and her parents are in good health. There is no family history of early deaths or of frequent or serious infections.

Since infancy she has had recurring staphylococcal infections of the skin leading to furunculosis, frequent abscess formation after cuts and abrasions and facial and postauricular dermatitis. Until tonsillectomy and adenotomy at the age of 6 years she had recurring upper respiratory tract infections and at the ages of 4 and 7 years she was treated in hospital for pneumonia. She had uncomplicated measles and chickenpox and a normal response to smallpox, as well as to BCG vaccination.

At the age of 11 years she was admitted to the University Clinic of Paediatrics after 5–6 days of fever, cough and respiratory distress. On admission she was found to have a severe bilateral interstitial pneumonia as manifested by diffuse infiltration in both lung fields, where a right-sided upper mediastinal mass was also noted.

Tracheal aspirates did not yield growth of pathogenic bacteria, fungi or virus. However, by microscopy it was found to consist of foam-like material containing cysts indistinguishable from *Pneumocystis carinii*.

Studies with a view to immune deficiency revealed a neutrophil granulocytosis of $13 \times 10^6/l$ in peripheral blood. Immunoglobulins in serum were IgG 13.5 g/l, IgA 2.8 g/l and IgM 1.5 g/l.

The NBT test did not show any reduction of NBT by the patient's granulocytes[1]. The ability of the granulocytes to kill *Staphylococcus aureus* 502 A was found to be significantly decreased[2].

A lymph node biopsy showed normal germinal centres and deep cortical areas but was infiltrated with pigmented lipid histiocytes as may be seen in CGD.

Skin test with PPD and *Candida albicans* (1:100) were positive and *in vitro* lymphocyte studies showed normal percentages (as well as normal absolute numbers) of T and B lymphocytes in peripheral blood. Also the transformation response of the patient's lymphocytes to the mitogens PHA and PWM as well as to the antigens PPD, *Staphylococcus aureus*, *Escherichia coli* and *Candida albicans* were normal. Complement factor C_3 and total haemolytic complement were also normal.

The patient was treated with Bactrim® 100 + 20 mg/kg per 24 h for 2 weeks, followed by Pentamidine 4 mg/kg per 24 h for another 2 weeks. This therapy was followed by the disappearance of the pulmonary infiltrates, but the mediastinal mass was still present and the patient remained febrile. Treatment with Bactrim® in the same dose as mentioned earlier was resumed and a series of 12 granulocyte transfusions were given over a 16-day period, each transfusion containing a median number of 3.0×10^9 granulocytes. The granulocytes were collected from normal, unstimulated ABO-compatible donors by means of a Haemonetics–30 blood cell separator. Citrated hydroxyethyl starch was used as an anticoagulant. After the first three transfusions the patient became afebrile and remained afebrile after discontinuation of transfusion therapy when the Bactrim® dose was reduced to 30 + 6 mg/kg per 24 h.

The size of the mediastinal mass, however, was unaffected by the transfusions and consequently surgical excision of the mass was performed under cover of three additional granulocyte transfusions. The granulocytes in this series of transfusions were obtained from HLA- and ABO-compatible donors because after the previous transfusions the patient had developed lymphocytotoxic antibodies. The mediastinal mass consisted of granulation tissue, which could be shown to contain pneumocystis organisms with Gomori's methenamine stain. The postoperative recovery was uneventful and the patient progressed well for 4 months thereafter on continued Bactrim® medication.

DISCUSSION

The lack of reduction of NBT and a decreased bactericidal capacity of the patient's granulocytes as well as the finding of pigmented lipid histiocytes in a lymph node biopsy is evidence for the diagnosis of CGD in this girl. Though mainly a disease of boys a recent review of 168 cases of CGD included 24 cases in girls, suggesting that in addition to X-linked transmission autosomal recessive transmission may also occur[3].

Infections in CGD are usually caused by catalase-positive bacteria such as *Staphylococci* and Gram-negative enteric bacteria or fungi[4]. *Pneumocystis carinii* infection is known to occur in premature infants, in immunosuppressed individuals and in patients with congenital defects of cellular and possibly humoral immunity[5], but to our knowledge infection with *Pneumocystis carinii* has not previously been reported in patients with CGD. The occurrence of this infection in our patient therefore might lead to suspicion of associated defects in immunity, but as mentioned we have found normal cellular and humoral immunity.

Bactrim® and Pentamidine are both reported to be effective in the treatment of *Pneumocystis carinii* infection[6], but failed to reduce fever and produce full recovery in our patient. Transfusion of granulocytes in infected, neutropenic patients appears to reduce mortality from infection[7]. Raubitschek in 1973 also reported a beneficial effect of granulocyte transfusions in a patient with CGD and aspergillosis[8]. In our patient the rapid reduction in fever during transfusion and Bactrim® therapy in contrast to the continued fever during Bactrim® and Pentamidine therapy alone also suggests an effect of granulocyte transfusions in CGD. The continued Bactrim® treatment is aimed at any remaining pneumocystis organisms. One might also speculate, however, that it could at the same time enhance the bactericidal activity of the patient's granulocytes, as it has been reported that at least sulfazoxazole may have this effect[9].

In summary this report presents another case of CGD in a female child, documents *Pneumocystis carinii* infection in this disease and suggests that transfusion of granulocytes may be of value in treating severe infections in patients with CGD.

References

1. Park, B. H., Fiknig, S. M. and Smithwich, E. N. L. (1968). Infection and nitroblue tetrazolium reduction by neutrophils. *Lancet*, ii, 532
2. Koch, C. (1974). Acquired defect in the bactericidal function of neutrophil granulocytes during bacterial infections. *Acta Pathol. Microbiol. Scand.*, 82 B, 439
3. Johnston, R. B. and Newmann, S. L. (1977). Chronic granulomatous disease. *Pediatr. Clin. N. Am.*, 24, 365
4. Lazarus, G. M. and Neu, H. C. (1975). Agents responsible for infection in chronic granulomatous disease of childhood. *J. Pediatr.*, 86, 415
5. Seto, D. S. Y. and Heller, R. M. (1974). *Pneumocystis carinii* pneumonia. *Pediatr. Clin. N. Am.*, 22, 690
6. Lau, W. K. and Young, L. S. (1976). Trimethoprim-Sulfamethoxazole treatment of *Pneumocystis carinii* pneumonia in adults. *N. Engl. J. Med.*, 295, 716
7. Herzig, R. H. *et al.* (1977). Successful granulocyte transfusion therapy for Gram-negative septicaemia. A prospective randomized controlled study. *N. Engl. J. Med.*, 296, 701
8. Raubitscheck, A. A. *et al.* (1973). Normal granulocyte infusion therapy for aspergillosis in chronic granulomatous disease. *Pediatrics*, 41, 230
9. Johnston, R. B. (1975). Enhanced bactericidal activity of phagocytes from patients with chronic granulomatous disease in the presence of sulphisoxazole. *Lancet*, i, 824

Discussion

P. ERNST (Copenhagen): Why do you have no rise in the activity of ADA in lymphocytes?

MEUWISSEN (Albany): Usually there is a 2–3-fold rise. We have recent data that showed most of the ADA is contained not in lymphocytes, but in cells that are adherent to plastic, are phagocytic and have the enzymatic markers of the monocyte. So, I think that probably that is where most of the activity occurs, not so much in lymphocytes.

ROOS (Amsterdam): I heard you say that granulocyte function might be affected in NP deficiency, may be not in ADA deficiency. We have had the opportunity to study the PMN function in a NP deficient patient from Dr DeLuca in Rome and found that granulocyte chemotaxis and release of lysosomal enzymes is not quite normal. Do you know of any such studies in the ADA deficiency?

MEUWISSEN: We have not done extended studies on the granulocytes in ADA deficiency nor has anyone else to my knowledge.

POLMAR (Cleveland): This morning Dr Pahwa stated that one of the ADA deficient patients that had a histocompatible bone marrow transplant donor required six bone marrow transplants. I was wondering, in your review of the literature, whether it is more difficult to get engraftment of histocompatible bone marrow in ADA deficient patients as compared to non-ADA deficient patients. Do you have any data on that?

PAHWA (New York): We did transplantation in three patients of severe combined immunodeficiency with ADA deficiency. The first patient required six bone marrow transplants. The second patient required three bone marrow transplants, and the third patient just required one bone marrow transplant and walked out in 6 weeks completely reconstituted for T and B cells. So, I don't think we have enough to draw conclusions.

POLMAR: We have not looked at neutrophil function in ADA deficient patients but many are neutropenic along with being lymphopenic. There is also a defect in platelet aggregation in ADA deficiency. I believe Dr Rosen and others in Boston have also found that. One is impressed with the many effects of the single enzyme defect, not only with regard to the immunological defect involving the lymphocytes but the bone defects, now platelet defects. One of the things that we noticed on successful enzyme replacement therapy was the rapidity with which hair growth occurred shortly after treatment. So, this is certainly a defect that involves many systems and not exclusively the immune system.

FABER (Copenhagen): Dr Meuwissen, would you comment on the late onset of symptoms in some of the children. One boy was actually well until he was vaccinated with living polio and then he died and was found to have had ADA deficiency.

MEUWISSEN: Yes, I tried to do that under the heading of immunological attrition. Initially, I thought that this might be an effect of loss of placental ADA activity in post-natal life: the ADA deficient baby is on his own and slowly loses immune function as toxic metabolites accumulate. But I'm not sure that this is what happens.

DISCUSSION ON CHAPTER 4 – ADENOSINE DEAMINASE DEFICIENCY: ENZYME REPLACEMENT THERAPY AND INVESTIGATIONS OF THE BIOCHEMICAL BASIS OF IMMUNODEFICIENCY

ANDERSON (Copenhagen): A technique has been suggested for correction of enzymatic deficiencies by perfusion of the blood past immobilized enzyme in a small chamber to be carried on the arm. Has this been tried?

POLMAR (Cleveland): No, but I think it is very likely that it would work.

SVEJGAARD (Copenhagen): I heard at the Birth Defects Meeting in Tennessee in June 1977 that there seems to be a tendency that the patients who did not respond to enzyme replacement therapy were those who had no enzyme in the blood, while those who responded had a small concentration of the enzyme.

POLMAR: At present only eight patients have been studied. I think it's likely that the severity of the enzyme deficiency will correlate with the severity of the immunological deficiency. But I don't feel that there's enough data yet to substantiate that. The biochemical changes which occur in patients who respond and those that do not respond are very similar. This is in support of the idea that there is an immunological component to irreversibility. One might correct the patient biochemically but when the therapy is initiated relation to the degree of irreversible immunological attrition would determine whether a patient will respond immunologically.

HIRSCHHORN (New York): Our patient does not show any correlation between the enzyme activity and the response.

CARSON (La Jolla): Your hypothesis is that these patients' cells form cyclic AMP more easily because they have a higher content of ATP. Did you ever measure the content of cyclic AMP?

POLMAR: The cyclic AMP has been measured in other cells particularly by others and is raised. We haven't looked at levels specifically in our patient prior to the time that therapy was started. Cyclic AMP has been found to be elevated in a number of patients with ADA deficiency. However, cyclic AMP is protein bound and is compartmentalized; merely the elevated level of cyclic AMP on a total cell basis is relatively meaningless. The functional data in terms of the differential inhibitory effects by beta-adrenergic stimuli or prostaglandins I think is far more significant in indicating a role for cyclic AMP than merely the elevated levels of cyclic AMP. I think the drug data are more impressive in terms of functional significance as to the role of cyclic nucleotides.

FABER (Copenhagen): Do you know of any of these two patients who did not respond. Were they treated with any drugs which might inhibit? I suggest that chloramphenicol which reduces the PHA stimulation and elevates the cyclic AMP, might interfere.

POLMAR: I cannot be sure of those particular patients. There were three patients that did not respond, two in Wisconsin, and one in Texas. I think the Wisconsin patients were not on chloramphenicol. The patients were clinically well and received transfusions for 4 weeks during a time that they were clinically well. So, I think that antibiotic administration is probably unlikely to be a complicating factor.

We were studying peripheral blood lymphocytes from a patient with ADA deficiency. I think one thereby gets a somewhat limited view of possible mechanisms. One might get abnormal development from precursor cells to identifiable mature lymphocytes. Cyclic AMP appears to be operative in the peripheral blood lymphocyte but may not be the mechanism which is operative in the conversion of precursors to more mature lymphocytes.

DISCUSSION ON CHAPTER 9 – SEVERE COMBINED IMMUNODEFICIENCY WITH B LYMPHOCYTES: A SELECTIVE DEFECT OF PRECURSOR T CELLS

ERNST (Copenhagen): How soon after bone marrow transplantation did you see restoration of recipient immune function?

GRISCELLI (Paris): We saw humoral reconstitution 4 months after bone marrow transplantation. Why do you ask this question?

ERNST: I was thinking of the fact that in experimental models as based on clinical experience it seems as if the graft-versus-host reaction is less pronounced in immunodeficiency syndromes. If we have a syndrome where in some cases we have recipient immune function ready to be expressed as soon as we have a helper function, we should actually be in a position where we have cells able to participate in a graft-versus-host reaction. So, I just wonder if we have this expression triggered very soon after transplantation.

GRISCELLI: I have to give more details. What we have observed is around 10–15 days after a bone marrow transplantation a rapid rise of IgM production occurs. 10 days later the IgM falls to the previous low level. But a second wave is seen several weeks or months later. This suggests that we have two phenomena. The first IgM increase can be due to an allogeneic effect during a mild graft-versus-host reaction characterized by a transient skin rash of 10 days, and an eosinophilia. The second wave is the result of a normal cooperation with fully mature T cells coming from the donor and the recipient B cells.

DISCUSSION ON CHAPTER 11 – ACTIVITY OF ADENOSINE DEAMINASE AND PURINE NUCLEOSIDE PHOSPHORYLASE IN LYMPHOCYTES OF MAN, HORSE AND CATTLE

HIRSCHHORN (New York): Together with Dr Green we have measured the content of phosphoribosylpyrophosphate (PRPP) in red cells and lymphocytes of an ADA deficient human. We found that the PRPP content of red cells is normal and that the PRPP content of lymphoyctes is no more than 20% reduced from normal.

TAX (Nijmegen): We have done some studies on PRPP metabolism not in lymphocytes but in erythrocytes of various patients and I think that it is not just the level of PRPP that is important since this compound has a high turnover.

HIRSCHHORN: We have measured also PRPP content, PRPP generation, and utilization in red cells and they have all been normal.

DISCUSSION ON CHAPTER 13 – IMMUNE FUNCTION IN DOWN'S SYNDROME

VALERIUS (Copenhagen): Which was the chemotactic agent that you used and were any of the patients which you had examined hepatitis–B antigen positive?

BJÖRKSTEN (Umeå): The chemotactic agent was zymosan activated serum of normal individuals. We looked for hepatitis–B antigen in most of the patients and none of them were positive.

WANDALL (Copenhagen): Do you know whether it is a cellular defect or it is the presence of a serum or plasma inhibitor which is responsible for your defective chemotaxis.

BJÖRKSTEN: It is a cellular defect because sera from Down's syndrome patients do not inhibit control neutrophils.

WANDALL: Have you tried to wash the cells, and do you get the same response?

BJÖRKSTEN: Yes, we have.

PAHWA (New York): Have you looked for a specific antibody formation in these patients?

BJÖRKSTEN: No, we have not.

PAHWA: It is possible that immunoglobulin may be normal, especially IgG, but one can have a defective rate of antibody production.

BJÖRKSTEN: Yes, there are indeed reports, or rather conflicting reports in the literature with regard to isohemagglutinins and to response to immunization. We did not look into that closely.

DISCUSSION ON CHAPTER 14 – MORPHOLOGICAL AND BIOCHEMICAL ALTERATION OF PMN FROM PATIENTS WITH INBORN ERRORS OF PHAGOCYTIC FUNCTION: A COMPREHENSIVE REVIEW

HIRSCHHORN (New York): Could you give us some idea of the clinical response of the patients with Chediak–Higashi syndrome to therapy?

BAEHNER (Indianapolis): It is difficult in small numbers of patients; we have three patients currently under evaluation. None of them have had infections. This is not conclusive. However, in a study by Dr Yell and associates at the NIH he has treated the beige mice with ascorbate and with a control group left off the ascorbate and has challenged them with a bacterial infection. His results show protection in those beige mice who are on ascorbic acid. One other point, is that the natural history of Chediak–Higashi is that these children end up with an accelerated phase of their disease, which is characterised by pancytopenia and hepato-spleno-megaly. Microscopic examination of the lymph nodes shows marked proliferation which resembles lymphoma. It is not clear whether we will be able to prevent the accelerated phase in which the patients succumb to overwhelming infection probably related to pancytopenia. *In vitro* early phases of killing are only at fault. With ascorbate we can correct only the functional defects. The morphogenic alterations are still present. We should continue morphometric evaluation; best mechanism for a evaluation of chemotaxis is to look at the cells as they move rather than to use some of the indirect methods.

DISCUSSION ON CHAPTER 15 – EXPERIMENTAL APPROACHES TO THE ROLE OF MONONUCLEAR PHAGOCYTES IN NON-SPECIFIC IMMUNITY

MADSEN (Copenhagen): Perhaps you could have stressed that macrophages are heterogeneous. They are certainly not like the neutrophil which is an end-cell. We have great difficulty in trying to do the same things that you do with granulocytes, with macrophages because they are so heterogeneous; it depends on where they are in the body as to how the macrophage functions, for example in the liver, peritoneum or in the lungs. Blood monocytes we can use for some of the functional tests that Dr MacPherson was talking about. You can of course do chemotaxis and bactericidal functions on monocytes. We have only 2–4% in the blood and this makes for difficulties. You have very beautiful systems for finding out how you kill off bacteria with neutrophils. As far as I know we still have no idea on how macrophages kill bacteria or viruses. Superoxide is a good candidate.

MacPHERSON (Oxford): I agree. It is so difficult in man where you only have the blood monocyte as a source of cells. We can look at the bactericidal mechanisms in this cell. It is quite clear that in the normal situation monocytes on their own are of little use in resistance to infection. If you have a low number of blood monocytes you may be able to kill bacteria such as *E. coli*. If you have a quantitative defective of polymorphonuclear leukocytes you will get infections. So, monocytes on their own can't cope. I agree again about the bactericidal mechanisms in macrophages. The enzyme systems that have been described are present also in polymorphs. Yet polymorphs are not very good at killing the organisms that macrophages can kill. I think that there are great differences.

ANDERSEN (Copenhagen): I have questions along the same line as Dr Madsen. Is phagocytosis always a reliable marker for all cells of the monocytic macrophage series? Is it possible sometimes to have cells in the blood which are so immature that they do not express there specific capacity?

MacPHERSON: It has been claimed this is so. It has also been claimed recently by Stewart that there are cells which will give rise to mononuclear phagocytic colonies *in vitro* and these cells are probably not phagocytic. So, it is possible. In fact we have some evidence of our own that there are cells which you cannot recognize in terms of phagocytosis, which are mononuclear phagocytes. Because this is a whole lineage of cells, starting with the stem cell and ending up with the giant cell or perhaps the epitheloid cell. They can appear in any state of differentiation.

The ones that are not phagocytic are peroxidase positive but they only develop esterase positivity when the colonies have developed to some extent.

DISCUSSION ON CHAPTER 17 – CHRONIC GRANULOMATOUS DISEASE: BIOCHEMISTRY AND OXYGEN METABOLISM

BAEHNER (Indianapolis): In a cell as complex as the PMN biochemical proof and morphological proof of the subcellular fractions is desirable. The implication here is that 5'-nucleotidase activity is marking the plasma membrane fraction. Do you have any morphological proof that indeed this fraction is a plasma membrane fraction?

SEGAL (Harrow): Obviously the most important thing in any subcellular fractionation is the reliability of your markers. 5'-nucleotidase is the classical marker for plasma membrane in various organelles such as liver. There is very low activity in neutrophils. We used two surface markers; we labelled the cells with fluorescamine which fluoresces when it binds to protein, and with the radioactive Bolton and Hunter reagent which covalently links to protein. Both of these markers are hydrolysed if they do not bind very rapidly. We then compared the distribution of the radioactivity, the fluorescence, and this enzyme activity and there was a very close co-distribution between these three things.

BAEHNER: Did you have any opportunity to do morphometric studies on your preparations?

SEGAL: No; it is very difficult to identify membranes as being plasma membranes by morphology. They could be endoplasmic reticulum membranes, for instance. A number of subcellular organelles have first been identified by their biochemical characteristics and then subsequently been shown to be present on morphological criteria.

ROMEO (Trieste): I have two comments. First, Baehner has shown that at pH 7 in the absence of manganese, the NADPH-dependent superoxide generation of CGD PMN is lacking. So, I do not think that you require a previous generation of superoxide in order to have an enhanced activity of the NADPH-dependent superoxide generation. Secondly, on the experiments with the SH-blocking reagents. When you react the cells with parachlormercuribenzoate you certainly have a block of the SH-groups on the surface of the cell which might impair the triggering of a stimulation. However, the disassociation between hydrogen peroxide and superoxide generation might be due to the fact that when you are measuring superoxide you have an excess of an exogenous protein added to the cells – a few milligrams of cytochrome C. As you know cytochrome C has a number of SH groups which might remove the blocking agents from the cell surface. So, when you stimulate the cells in the presence of cytochrome C you have cells which have their full complement of SH groups. When cells are stimulated in the absence of cytochrome C to measure hydrogen peroxide production and oxygen consumption, then the SH reagents might exert there activity.

SEGAL: I agree that it has been shown that in the absence of manganese or cyanide the reduction of cytochrome C is present in normal neutrophils and absent in chronic granulomatous disease. However, it is still a very messy system and it still contains the zymosan which has been used as an initiating stimulus.

ROOS (Amsterdam): First the cells are stimulated with zymosan for a couple of minutes. Then they are disrupted. Then you do a mild centrifugation to get rid of whole cells and zymosan. After that you do a $27000 \times g$ centrifugation to collect your membranes and whatever else there may be. In that preparation the NADPH oxidase activity is measured. Therefore, I don't think that there will be any zymosan left in that preparation; you will have got rid of it in the first stage.

SEGAL: I think that it's very important to know this and it seems to me if the zymosan has been phagocytized and then homogenized there must be some of it around. As far as the PC–PSA inhibition of peroxide production but not of superoxide production, they also found that killing was not inhibited by PC PSA whereas peroxide production was.

BAEHNER: To continue on this same point. My prediction would be that since hydrogen peroxide was measured by the formate oxidation method, this probably gives you false results. It should be repeated with a better more specific method. I have another question for you. Since you are looking at a system that is activated upon phagocytosis, what happens to the activity of your enzyme when you use activated cells? Is it stimulated by the presence of particles or not?

SEGAL: This is a common criticism. My point is that if you have an inborn error of metabolism and an enzyme which is found to be missing under resting conditions then there is rarely a need to find it missing under phagocytosing conditions. Many complications arise when one starts looking for an enzyme by these methods in activated cells because you are changing the properties of a membrane. You don't know what you are doing to the density of the membranes during the various subcellular fractionation procedures. The next point is this business of activation of the enzyme. An enzyme can itself be activated by a conformational or similar intrinsic change, but can also be activated by changes, physicochemical changes in the surrounding environment and these might not be reflected by changes in activity in an *in vitro* assay.

PAHWA (New York): It has been shown that KX–antigen is normally present in white cells as well as in red cells. In patients with chronic granulomatous disease the KX–antigen is absent in white cells while it is present in red cells. I'm just wondering the deficiency or absence of KX–antigen on the white cells may be a triggering mechanism.

WEENING (Amsterdam): I thought that the KX was only found in the x-linked form and not in the recessive form. It is not a common part in this activation.

SEGAL: It seems very likely that the plasma membrane is totally abnormal in these patients, the lack of that one antigen is evidence. There is other evidence that degranulation might be delayed in these patients and that the phagocytic vacuoles might not be of normal size. It is very likely that if a membrane enzyme is located within an abnormal membrane its activity might be compromised.

DISCUSSION ON CHAPTER 18 – THE PROTECTIVE ROLE OF GLUTATHIONE

WEENING (Amsterdam): I would like to add that the mechanism of neutrophil stimulation is not an increase in glutathione reductase activity. We have assayed the activity of this enzyme in more than a dozen of such preparations and we completely found the activity is normal; there is no activation at all.

ROOS (Amsterdam): Well, that adds to what we found, thank you.

SEGAL (Harrow): It seems very likely to me that there are two processes: superoxide production which is normal in these patients, and hydrogen peroxide production which is initially normal and then stops. What probably happens is that superoxide is not converted to hydrogen peroxide because of a drop in the intracellular glutathione concentration. I think the way to investigate this would be to measure the relationship between superoxide and hydrogen peroxide production and intracellular glutathione levels.

ROOS: I agree with your last conclusion that we should measure the amount of glutathione in the cells and what we expect to find is that it drops and stays low and then in that situation I expect that you can get damage of the cell. I must admit that we have tried once to do that and we did not see that expected drop. We are going to repeat that in a few weeks. The explanation may be that our method of measuring GSH is not perfect. It is also possible that the level of GSH stays high and that our theory is completely wrong. I just want to add one more thing to your point of view. You say that you need another reaction for conversion of superoxide to hydrogen peroxide. I think that many physical chemists will tell you that superoxide is such a very highly reactive compound, you don't need anything to make it react. It is so very active that it will immediately be converted to another product. If any proteins are around you will get hydrogen peroxide. I really think that the removal of superoxide by cytochrome C is a very effective method of protecting a cell against oxidative damage by superoxide. The patients were not clinically affected and not unduly prone to infection. We discovered this abnormality because one of these children developed haemolytic anaemia and we measured the glutathione reductase activity and found it to be abnormal. But as to infections in these children, they are absent and the children are quite healthy, which is strange in comparison with the situation in glutathione peroxidase deficiency. It may be explained by the fact that there is a slightly better chance to deduct by measurement of hydrogen peroxide in these cells as compared to the peroxidase deficient cells.

DISCUSSION ON CHAPTER 19 – DEFECTIVE INITIATION OF THE METABOLIC STIMULATION IN PHAGOCYTIZING GRANULOCYTES

MEUWISSEN (Albany): I was wondering what types of bacterial infections did these children have?

WEENING (Amsterdam): These patients had trouble with staphylococci and with *Candida albicans*. The first boy died from severe lung infections and other patients have trouble with candidiasis of the esophagus. The third boy had abscesses which were mainly staphylococcal.

HANSSON (Lund): For an explanation of your findings would it be possible that the C_3 receptor could be engaged. You have a purified IgG on the latex particles and you have the serum opsonized plate which would contain IgGs and a lot of different complement factors.

WEENING: Well, on the various particles there is not only IgG bound but also a little bit of C_3 and the IgG complexes are more heavily loaded with IgG but still there is some complement on it. We use human pooled serum. So, we never found that the combination of some C_3 on the latex particles inhibits the respiratory burst. So, I have to imagine that would be the case in these experiments.

MEUWISSEN: Where does the oxygen come from in the first place? Secondly, do you then conclude that hydrogen peroxide is not important for killing of, at least, zymosan?

WEENING: No, I hope that I don't give you that impression. We wondered why in our experiments the oxygen consumption was defective. But later on it was clear that it was due to the experimental conditions. We measured oxygen consumption in the presence of serum and we measured H_2O_2 without serum because the H_2O_2 is degraded in that medium. So, we had to pre-opsonize the particles; so we are measuring under two different conditions. That is the explanation of the oxygen consumption and present H_2O_2 production. When you repeat the experiments and do oxygen consumption in the presence of IgG-coated latex particles you find a perfectly normal oxygen consumption.

DISCUSSION ON CHAPTER 20 – MODIFICATION OF GENETIC EXPRESSION IN PHAGOCYTES

BAEHNER (Indianapolis): I have a belief that perhaps the iodination reaction in PMNs is more dependent upon the myeloperoxidase content of the cell than the hydrogen peroxide *per se*. In view of your demonstration that the anti-oestrogen drug increased myeloperoxidase activity in the cells, I wonder if you have had the opportunity to do functional studies such as iodination to see if there is any enhanced iodination or perhaps bacterial killing in the cells under these conditions?

HARKNESS (Harrow): I think we need to look very carefully at bacterial killing. There is no simple linear relationship between an enzyme activity and a biological function unless the enzyme activity is perhaps less than about 10% of the normal control mean activities.

BAEHNER: Some time ago we reported some studies on human monocytes which contain about 1/3 of the myeloperoxidase activity present in human PMNs. We used two labels, looking at ^{131}I-iodination of ^{14}C labelled bacteria, there seemed to be some correlation in that study. There was a close parallelism between the iodination per bacteria ingested and the myeloperoxidase content of the cells. It may be of some interest to look at that. I would agree with you that it may not be a one to one relationship in all cases.

HARKNESS: I think your method may be very useful.

DISCUSSION ON CHAPTER 21 – NEUTROPHIL GRANULOCYTE CHEMOTAXIS IN REVERSIBLE BOYDEN CHAMBER

MADSEN (Copenhagen): I would just like to make the comment that you can use these chambers for blood monocytes but it takes longer, 5 hours. You will have to turn the chambers after about $2\frac{1}{2}$ or 3 hours and one gets the same sort of result with casein. But you cannot use *E. coli* extracts for monocytes. It is not chemotactic.

BJÖRKSTEN (Umeå): By shortening your incubation time, you might possibly avoid the loss of cells.

VALERIUS (Copenhagen): I have tried that and it seems to me that the cells start to detach from the filter surface as soon as they arrive.

DISCUSSION ON CHAPTER 22 – SIMPLIFIED TESTS FOR LEUKOCYTIC FUNCTION

ROOS (Amsterdam): Did you use the patients own serum in your bactericidal test?

OLLING (Gothenburg): No, pooled normal human serum. AB Rh-positive serum was used.

ROOS: Then don't you think that in a screening test this should be included because there may be serum factors missing?

OLLING: Yes, but I think this would very much depend on the strain of bacterium you use. I would guess that the killing of some kinds of bacteria would depend on the serum used.

ROOS: I recognize that it is a difficult problem. But still this is an area in which defects have been found and we must be aware that they can occur. It is extremely difficult to include all the different kinds of bacteria.

OLLING: Then you need two tubes for each patient, one for serum and one for leukocytes.

ROOS: Certainly, if you want to differentiate between cellular and humoral defects.

SEGAL (Harrow): Just one point about screening for chemotactic defects. I think that all these *in vitro* tests are only really screening the efferent loop of the chemotactic response. Very little is known about the afferent loop. In other words, the release of mediators from the site of inflammation and the attraction of neutrophils to it. We found an *in vivo* skin-window technique in which you have abraded the skin and put a little chamber on containing the patient's own serum very useful. We measure the rate of accumulation of neutrophils in the fluid in the chamber and, think that we have found a major defect in Crohn's disease.

DISCUSSION ON CHAPTER 23 – ANTIGEN-INDUCED NEUTROPHIL DYSFUNCTION IN A PATIENT WITH CHRONIC ECZEMA, RECURRENT "COLD" STAPHYLOCOCCAL INFECTIONS AND HYPERIMMUNOGLOBULINAEMIA E.

POLMAR (Cleveland): Did you try to reverse the effect of the patient's serum either by absorbing the IgE out with an anti-IgE immuno-absorbent or perhaps if the mechanism requires histamine in treating the serum with a diamine oxidase.

SCHOPFER (St Gallen): No, we did not try this but chemotaxis was depressed in the absence of serum. IgE absorbs to the basophils in the leukocyte preparation.

POLMAR: Then diamine oxidase added to the cells would have permitted normal function.

ROMEO (Trieste): A point I might add is that *in vitro* studies have shown that histamine does not effect the metabolic concomitants of phagocytosis. So, the oxygen dependent killing mechanism is not impaired. As far as the release of histamine is concerned I think that very high concentrations of histamine inhibit chemotaxis and phagocytosis.

SCHOPFER: There was no killing defect, but a defect at another level in the leukocyte. Histamine in small concentrations can effect white blood cell enzyme release when there is no killing defect.

DISCUSSION ON CHAPTER 24 – LACK OF MYELOPEROXIDASE-MEDIATED IODINATION IN GRANULOCYTES FROM A PATIENT WITH GENERALIZED PUSTULAR PSORIASIS

BAEHNER (Indianapolis): Did you have any opportunity to do the iodination study in normal cells that were treated with cyanide or azide to compare the degree of iodination to that which you have observed in your patient with deficiency of myeloperoxidase?

STENDAHL (Linköping): The iodination activity in cyanide and azide treated cells is very low in normal cells.

BAEHNER (Indianapolis): Even lower than was observed in the patient?

STENDAHL: Well, it is almost impossible to differentiate at that level because in this patient it is completely lacking. The figure I showed is really too high. They have no iodination activity linked to the myeloperoxidation.

BAEHNER: In the patients with a congenital deficiency of myeloperoxidase there is still catalase present. At low substrate concentrations of hydrogen peroxide it is conceivable that the catalase could be functioning as a peroxidase; in that way killing bacteria. That may be an explanation for your *in vitro* studies on bacterial killing, where you show that the cyanide and azide treated normal cell had a more profound killing defect than did the myeloperoxidase deficient patient.

STENDAHL: I have not tried to evaluate the difference between the cyanide treated normal cells and the cells of this patient.

ROMEO (Trieste): I don't expect catalase activity to be involved.

DISCUSSION ON CHAPTER 25 – FUNCTIONAL CHARACTERISTICS OF NEUTROPHIL GRANULOCYTES FROM CHILDREN WITH RECURRENT RESPIRATORY INFECTIONS

ANDERSEN (Copenhagen): You mentioned the possibility that recurrent infections might influence your results.

WANDALL (Copenhagen): Yes, in the serum dependent phagocytosis.

ANDERSEN: Did you evaluate some of the patients repeatedly to see if the length of a symptom-free period would effect your results?

WANDALL: We have re-evaluated one of the opsonin defects and found a normal value in the second investigation. One of the three patients with chemotactic defects has been studied 3–4 times at monthly intervals and every time there has been a decreased chemotactic function.

KOCH (Copenhagen): So, that you think you have an intrinsic defect of chemotaxis which is not serum related since these cells are washed.

WANDALL: It may be an intrinsic or it may be a cell-associated defect.

BAEHNER (Indianapolis): I think that a very careful controlled evaluation of children with infections is necessary. We are using selected tests. Dr Quie has made the statement that he feels that chemotactic disorders either primary of the cell or secondary to defective serum chemotactic factor will probably turn out to be the most frequently occurring disorders of non-specific immunity related to the neutrophil. I would agree with that. One point to be made is that despite a chemotactic defect these patients may be able to form a pustule or in other words to move enough granulocytes into the area of an infection. However, in larger groups of patients with disorders such as hyper-IgE syndromes the neutrophils ofter arrive late to the area of infection; there is a late accumulation of granulocytes but they do eventually form pus. The fact that the patient mounts a pyogenic response doesn't necessarily rule out the possibility of a chemotactic disorder. Evaluation of chemotaxis should be done in all patients who are considered to have a primary immunodeficiency of the phagocytic cells, particularly the neutrophil.

WANDALL: I would like to make one comment. Dr Boxer some years ago found that the Rebock-window turned out to be more sensitive in detecting chemotactic disorders than related *in vitro* techniques.

DISCUSSION ON CHAPTER 26 – *PNEUMOCYSTIS CARINII* INFECTION IN A GIRL WITH CHRONIC GRANULOMATOUS DISEASE TREATED WITH TRANSFUSIONS OF GRANULOCYTES

PAHWA (New York): We had a case of chronic granulomatous disease who while on artificial respiration developed an infection with pneumocystis which we treated effectively with Bactrim. I agree with you that no cases have so far been reported in the literature.

MEUWISSEN (Albany): I think that your paper is relevant to the frequent occurrence of pneumocystis in prematures and newborns. We have always assumed such infections were due to undeveloped T- and B-cell immunity but prematures and newborns, particularly if they are sick, have also 'defects' in the polymorphonuclear leukocyte systems which might render them less resistant to infection.

BAEHNER (Indianapolis): Unfortunately, we've had a vast experience with pneumocystis in our institution. There is a paper in *The Journal of Pediatrics* a few months ago by Wolff and co-workers which reported on 21 cases of pneumocystis in our leukaemic population of children who developed their disease between the fourth and tenth week after the initiation of cytotoxic therapy. In these patients total granulocyte count was normal. Yet, they had pneumocystis proven in all cases by open lung biopsy. I would agree from your studies that there may be some failure of phagocyte function but I'm not totally convinced that the granulocyte is important, I still believe that the most important immune system here is probably the lymphocyte and macrophage. There is another piece of evidence. Pneumocystis is very difficult to culture *in vitro*. Dr Hughs at St Jude Hospital now at Johns Hopkins has tried and has not been able to get it through a life cycle. It can be isolated in rats that are given steroid therapy; such rats developed pneumocystis at about 6 weeks. In studies where pneumocystis was isolated and then injected into rabbits to make an antibody and then exposed to macrophages one can show that the addition of specific, anti-pneumocystis antibody enhanced the ingestion of the organism by the macrophages. So, that points indirectly to the involvement of the macrophages in host resistance to this disease.

PEDERSEN (Copenhagen): I think Dr Hughs recorded successful culture of the organism a few months ago in *Pediatric Research*, using cell cultures of fetal lung fibroblasts.

MEUWISSEN: It may have been the macrophages that were enzyme deficient; did you give any macrophages?

PEDERSEN: In the peripheral blood the monocyte count was normal, which was around 4%.

VALERIUS (Copenhagen): You are right that the granulocyte transfusions did contain a number of mononuclear cells. So, it could possibly be those that were responsible for the clinical effect. It wasn't a granulocyte transfusion but a monocyte transfusion we actually gave.

SECTION FOUR

Screening for Immunodeficiency

Round Table Discussion

V. Faber: Within our area of discussion, some important questions are:

(1) What is the incidence of primary immunodeficiency?

(2) Which groups at risk should be investigated for primary immunodeficiency?

(3) Which laboratory methods should be used for screening?

V. Andersen: As an introduction we want to present some data and suggestions. The data are from Denmark, which has 5 million inhabitants and a declining birth rate of about 60 000 births per year. We do not know the number of deaths in childhood from infection without serious underlying disorder like congenital heart disease, but in the first year of life there are maybe 50 per year in Denmark.

How many cases of primary immunodeficiency are diagnosed per year in Denmark? This is also not known. However, Table 1 shows patients known to the University Hospital of Copenhagen, which is the hospital in Denmark that has most actively investigated primary immunodeficiency, in particular the Department of Infectious Diseases. So these are patients known during a 5-year period to the study group on immunodeficiencies which has grown up around this department. There is certainly selection before the patients are referred to us. For example, the agammaglobulinaemia group is large because these patients are treated in the paediatric departments that have diagnosed these disorders. Other major groups are severe combined immunodeficiency, chronic granulomatous disease and common variable immunodeficiency, which is a cover name for a multitude of conditions. In all, there have been 63 patients during a period of 5 years, but how large a fraction this constitutes of the total number in Denmark we do not know. So, my first question is: What do we know about the incidence of primary immunodeficiency and the relative importance of the various diagnostic categories?

I think there is one more question to be asked in relation to Table 1. In which cases will the patient benefit from the proper diagnosis being made? All cases of severe combined immunodeficiency should be diagnosed as soon as possible for further investigation and treatment; bone marrow

TABLE 1   Cases of primary immunodeficiency diagnoses over a 5-year period

	Number of patients
Severe combined deficiency	9
DiGeorge's syndrome	2
Wiskott–Aldrich syndrome	2
Ataxia–telangiectasia	4
T lymphocyte deficiency	
combined with deficient chemotaxis	3
combined with Fanconi anaemia	2
Agammaglobulinaemia	8
IgA deficiency with infections	7
Common variable immunodeficiency	10
Schwachman's syndrome	2
Chronic granulomatous disease (CGD)	9
Deficient chemotaxis	2
Cyclic neutropenia	4
Total	64

transplantation should be done when a compatible bone marrow donor can be found. Enzyme replacement therapy should be attempted in ADA deficiency. Patients with DiGeorge's syndrome should have thymus transplantation. Of the patients with Wiskott–Aldrich syndrome, maybe half seem to benefit from treatment with transfer factor. Patients with agammaglobulinaemia should have an adequate plasma IgG concentration maintained during substitution therapy, and long-term treatment with sulphamethoxazole plus trimethoprim should be considered. As to chronic granulomatous disease, the proper choice of antibiotics depends on knowledge of the diagnosis.

We think that the present stage of our knowledge and techniques does not justify screening of the newborn at large for immunodeficiency. My second question is: Which groups at risk should be investigated for immunodeficiency? Among the top priority groups are:

(1) children and young adults with unusual or unusually frequent infections;

(2) members of families with immunodeficiency;

(3) children with metabolic defects.

As to the last group I will emphasize to our biochemical colleagues that few metabolic defects and few chromosomal defects have been examined for their effects on the immune system although studies within both fields have been reported at this meeting.

An important point is: To what degree does infection influence the laboratory results and maybe invalidate them as regards the diagnosis of primary immunodeficiency? I think it is known that all the tests that have been discussed may be influenced by the presence of infection. So the third question is: To what degree should active infection eliminate patients from screening?

In summary these three questions are:

(1) What is the incidence of the various immunodeficiency disorders?
(2) Which groups at risk should be investigated for immunodeficiency?
(3) How are the results influenced by infection?

R. Pahwa: In the United States it is difficult to estimate the incidences because most of the cases we get are referred. In 3 years we have seen 12 cases of severe combined immunodeficiency. I think that about 150 cases of severe combined immunodeficiency have been diagnosed in the United States.

S. H. Polmar: A workshop in Lansing, Michigan, in about 1975 gave estimates fairly close to that of Dr Pahwa. During a 2-year period, 175 new cases of severe combined immunodeficiency occurred in various centres in the USA.

The incidence is low; a reason for finding these patients is as experiments of nature; inborn errors of metabolism give us an opportunity to uncover mechanisms which may then be applied not only to the patient himself or herself, but to other disease processes.

R. L. Baehner: In childhood, 24 to 26 cases of leukaemia are diagnosed per million children on an annual basis. The incidence for immunodeficiencies is probably lower. But I would agree with Dr Polmar's statement of their scientific value.

Another problem is the granulocyte disorders. The patients with neutropenias of the Kostmann type that was originally described in Scandinavia generally have severe neutropenia and recurring infections, but for the most part do not have problems in the newborn period. Chronic granulomatous disease was recently reviewed by Dr Johnston[1]; he found 162 cases described in the world literature during the last decade. Again, those patients generally do not get into difficulty in the neonatal period, but their infections start in the first few months of life.

As regards granulocyte dysfunction, if we are going to 'screen' in the newborn period do we have to know of transient abnormalities? We know on the basis of studies which have been done in the United States and in

England that the newborn has a primary chemotactic defect of the granu-locyte, and it has recently been shown that the monocyte is also defective in the chemotactic response. Dr Rosen and others have shown that the factor B of the alternative complement pathway is diminished in over 50% of cord blood samples and that there is also a functional defect in opson-ization in the newborn. So we have a large number of newborns who have a defect of their serum system as well as of their cellular system; these defects are transient, clearing after the neonatal period.

It seems that it is the patients with combined immunodeficiency who need to be defined quite early in life.

S. H. Polmar: One would have to consider first the children from a family with a previously affected child. In children without a family history of immunodeficiency, how many infections are significant? Are mild upper respiratory tract infections significant? On of the problems is the vari-ability of presentation and of the age at onset. In severe combined immuno-deficiency the presenting symptoms may be quite mild at times, without infection until close to the end of the first year of life. The symptoms are often upper and lower respiratory tract infections. Any patient with *Pneumocystis carinii* or persistent pulmonary infiltrate in the first year of life that turns out to be *Pneumocystis* has a 90% chance, at least in the United States, of being immunodeficient, mostly with severe combined immunodeficiency; besides, the chronic diarrhoeas in early childhood with general failure to thrive may be a sign of immunodeficiency. I have had difficulty in trying to make a formula for house staff to say at what point you consider the diagnosis, but the overall clinical situation can provide useful information.

R. Hirschhorn: By screening, do we mean screening of healthy newborns? What are the criteria for screening? I think Dr Baehner mentioned an important criterion, namely that you have a form of therapy which is more effective if made available before the onset of clinical symptoms that allow you to make a diagnosis without 'screening'.

If screening allows you to perform prenatal diagnosis in a family then one would like to be able to detect heterozygotes. This is clearly not feas-ible in this series of disorders. In order to propose screening for hetero-zygote detection one needs a high gene frequency in a particular population which is not yet apparent for any of the immunodeficiencies.

If you are talking about screening of children who present with clinical symptoms, I do not think you are talking about screening. You are dis-cussing the clinical criteria for further investigation. The remaining area for discussion would be the investigation of families in which a previous child has died with a diagnosis of one of the disorders of immunodeficiency, or in which the history is compatible with such a diagnosis.

H. Bickel: I think the word is 'selective screening' – in families where there is great likelihood that the diseases exist. The very first remarks suggested that population-wide screening probably is not yet feasible. I would agree. The European Council some years ago, and next year the International Symposium of Screening, are trying to decide which diseases justify population-wide screening. Frequency, methods and treatment are important factors influencing these disorders. Already it may be justifiable to throw out some diseases where screening had been applied. For instance homocystinuria screening may not be as effective as it should be, whilst screening for hypothyroidism, I think everybody agrees, should be started at once. There is one danger; there are some diseases for which screening is incomplete due to lack of organization. For instance, very good methods are available for galactosaemia screening, but there are large parts at least in Europe, including my own country, where there is no screening on a population-wide basis for galactosaemia.

Now as to immunodeficiency, I am no specialist, but it seems that talk about frequency of immunodeficiency is premature. We have seen in other inborn errors that we needed millions of samples before we could estimate frequency; possibly, as in maple syrup urine disease, some cases may even have died before screening can detect them.

Another argument against population-wide screening is the absence of good therapeutic methods. The methods that have been mentioned are with one or two exceptions still difficult. It is not very beneficial to diagnose something which you cannot then treat properly, for instance muscular dystrophy. In the United States and in Germany, screening for muscular dystrophy has been proposed.

Genetic counselling has been proposed as a basis for screening. I am not in favour of screening only for genetic counselling. I must be sure there is a real chance that successful treatment is well on the way.

D. N. Raine: I would like to put some points which would help counteract the arguments against screening. First of all you have to decide whether it is healthy neonatal screening or whether it is going to be in a selected population. I agree with what Dr Hirschhorn said, except that I think if you decided to screen every child on its first infection, this could be regarded as a form of screening. But before deciding to do that, you need to consider the tests you are going to use and their coverage. Screening tests should always have false-positives and should never have false-negatives. If you embark on a screening programme with a test that will miss certain diseases then you should make this known and admit that you are not screening for those diseases. It is wrong to lead the public to believe that they are being checked for a condition that your test will not detect.

The question of whether there is a treatment available has been mentioned. I would put it differently. It is the management of the disease you want to know about. You may not be able to cure it but are you able to treat it better because you knew about it sooner? Are you able to prevent irreversible damage because you treated it from the outset?

I would include genetic counselling as part of the management and part of the justification for a screening programme.

It seems to me that at the present time you cannot make sound decisions on screening for immunodeficiency until you have done a very substantial further study. In a previous discussion, I said that there are some questions that cannot be answered without doing an experiment on a million people. This is something that it is important for the investigator to realize. He must have thought out his experiment sufficiently well to justify doing it on a million people. If his expectations are not realized, he must have the courage to stop his experiment and try something different or go back to where he was before.

Now the question of the relationship between the profession and the public. We have learned the hard way that the smallest part of any screening programme is the laboratory work. This is usually easy, you know how to do it, you have confidence in the people who are going to be involved in it. But your troubles start the moment your results go out of the laboratory, assuming you have overcome the troubles about the specimens coming into your laboratory. You have to give the personnel involved a training programme, you have to educate them on how to discuss and answer the questions the parents will ask.

When you have produced your results you must know how this is received by the public. Again from our own experience, we set up the Scriver screening methods for amino acid disorders which picks up phenylketonuria and several other things. If anyone phoned us I always encouraged laboratory staff to give the appropriate amount of information. If we ever needed to do more than a second test on the baby we arranged for the parents to come to the clinic and have an informed discussion, so we have tried not to increase the anxiety that this might have given parents. But we did a survey after about 5 years on the public reaction to this and we were horrified at the anxiety that was being generated. In *Medico-Social Aspects of Inherited Metabolic Diseases*, which is published in The Society's series of monographs, several of the chapters give real observations and data on the anxiety that can be generated in the public with a wll-justified screening programme that is known to produce good results as in the case of phenylketonuria.

V. Andersen: I think that it is most valuable for us all to hear about the experience of many years of screening. I wonder if Dr Meuwissen has any comments on the groups at risk that should be investigated.

H. Meuwissen: Maybe I could comment on the ADA screening. Dr Hirschhorn mentioned the maximum figure for ADA deficiency of 1 in 100 000; probably the figure is lower. We have now screened about 700 000 newborns and found the same child that Dr Hirschhorn found one year ago; this is an example of an experimental screening programme which we found was not worthwhile, at least in New York State; we know that the incidence may be different in various parts of the country.

R. Hirschhorn: I know from my own experience that in addition to the child in whom we detected ADA deficiency we lost another to follow-up. That is why my figures were a little higher. I was wondering how complete was the survey in New York State and what is the incidence of those lost to follow-up?

H. Meuwissen: I do not know the precise figures. But Dr Carter who was running the survey tells me that it is complete. We get the blood spots from the hospitals as for phenylketonuria screening.

R. Hirschhorn: How many that were negative for ADA on screening were confirmed by follow-up?

H. Meuwissen: We had six with no ADA activity on the newborn screening programme. Four of these were followed up by whole blood investigation 6 weeks later and had normal ADA. There was one lost to follow-up, thus one ADA-deficient child was found in New York City whom you are now following.

R. Hirschhorn: Another child was lost to follow-up in New York City. That gives a maximal incidence of three in 700 000 which is about 1 in 200 000.

D. N. Raine: ADA deficiency is only one of the diseases of interest. What you should be thinking about is a screening test which will take in as many diseases as can be covered with specificity.

R. Hirschhorn: For newborn screening I think ADA deficiency and NP deficiency are the only diseases relevant to the discussion; for NP there is no screening method. I think one could be developed.

R. Pahwa: When talking about screening we should define the resources. If resources are available I think it is a good idea to screen the whole population. If the resources are not available I think we should screen selected groups of patients.

I have a few more suggestions to add to the list of indications for screening.

(1) Repeated abortions with a family history of immunodeficiency; histological examination of aborted fetuses especially thymus and the lymph nodes, by a pathologist who is aware of immunodeficiency, may reveal evidence of immunodeficiency.

(2) Patients with partial DiGeorge's syndrome, in which there is a partial defect of the T cell system, may be followed by endocrinologists or cardiologists; I think that any child who in the neonatal period presents with hypocalcaemia or has a right-sided heart defect should be investigated for T cell deficiencies.

(3) Routine chest X-ray during the first year of life may be useful. It should be specifically asked whether the thymus shadow is present. Recently at the Cornell Medical Center, we had a patient with DiGeorge's syndrome who was discovered by chest X-ray. The pathologists were alerted and in their autopsy material found two additional patients with DiGeorge's syndrome.

(4) The paediatrician should be suspicious of patients with more than three recurring infections, especially if chronic diarrhoea or fungal infection is present. The value of recording the absolute concentration of lymphocytes in the blood should be stressed, since lymphocytopenia is an additional clue to several immunodeficiency disorders.

(5) Finally, congenital deficiency syndromes or birth defects should prompt immunological investigation; for example, we have heard that patients with Down's syndrome have defects of chemotaxis.

P. Platz: One phenomenon has been noticed in many places, that diagnoses of immunodeficiency disorders tend to cluster around people with special interest in this field. So I think that we have not reached the point where we can discuss true incidence. One of the important first steps might be to increase the knowledge and interest among general practitioners and in paediatric departments.

V. Faber: By my counting, we have mentioned eight groups at risk for immunodeficiency which should be investigated. What about other groups? Could we suggest any other inborn errors of metabolism, which might justifiably be investigated for immunodeficiency?

H. Bickel: That is difficult to answer; there are some inborn errors of metabolism which tend to have infections. But they are often diseases which are severe such as maple syrup urine disease or methylmalonic acidaemia. In phenylketonuria it has been said that infections are more frequent, but this is not my own experience. When the patients are treated properly, they have no more infections than others. But in diseases like maple syrup urine disease I feel sure the immunological investigation should be of interest because we have frequently seen chronic pyelo-nephritis.

S. Cahalane: I wonder if some member of the panel might discuss the natural history of the disorders for which we are screening. The lessons which have been learned from wide-scale screening of newborns have shown that the classical disorders are not what we are detecting. This has emerged from the phenylketonuria/hyperphenylalaninaemia situation. The people who are interested in immunodeficiency diseases must also satisfy themselves that the conditions for which they are screening are the conditions they are encountering clinically. This is a great difficulty. I am for going ahead with research if you can screen without additional trouble as you can with the ADA test on newborn blood already collected. But do we know enough about the natural history of, for example, severe combined immunodeficiency to say that when the diagnosis is established you must intervene with radical treatment?

R. Pahwa: We know that in patients with DiGeorge's syndrome, you can completely correct this disorder by thymus transplantation. In patients with severe combined immunodeficiency where we have matched siblings I think the success of bone marrow transplantation is usually above 70%. The difficulty comes when we do not have a matched sibling. I think that it is important to study immunodeficient patients in depth, so that in the future we can treat common disorders.

S. H. Polmar: It should be clear that when we talk about immunodeficiency diseases, this means at least 36 different disorders; screening for 36 diseases is difficult. A lymphocyte stimulation test, which on 1 million people would cost something like 30 million dollars, would miss a large proportion of the immunodeficient patients. Neutrophil functional tests would also be costly. I think non-selective screening for immunodeficiency diseases in general is clearly impractical, until we identify more biochemical defects that can be easily screened for and that are worthwhile screening for. The relatively easy screening for ADA deficiency has been non-rewarding.

R. Hirschhorn: What of the disorders that are currently being screened for on a population basis and what are the frequency figures for those disorders?

H. Bickel: That is a difficult question because you will need millions of people before you will know something about frequency. One can say that hypothyroidism, although we do not have much material, seems to be frequent: 1 in 3000 or 1 in 4000. Phenylketonuria is different from one country to another: 1 in 6000 in Ireland, 1 in 7000 in Western Germany, 1 in 15000 in Switzerland, 1 in 15–20000 in America. In Finland there are practically none. For galactosaemia the frequency is 1 in 20 000 to 1 in 30 000. The rarer diseases may be rare because the methods of detection are not good enough. I personally think that there must be more homocystinuria than we have detected by screening by an increased methionine level; we need a better screening method for this condition. I personally think that maple syrup urine disease is more frequent than 1 in 200 000.

R. Hirschhorn: Would you say that we have enough data to provide a reliable estimate of the one disorder causing immunodeficiency that we have screened for, namely ADA deficiency? Are you satisfied with the incidence of 1 per 200 000?

H. Bickel: No, you must have millions of children tested. The rarer the disease the bigger must be the number screened to provide a reliable estimate.

H. Meuwissen: Would you be happy if we stop screening for ADA deficiency?

H. Bickel: I do not want to answer that question directly.

D. N. Raine: I will answer it. I am convinced that it is important that some informed groups go on screening on as wide a basis as possible for these diseases. Otherwise you will make irrevocable decisions on a wrong basis.

I would like to comment on Mrs Hirschhorn's questions which cannot be answered in an absolute sense. It depends on what the circumstances are and what is the screening test. For example, Phenistix is cheap and simple. But as soon as we converted to the Guthrie test we probably increased cost and complexity 10-fold but at that time we got more justification. It may be advisable to rethink the problem by looking at the diseases which you want to detect and develop a more comprehensive screening test.

It was said that only ADA and NP deficiency could be recognized at birth. If any of these lymphocyte functional defects are really enzyme deficiencies you should be able to detect them at birth even though they are not manifest clinically; at present you might be able to detect them now only with the most elaborate laboratory resources. But it is amazing what is being done for, say, mass screening for phenylketonuria and for sickle cell disease once someone has recognized the need to have a mass approach to a particular problem.

I. Smith: I do not think that Dr Cahalane's question has been answered. The point was that a test which seems to be specific for a disease at the time when you first describe the disease may turn out to be a test which is always positive in that disease but may also be positive in other diseases. You detect these in a screening programme because all you have done is to apply your test to a classical disorder. This is the experience in inborn errors.

H. Bickel: The answers seem to come from phenylketonuria or galactosaemia. You will just have to experiment and determine which are the variants and which are the classical diseases. We are only now determining the difference between the classical phenylketonuria and the variants.

R. Hirschhorn: The one child picked up on screening for ADA deficiency may be a 'variant' because he is perfectly healthy.

V. Faber: Can we turn to the immunological investigations at various levels of complexity, and then to the prolems of phagocytes?

V. Andersen: The following are our suggestions for initial tests and the more centralized tests for deficiencies in various parts of the immune sys-

TABLE 2   Laboratory screening: T lymphocytes

	Quantity	Function
Initial	Total lymphocyte concentration and morphology Size of thymus (X-ray)	Delayed hypersensitivity skin tests
Centralized	Concentration of E-rosetting lymphocytes	Lymphocyte transformation Lymphokine production Contact sensitization (DNCB, NDMA)

tem: Table 2 shows investigations on T lymphocytes. All physicians caring for patients who may have a primary immunodeficiency should evaluate the total lymphocyte concentration in the blood, chest X-ray with special regard to the thymus and delayed hypersensitivity skin tests. More centralized tests would be quantitation of E-rosetting lymphocytes and the various tests of T lymphocyte function including contact sensitization.

As regards B lymphocytes (Table 3), initial studies would involve determination of the immunoglobulin classes by quantitative immunoelectro-

TABLE 3   Laboratory screening: B lymphocytes

	Quantity	Function
Initial	Concentrations of IgM, IgA, IgG	Isohaemagglutinins
Centralized	Concentration of membrane-Ig-bearing lymphocytes Secretory IgA	Antibody titres following immunization

TABLE 4   Laboratory screening: Phagocytes

	Quantity	Function
Initial	Concentrations of neutrophils and monocytes + morphology	
Centralized		NBT test Chemotaxis Phagocytosis Bactericidal capacity

TABLE 5 Laboratory screening: Complement

	Quantity	Function
Initial		Total haemolytic complement
Centralized	Concentration of individual components	Performance of patient's serum + single complement components

phoresis according to Laurell and isohaemagglutinins. Enumeration of B lymphocytes, concentration of secretory IgA and of antibody titres in serum after various stimuli are centralized tasks.

For neutrophil granulocytes and for monocytes–macrophages, there is not much one can do in the periphery as yet, apart from counting them and looking at their morphology. The functional phagocyte tests will have to be done in a centralized fashion.

For the complement system (Table 5), total haemolytic complement is a screening test that will not pick up all defects, but all other complement tests are at present centralized.

R. L. Baehner: For diagnosis of phagocyte dysfunction, we have tried to decide what we could consider to be an adequate 'screening' evaluation of a patient with an immune dysfunction. We estimate that the cost of such an evaluation would be in the range of 400 to 500 dollars. We would include in this a white blood cell count and a differential; absolute lymphocyte counts and absolute granulocyte counts are important. Secondly immunoglobulins should be quantitated, a simple serum electrophoresis is inadequate. Total haemolytic complement would probably be an adequate test.

For neutrophil function, a chemotactic assay using the Boyden chamber technique should evaluate both the cellular aspects and the serum of the patient. As regards primary disorders of phagocytic ingestion, and we know of at least the one baby that was described by Boxer and colleagues[2]; this baby had a leukaemoid reaction with leukocyte counts approaching 50 000 μl. Leukaemoid reactions could be one sign, perhaps, of a problem of mobilization of the granulocytes out of the vascular tree into the extravascular areas. If we are going to use a phagocytic evaluation, my own preference is the Oil Red O study of Stossel. The NBT test is one of a variety of tests that screens for the oxidative potential of a cell. The NBT test could be combined with an opsonic zymosan system, so that you could evaluate the alternative complement pathway at the same time. By combining the NBT test with the zymosan system, you may be able to evaluate phagocytic ingestion as well as alternative complement opsonic function and the oxidative potential of the cell, provided that you use patient serum in the system. A bactericidal assay is somewhat difficult to perform if it is not done on a routine basis. We feel that this is possibly the ultimate test. I like to use the patients' own infecting bacteria with their own serum in the system and their own granulocytes.

For lymphocyte function, skin test reactivity would be one measure of delayed hypersensitivity and the lymphocyte phytohaemagglutinin response a second functional assay; you heard that there is not always a close correlation between the two tests. Then finally perhaps a peroxidase stain. So, it costs about 500 dollars to investigate a patient at least in the United States. We would not embark on such a series of tests on every patient but only on selected cases with some consideration of the type of infection. If there is a primary pyogenic infection where we know the granulocyte and the humoral mechanisms are most important, we would select out tests of granulocytes and humoral mechanisms. If we think that we are dealing with a patient who has a disorder predominantly of the lymphocyte–macrophage system, we would first move toward those tests.

D. Roos: I agree with Dr Baehner's remarks. Perhaps you could omit the phagocytosis assay because defects are rare. Perhaps you have to determine the concentration of white blood cells serially. As we have heard, in ADA deficiency lymphocytopenia is not present in the first three months of life.

B. Bjorksten: One should look for folic acid defects in patients with chronic infectious disease.

R. Hirschhorn: One comment, since this was a metabolically oriented conference dealing with immunodeficiencies; I would like to add to that list of tests an evaluation of adenosine deaminase, purine nucleoside phosphorylase, vitamin B_{12}, if that is absent, transcobalamin too, and orotic acid.

V. Faber: Thank you all for your contentions. I hope that we have provided some impression of what we intend to do in the next 5 years.

Discussion references

1. Johnston, (1977). *Ped. Clin. N. Am.*, 24, 365
2. Boxer *et al.* (1974). *N. Engl. J. Med.*, 291, 1093

Index